Pocket Guide to Advanced Endoscopy in Gastroenterology

Springer Nature More Media App

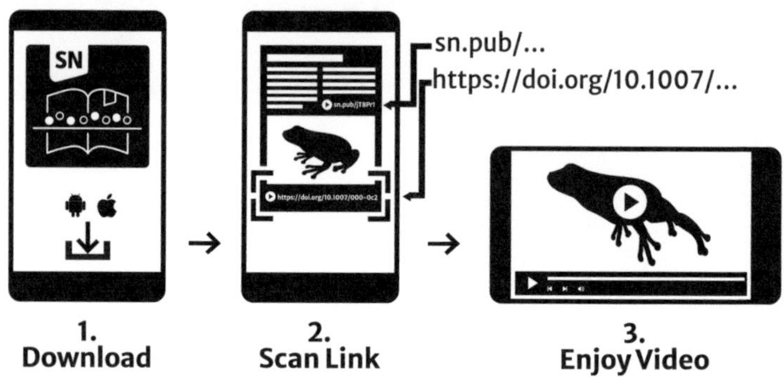

Support: customerservice@springernature.com

Adrian Săftoiu

Editor

Pocket Guide to Advanced Endoscopy in Gastroenterology

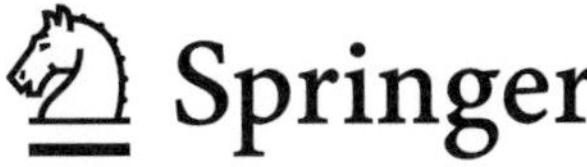

Springer

Editor
Adrian Săftoiu
Department of Gastroenterology and Hepatology
Elias Emergency University Hospital
Carol Davila University of Medicine and Pharmacy
Bucharest, Romania

This work contains media enhancements, which are displayed with a "play" icon. Material in the print book can be viewed on a mobile device by downloading the Springer Nature "More Media" app available in the major app stores. The media enhancements in the online version of the work can be accessed directly by authorized users.

ISBN 978-3-031-42078-8   ISBN 978-3-031-42076-4   (eBook)
https://doi.org/10.1007/978-3-031-42076-4

This Springer imprint is published by the registered company Springer Nature Switzerland AG
The registered company address is: Gewerbestrasse 11, 6330 Cham, Switzerland

Paper in this product is recyclable.

Foreword

Gastrointestinal endoscopy (GIE) has undergone a huge development during the last 30–40 years mainly due to improvements in technology combined with new creative innovations. Even though the endoscopic platform is unchanged the usefulness and functionality has undergone a breakthrough: The flexibility and handling of the endoscopes have markedly improved, resulting in an improvement in image quality that allows even the tiniest details to be visualized due to higher image resolution, new computerized image filters and new software allowing for structure enhancement and characterization, and development of new dedicated specialized endoscopes including the combination of image technology such as endoscopic ultrasound or confocal laser endomicroscopy. In addition to this, innovative micro-tools that can be introduced via the instrument channel or mounted on the endoscope as well as new pharmaceutical products for application through the endoscope either the standard version or an EUS endoscope have further expanded the applicability in a variety of diseases within and outside the GI tract. These developments have paved the way for minimally invasive diagnostics and therapies and in many ways challenged or even replaced traditional surgery. GIE has become a cornerstone in modern gastroenterology both for diagnosis and for therapy for most GI diseases but also in many other conditions where the GI tract or adjacent organs or regions are involved.

The present book is a pocket guide to advanced endoscopy in gastroenterology. The book is a condensed description of almost all conditions and diseases of the GI tract but at the same time gives the reader a comprehensive overview of the role of endoscopy in upper GI tract diseases, lower GI tract diseases, pancreatico-biliary diseases, and liver diseases. Furthermore, it covers all that is important to know regarding different types of endoscopes, construction of an endoscopy unit, examination techniques, sedation, and monitoring of the patient. One of the key questions is of course whether the endoscopic procedure makes any diagnostic or therapeutic gain for the patient. This topic is nicely overviewed focusing on the clinical impact of GI endoscopy within gastroenterology, hepatology, surgery, and bariatrics.

The book is enriched by more than 400 original images and accompanied by instructive videos. The work done by the authors is the result of many years of clinical experience mixed with firm scientific evidence within their fields of expertise. I believe that this book will not only become a reference guide for residents and trainees but also for specialists in gastroenterology, hepatology, pancreatology, and surgery, who want to get a good overview of endoscopy techniques.

Peter Vilmann
Department of Clinical Medicine
University of Copenhagen
Copenhagen, Denmark

Contents

Part VI Upper Gastrointestinal Tract

Part VII Lower Gastrointestinal Tract

Part VIII   Pancreatico-Biliary Diseases

Part IX   Liver Diseases

Part I

Introduction

The Future of Digestive Endoscopy

1

Adrian Săftoiu

In medicine, predictions are extremely risky, especially for a minimally invasive technique that has revolutionized gastroenterology in the last 50 years. Recently developed, a series of disruptive techniques seem to "threaten" flexible endoscopy, a technique defined in the current context of diagnosis and treatment of gastroenterological and hepato-bilio-pancreatic diseases

1.1 Single-Use Endoscopes

- Types of single-use endoscopes:
  - Due to the issues generated by disinfection/sterilization, duodenoscopes were the first to be launched on the market, the cost of use being prohibitive for the time being.

A. Săftoiu (✉)

Department of Gastroenterology and Hepatology, Elias Emergency University Hospital, Carol Davila University of Medicine and Pharmacy, Bucharest, Romania

3

A. Săftoiu (ed.), *Pocket Guide to Advanced Endoscopy in Gastroenterology*, https://doi.org/10.1007/978-3-031-42076-4_1

1.2   Miniaturization and Wireless Devices

- Types of miniaturized devices [1]:
  - Ultrathin endoscopes are already used in various clinical applications.
        Transnasal endoscopy.
        Cholangioscopy.
        Fistuloscopy.
  - Single-fiber endoscopes are under development, with miniaturization increasing patient comfort and acceptability of intracavitary procedures.
  - Endoscopic videocapsule involves miniaturization and remote ("wireless") transmission of images.

1.3   Endoscopic Robots

Different types of endoscopic robots are being evaluated, to improve standard diagnostic procedures or increase the precision of therapeutic interventions [2, 3]:

- Guided locomotion endorobots.
- Capsules directed externally in magnetic field.
- Externally coupled "tethered" capsules.
  - Pneumatically guided.
  - Guided by water jet.
  - Magnetically guided.
- Endorobots with surgical instruments.
- Operative instruments (dissectors, graspers, clips, electrodes, loops, needles, etc.).
- Useful in repetitive, long procedures.
  - Endoscopic submucosal dissection.
  - Endoscopic gastroplasty.

1.4   **Endoscopic Surgery**

Flexible endoscopy has gradually become a complementary technique to laparoscopic/robotic surgery, with multiple clinical applications [4, 5]:

- "Third space" endoscopy procedures performed by penetrating the submucosal plane:
  - POEM (PerOral endoscopic myotomy) procedures for achalasia, with/without fundoplications (F-POEM).
  - Derivative procedures Z-POEM (Zencker diverticulum)/ G-POEM (refractory gastroparesis).
  - STER procedures (submucosal tunneling endoscopic resection) for submucosal tumors.
- Endoscopic procedures combined with laparoscopic ones such as CELS (combined endoscopic laparoscopic surgery):
  - Laparoscopic-assisted enteroscopy.
  - Laparoscopic-assisted polypectomy (difficult polyps).
  - Resections of submucosal tumors.
- NOTES (natural orifice transluminal endoscopic surgery) endoscopic procedures that involve passing the endoscope into the peritoneal cavity:
  - Transgastric peritoneoscopies.
  - Transgastric/transvaginal appendicectomies.
  - Transvaginal cholecystectomies.
  - Transanal sigmoidectomies.
- Procedures similar to digestive anastomoses.
  - EUS-guided drainage of pseudocysts/abscesses.
  - EUS-guided bilio-pancreatic drainages (choledoco-duodeno-, hepatico-gastro-, cholecysto-gastro-, pancreatico-gastro-).
  - EUS-guided gastrojejunal anastomoses (GJA).
  - EDGE procedures (EUS-directed transgastric Endoscopic retrograde cholangiopancreatography).

1.5 Molecular Endoscopy

- Early detection of premalignant/malignant lesions and assessment of prognosis by microscopic examination of the gastrointestinal mucosa after topical/systemic application of contrast agents [6, 7]:
- Fluorescein is the only FDA-approved human fluorophore used in vivo in confocal laser endomicroscopy (CLE).
- Alexa-fluor 488 or fluorescein isothiocyanate (FITC) are used to label molecular targets with emission at 488 nm (Fig. 1.1), and indocyanine green (ICG) with emission in the near-infrared spectrum (NIR) at 665–900 nm [8].
- Clinical applications include:
  - Detection of high-grade dysplasia/early adenocarcinoma in Barrett's esophagus.
  - Detection of intestinal metaplasia/early gastric adenocarcinoma.
  - Assessment of ulcerative colitis/Crohn's disease.
  - Detection of colonic adenomas (including serrated adenomas) or early colonic adenocarcinoma.
  - Evaluation of prognosis in advanced cancer.

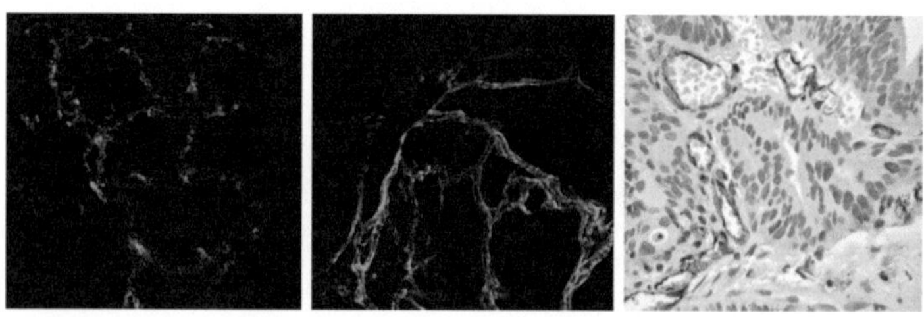

Fig. 1.1 *Ex vivo* confocal laser endomicroscopy with anti-CD31 antibodies labeled with alexa fluor 488 (**a**—normal appearance of vessels regularly surrounding colonic crypts, **b**—colonic adenocarcinoma), compared to immunohistochemical appearance (**c**—colonic adenocarcinoma, col. HE + CD31)

1.6   Artificial Intelligence

Artificial intelligence techniques using neural networks have recently been used in the field of digestive endoscopy, especially after the introduction of "deep learning" techniques using convolutional neural networks (Fig. 1.2) [9]:

- Computer-aided detection systems (computer-aided detection—CADe).
  - Detection of digestive bleeding.
  - Detection of diminutive colonic polyps [10].
  - Early digestive cancer detection.
- Computer-aided characterization/diagnosis/prognosis systems (computer-aided diagnosis—CADx).
  - Differentiation of neoplastic/hyperplastic polyps based on NBI/i-SCAN appearance (see Chap. 6).
  - Early diagnosis and delimitation of eso-gastroduodenal/colorectal cancers.
  - Diagnosis of inflammation in ulcerative colitis/Crohn's disease to assess remission.
  - Differentiation of focal pancreatic tumors according to EUS appearance.

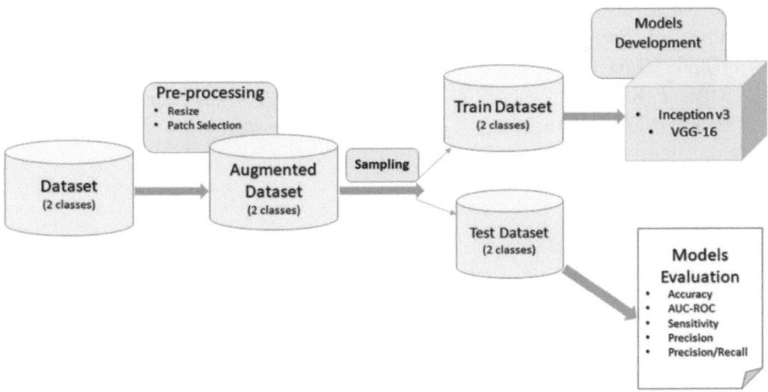

Fig. 1.2 Deep learning model for the use of convolutional neural networks for computer-assisted diagnosis

References

1. McGoran JJ, McAlindon ME, Iyer PG, Haidry R, Lovat LB, Sami SS. Miniature gastrointestinal endoscopy: now and the future. World J Gastroenterol. 2019;25:4051–60.
2. Boskoski I, Costamagna G. Endoscopy robotics: current and future applications. Digestive Endoscopy. 2019;31:119–24.
3. Martin JW, Scaglioni B, Norton JC, et al. Enabling the future of colonoscopy with intelligent and autonomous magnetic manipulation. Nat Mach Intell. 2020;2:595–606.
4. Surlin V, Săftoiu A, Rimbaş M, Vilmann P. Notes—"state of the art" surgical gastroenterology: the beginning of the voyage. Hepatogastroenterology. 2010;57:54–61.
5. Arezzo A, Zornig C, Mofid H, et al. The EURO-NOTES clinical registry for natural orifice transluminal endoscopic surgery: a 2-year activity report. Surg Endosc. 2013;27:3073–84.
6. Karstensen JG, Klausen PH, Saftoiu A, Vilmann P. Molecular confocal laser endomicroscopy: a novel technique for in vivo cellular characterization of gastrointestinal lesions. World J Gastroenterol. 2014;20:7794–800.
7. Ahmed S, Galle PR, Neumann H. Molecular endoscopic imaging: the future is bright. Ther Adv Gastrointest Endosc. 2019;12:1–15.
8. Ciocâlteu A, Săftoiu A, Cârţână T, et al. Evaluation of new morphometric parameters of neoangiogenesis in human colorectal cancer using confocal laser endomicroscopy (CLE) and targeted panendothelial markers. PLoS One. 2014;9:e91084.
9. Săftoiu A, Vilmann P, Gorunescu F, et al. Efficacy of an artificial neural network-based approach to endoscopic ultrasound elastography in diagnosis of focal pancreatic masses. Clin Gastroenterol Hepatol. 2012;10:84–90.e1.
10. Mori Y, Kudo S. Detecting colorectal polyps via machine learning. Nat Biomed Eng. 2018;2:713–4.

Part II

Integrated Endoscopy Units

Infrastructure of the Endoscopy Unit

2

Adrian Săftoiu

2.1 Estimated Flow

Modern endoscopy units have a complex infrastructure and allow multidisciplinary team activities [1–5]

- 1000–1500 patients for each room.
- At least 2–4 examination rooms +1–2 interventional rooms (EUS/ERCP, etc.).
- Flexibility to adapt to emergencies.
- Possibility of extension with two more rooms (for screening/ polypectomies, etc.) (Fig. 2.1).

A. Săftoiu (✉)
Department of Gastroenterology and Hepatology, Elias Emergency University Hospital, Carol Davila University of Medicine and Pharmacy, Bucharest, Romania

A. Săftoiu (ed.), *Pocket Guide to Advanced Endoscopy in Gastroenterology*, https://doi.org/10.1007/978-3-031-42076-4_2

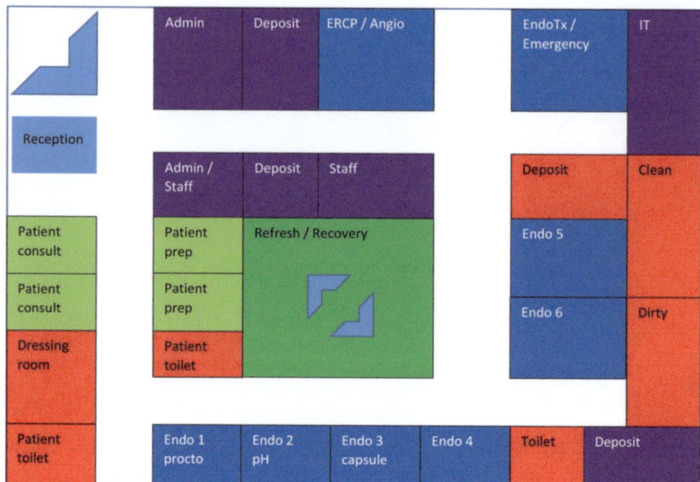

Fig. 2.1 Flows in the endoscopy unit

2.2 Functional Circuits

- Waiting room.
- Patient preparation room.
- Pre-procedure consultation office.
- Endoscopy examination room.
  - O_2, CO_2, compressed air (suction).
  - Blood pressure (BP), heart rate, O_2 saturation (continuous monitoring).
- Post anesthesia room—refresh.
  - Minimum three beds for a room.
- High-grade disinfection of endoscopes + sterilization of consumables (preferably single use).
  - Automatic washing machines,
  - In-out circuits, dirty-clean,
- Separate storage room + transport with dedicated tanks (Fig. 2.2).

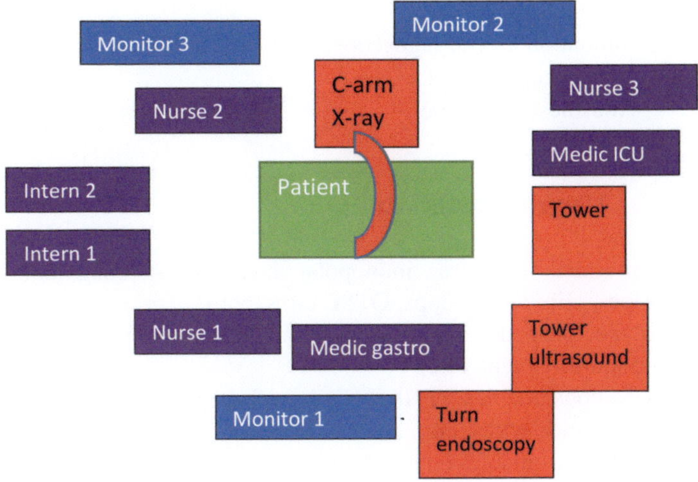

Fig. 2.2 The disposition of endoscopy equipment

2.3   Other Rooms

- Doctors' offices + nurse's office.
- Registration offices/technical support + IT.

2.4   Equipment

- High-definition (HD) endoscopy towers.
  - Dx and Tx gastroscope.
  - Colonoscope.
  - Linear/radial echoendoscope.
  - Tx duodenoscope (ERCP).
  - Pediatric enteroscope/colonoscope.
- Digital radiology equipment.
  - For EUS/ERCP/dilation, etc.
  - Mobile radiology table.

- Emergency equipment.
  - Intubation kit (laryngoscope, etc.).
  - Ambu bag, O_2 masks.
  - Anesthesia machine.

2.5 Usual Consumables

- Hemostasis (needles, monopolar and bipolar coagulation probes, clips, endo loops, OTSC clips, etc.)
- Polypectomy (different size, oval and hexagonal loops, mono- and multifilament, etc.)
- EUS consumables (FNA/FNB needles, plastic and metal stents, guide wires, etc.)
- ERCP consumables (sphincterotomies, guide wires, extraction baskets and balloons, dilation balloons, plastic and metal stents, dilators, etc.)
- Video endoscopy capsule.

2.6 Staff

- Two full-time doctors/each room.
- Three nurses for one doctor (3:1).
- An IT technician.
- An anesthesiologist/unit.
  - Anesthesia nurses for NAPS.
- Reception and technical secretary.

References

1. Burton D, Ott BJ, Gostout CJ, DiMagno EP. Approach to designing a gastrointestinal endoscopy unit. Gastrointest Endosc Clin N Am. 1993;3: 525–40.
2. Mulder CJJ, Jacobs MAJM, Leicester RJ, et al. Guidelines for designing a digestive disease endoscopy unit: Report of the World Endoscopy Organization. Dig Endosc. 2013;25:365–75.

3. Valori R, Cortas G, de Lange T, et al. Performance measures for endoscopy services: A European Society of Gastrointestinal Endoscopy (ESGE) Quality Improvement Initiative. Endoscopy. 2018;50:1186–204.
4. Lennard-Jones JE, Williams CB, Axon A, et al. Provision of gastrointestinal endoscopy and related services for a district general hospital. Working party of the Clinical Services Committee of the British Society of Gastroenterology. Gut. 1991;32:95–105.
5. Lennard-Jones JE. Staffing of a combined general medical service and gastroenterology unit in a district general hospital. Gut. 1989;30:546–5.

Deconstructing the Endoscope

3

Irina F. Cherciu Harbiyeli

3.1 Anatomy of the Endoscopy System

- Endoscope.
- Video processor.
- Light source.
- Video recorder.
- Suction system.
- Electrosurgical generator unit.
- Trolley with hanger + monitor.

The endoscope is a flexible instrument facilitating the illumination and visualization of the lumen of hollow organs. It incorporates the following:

- A proximal end (control section).
- An insertion tube.
- A distal end (tip).

I. F. Cherciu Harbiyeli (✉)
Research Center of Gastroenterology and Hepatology Craiova,
University of Medicine and Pharmacy of Craiova, Craiova, Romania

© The Author(s), under exclusive license to Springer Nature Switzerland AG 2023
A. Săftoiu (ed.), *Pocket Guide to Advanced Endoscopy in Gastroenterology*, https://doi.org/10.1007/978-3-031-42076-4_3

3.2   The Proximal End [1, 2]

- Includes the control unit.
- Held in the left hand of the endoscopist (Figs. 3.1 and 3.2).
- Used to maneuver the endoscope and introduce accessories.
- The twin dials help maneuver the tip.
    - Larger dial (deflects the tip up/down).
    - Small dial (left/right lateral control).
    - Ultra-thin specialized endoscopes may have only a single dial (up/down angulation).
    - Duodenoscopes (utilized for ERCP) and linear echoendoscopes carry a supplementary dial for maneuvering the elevator.

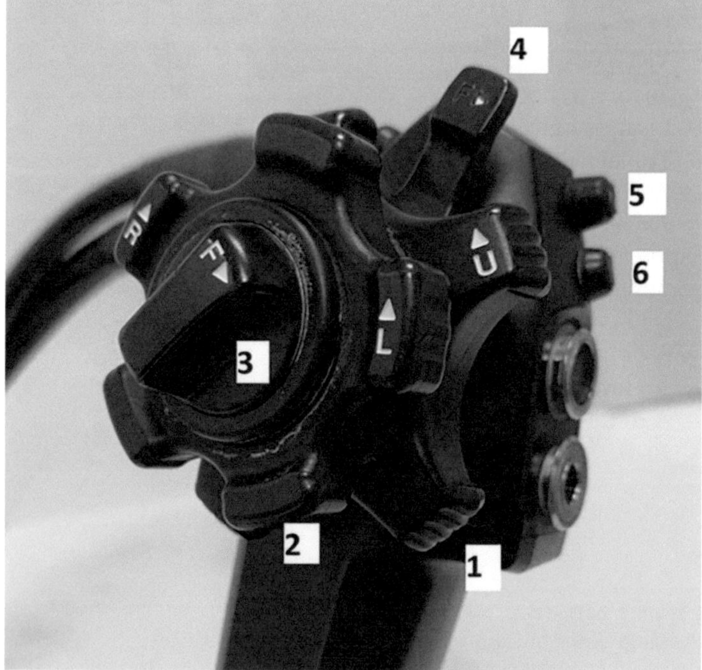

Fig. 3.1 The proximal end of the endoscope: 1—large dial (up/down control), 2—small dial (left/right control), 3—small wheel lock lever, 4—large wheel locking lever, 5 and 6—buttons for storing images, other functions

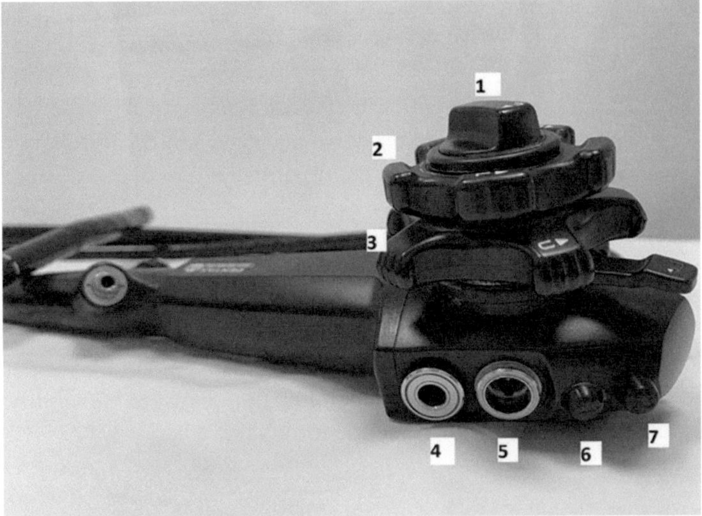

Fig. 3.2 The proximal end of the endoscope: 1—small wheel lock lever, 2—small dial (left/right control), 3—large dial (up/down control), 4—button with dual air/water insufflation function, 5—suction button, 6 and 7—buttons to record/store images; other functions

- An additional rotatable dial might be incorporate in colonoscope for controlling the variable-stiffness function of the insertion tube.
- Front openings accommodate specially designed buttons.
  - Suction button.
  - Button with dual functions of air/water insufflation.
  - Buttons to save images, switch the NBI/i-SCAN mode, etc.

3.3   The Insertion Tube [1, 2]

- Contains multiple layers of polymers that confer durability along with flexibility.
- It accommodates a "working channel" of variable diameters, which permits the passage of endoscopic accessories.
- Involved in applying suction and insufflation.

- Guides a jet of water toward a target within the lumen, the "power wash" function is used for cleaning debris.
- Angulation wires.
  - Run along the length of the insertion tube.
  - Are connected to the up-down and right-left control dials.
  - Allow to flex−/retroflex the tip of the endoscope.
- Spiral metal bands.
  - Facilitate the ability to torque.
- Certain endoscopes conceal devices to create variable stiffness of the insertion tube.
  - The rigidity does not extend to the distal 15–20 cm.
- The art and science behind designing the insertion tube resides in obtaining the optimum combination between flexibility, elasticity, column strength, and torquing ability.

3.3.1   Tip of the Endoscope [1, 2]

- The widest opening is a port of the working channel for passage of various endoscopic accessories.
- Allows the air/water insufflation/aspiration.
- The objective lens might be forward-viewing, oblique, or side-facing.
- The "light source" dispatches light into the field of view.
- The charge-coupled device (CCD) unit:
  - Sets up an integrated system with the objective lens.
  - Allows transmission of images directly into the image processor through an "umbilical cord" (connector).

3.4   Image Processing [3]

- Electronic images are sent to a video monitor.
- Real-time automatic detection systems are available for increasing adenoma detection rates.
- High-magnification endoscopes perform optical zoom.
- Digital magnification enlarges the image on the display, reduces pixel density and therefore decreases the image quality.
- Details regarding enhanced imaging techniques in Part 3, Chap. 7.

3.5 Modalities to Increase the Visualization Field [4, 5]

- Additional imaging devices (Fuse® Full Spectrum Endoscopy® platform, EndoChoice Inc., Alpharetta, GA, USA) or cameras with extra wide view (Extra-Wide-Angle-View Olympus colonoscope, Tokyo, Japan), with angles between 170 and 330° to allow visualization of mucosa behind the folds.
- Accessories that can flatten the haustral folds for inspection (attached to the tip of the endoscope or passed through the working channel).
  - NaviAid G-EYE colonoscope (Smart Medical Systems Ltd., Ra'anana, Israel)—permanently integrated balloon system for straightening colon folds, centralizing the image, and reducing bowel slippage.
  - Endocuff (Arc Medical Design Ltd., Leeds, United Kingdom)—accessory mounted on the distal tip of the endoscope with multiple soft fingerlike projections that can flatten the haustral folds.
  - Third Eye Retroscope (Avantis Medical Systems, Sunnyvale, CA, USA)—a retroflexed video camera system passed through the working channel of the endoscope, functioning as a rear-view mirror.

3.6 Technical Perspectives [5]

- The ideal endoscope:
  - A single-use, super-flexible, multidimensional, self-propelled tool for a pain free procedure and with no sedation.
  - Enables an elective increase in rigidity to allow a stable position during therapeutic maneuvers.
  - Has a small caliber and adequate size working channels to easily employ/exchange all of the endoscopic accessories.

- Improving real-time image processing programs to assist in lesion detection and characterization through artificial intelligence techniques.
- Dedicated endoscopy robotic platforms to additionally boost the 3D imaging of intraluminal and transmural advanced procedures [5].

References

1. Kurniawan N, Keuchel M. Flexible gastro-intestinal endoscopy—clinical challenges and technical achievements. Comput Struct Biotechnol J. 2017;15:168–79.
2. Kochman M, Swain P. Deconstruction of the endoscope. Gastrointest Endosc. 2007;66:677–8.
3. Gkolfakis P, Tziatzios G, Dimitriadis GD, Triantafyllou K. New endoscopes and add-on devices to improve colonoscopy performance. World J Gastroenterol. 2017;23:3784–96.
4. Varadarajulu S, et al. GI endoscopes—report on emerging technology. Gastrointest EndoscGastrointest Endosc. 2011;74:1–6.
5. Gralnek IM. Emerging technologies in colonoscopy. Dig Endosc. 2015;27:223–31.

Types of Flexible Endoscopy

4

Irina F. Cherciu Harbiyeli
and Bogdan S. Ungureanu

4.1 Gastroscope [1]

- Diagnostic and therapeutic endoscopes (with enlarged/dual working channels).
- *Narrow-caliber/ultra-slim endoscopes.*
  - A diameter ranging from 4.9 to 6 mm (can be introduced transnasally/transorally).
  - The accessory channel is relatively narrow (2 mm).

4.2 Colonoscope [1, 2]

- Designed to minimize loop formation (Fig. 4.1).
  - The distal end is rather soft and flexible to permit the negotiation of angulations/curves.
  - The proximal end is comparatively stiffer and slighter flexible to decrease loop formation.
  - Due to elasticity, it straightens when pulled back.

I. F. Cherciu Harbiyeli (✉) · B. S. Ungureanu
Research Center of Gastroenterology and Hepatology Craiova,
University of Medicine and Pharmacy of Craiova, Craiova, Romania

© The Author(s), under exclusive license to Springer Nature Switzerland AG 2023

A. Săftoiu (ed.), *Pocket Guide to Advanced Endoscopy in Gastroenterology*, https://doi.org/10.1007/978-3-031-42076-4_4

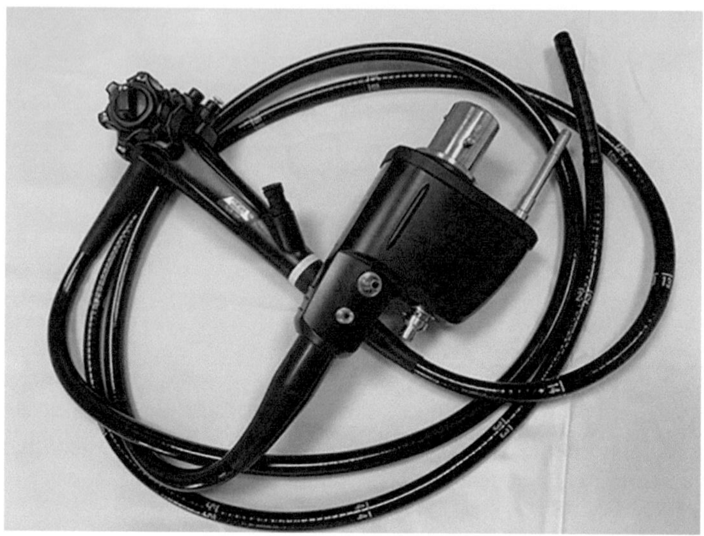

Fig. 4.1 Standard colonoscope, with fixed stiffness

- The variable-stiffness colonoscope.
    - Used to stiffen the proximal 40–50 cm.
    - Improves cecal intubation rates with less discomfort.

4.3   Enteroscope [1, 2]

- Characteristics.
    - Forward-viewing endoscope, considerably longer.
    - Comprises devices ("overtube," inflatable balloons) designed for the intubation of the jejunum/ileum.
    - Performed anterograde/oral or retrograde/anal.
- *Balloon-assisted enteroscope* utilizes an overtube with a single- or double-balloon system mounted at the distal end:
    - Examination of the small intestine on large portions.
    - The balloons anchor alternately the endoscope and the overtube to facilitate the pleating of the bowel.
- *Spiral enteroscope.*
    - Do not engage balloons, but an overtube with external spirals that folds the small bowel as it rotates.

- *Push enteroscopy.*
  - Do not rely on balloons or overtubes.
  - Assessment limited to the upper GI tract.
  - Adult/pediatric colonoscopies/enteroscopes.

4.4   Duodenoscopes [3]

- Specialized endoscopes used primarily for ERCP (Figs. 4.2 and 4.3).
- Side-viewing for looking at the major duodenal papilla en face.
- A lever is used to maneuver the elevator, hence:
  - The doctor may angle the accessories.
  - It facilitates access to the bile/pancreatic duct, which is helpful for cannulation of the papilla.
- Cholangioscopes (SpyGlass Direct Visualization System, Boston Scientific Corp, Natick, MA, USA) are devices that can be passed throw the working channel of the duodenoscope into the biliary/pancreatic duct for real-time visualization and sampling of the mucosa, for the treatment of lithiasis and strictures.

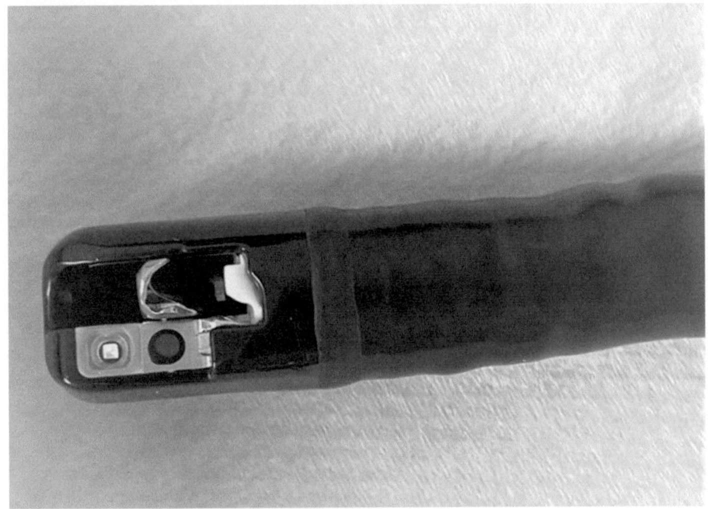

Fig. 4.2 Details of a side-viewing duodenoscope, with elevator used for the angulation of accessories inserted through the papilla

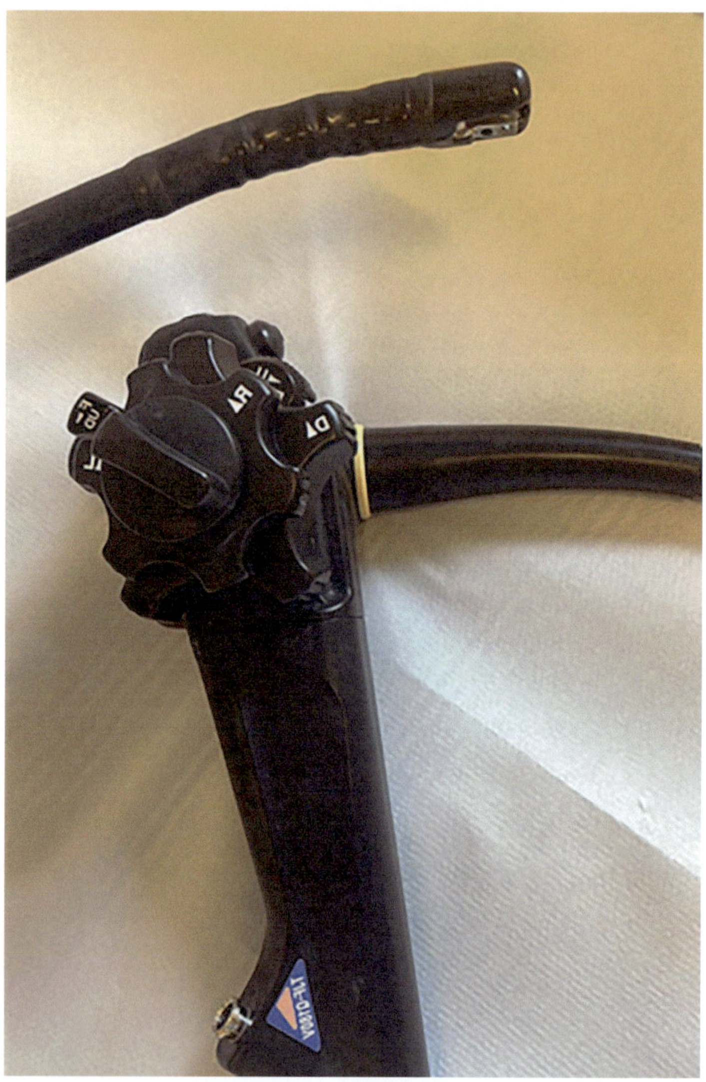

Fig. 4.3 Side-viewing duodenoscope, dedicated to ERCP

4.5   Echoendoscope [2, 3]

- Allows the examination of the GI wall and extra-luminal structures, combining ultrasound with endoscopy.
- *The ultrasound transducer* at the tip (Fig. 4.4):
  - Differentiates echoendoscopes from the standard endoscopes.
  - Contains piezoelectric crystals→convert electrical energy into sound waves→travel through the wall of the GI tract→get reflected back to the transducer→reconverts it to electric signals→processed for creating an EUS image.
- Scanning frequencies: 5–12 or 20 MHz (miniprobes).
  - Higher frequencies enhance the resolution and reduce depth of penetration.
  - Lower frequencies utilized for imaging distant structures.
- Doppler signal assessment allows the identification and avoidance of vascular structures.
- *Curvilinear echoendoscope.*
  - Produces an image parallel to the insertion tube.
  - Visualizes structures in the 100–180° range.
  - Allows real-time visualization of EUS needles.
  - Can be used for diverse guided/assisted EUS interventions (Fig. 4.5).
- *Radial echoendoscope.*
  - Produces an image that is perpendicular to the insertion tube.
  - Provides an ultrasonographic 360° view.
  - Cannot be used for therapeutic procedures.

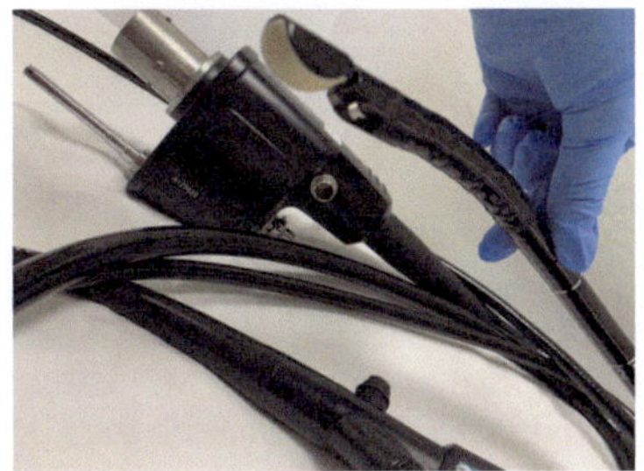

Fig. 4.4 Side-viewing echoendoscope, dedicated EUS-FNA

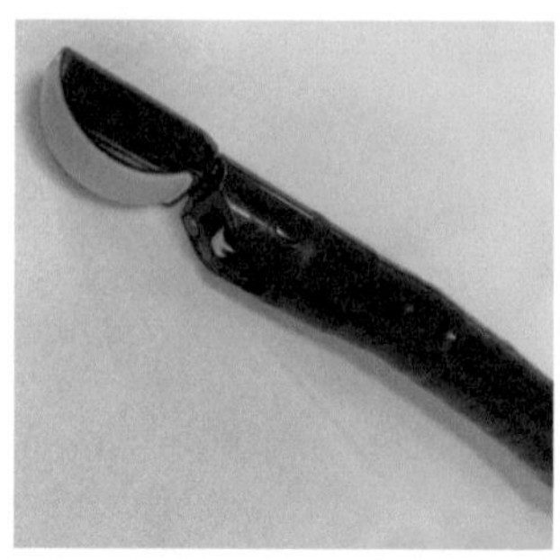

Fig. 4.5 Linear echoendoscope, dedicated EUS-FNA, with elevator used for the angulation of the accessories introduced through the biopsy channel

4.6   Capsule Endoscope [1]

- Made of:
  - A clear plastic dome.
  - Compact lens system.
  - Illumination white LED.
  - High-resolution CCD (to capture images).
  - Battery.
  - Antenna.
- Activated after removal from the magnetic holder.
- Can be swallowed or endoscopically positioned in the stomach/small intestine (proximal).
- Disposable and designed to be excreted.
- The endoscopist/endoscopy nurse can:
  - Review all the images in multiple/single frames, inspecting for mucosal lesions.
  - Calculate the transit time of the capsule (see more about capsule endoscopy in Chap. 5).

References

1. Kohli DR, Baillie J. How endoscopes work. In: Chandrasekhara V, Elmunzer BJ, Khashab MA, Muthusamy VR, editors. Clinical gastrointestinal endoscopy. 3rd ed. Amsterdam: Elsevier; 2018. p. 24–31.e2.
2. Kurniawan N, Keuchel M. Flexible gastro-intestinal endoscopy—clinical challenges and technical achievements. Comput Struct Biotechnol J. 2017;15:168–79.
3. ASGE Technology Committee, Komanduri S, Thosani N, Abu Dayyeh BK, et al. Cholangiopancreatoscopy. Gastrointest Endosc. 2016;84:209–21.

Capsule Endoscopy

5

Vlad-Florin Iovănescu and Adrian Săftoiu

5.1 General Principle

- Diagnostic method that allows endoluminal evaluation of the gastrointestinal tract by recording sequential images captured by a pill-like device that is swallowed and moves with peristalsis.
- The capsule endoscopy consists of a miniature video camera, a light source (LEDs), a transmitter, and a battery incorporated in a plastic housing measuring an average of 2–3 cm.
- Two types of capsules available:
  - Capsules that record the images onto the internal memory. The capsule has to be retrieved from the stool.
  - Capsules that transmit the signal wirelessly to a series of sensors applied to the patient's body which are connected to a device that allows live-image viewing and storage.

V.-F. Iovănescu (✉)
University of Medicine and Pharmacy of Craiova, Craiova, Romania
e-mail: vlad.iovanescu@umfcv.ro

A. Săftoiu
Department of Gastroenterology and Hepatology, Elias Emergency
University Hospital, Carol Davila University of Medicine and Pharmacy,
Bucharest, Romania

© The Author(s), under exclusive license to Springer Nature
Switzerland AG 2023
A. Săftoiu (ed.), *Pocket Guide to Advanced Endoscopy in
Gastroenterology*, https://doi.org/10.1007/978-3-031-42076-4_5

- Dedicated software is used for analyzing the retrieved images.
  - Software postprocessing allow image enhancement such as red spot detection (for easier identification of hemorrhagic lesions/active bleeding).
- Non-most commonly used for assessing small bowel pathology.
- Different systems also available for visualization of esophagus, stomach, and colon.
  - Esophagus and stomach capsules usually indicated when a patient refuses to undergo upper gastrointestinal endoscopy.
  - Colon capsules used in patients with an incomplete colonoscopy due to inadequate bowel preparation and when complete colonoscopy is not technically feasible [1].

5.2   Preparation

- Fasting is recommended 12 h before the examination.
- Preparation with 2 L polyethyleneglycol (PEG) solutions prior to capsule ingestion is recommended by European guidelines [2].
- Optimal timing is not established.
- Use of antifoaming agents (e.g., simethicone) is advised.
- Prokinetics are not routinely recommended; however, may be used in particular cases (e.g., diabetic neuropathy) if the capsule fails to progress beyond the stomach for 30–60 min as observed by real-time viewing.

5.3   Indications

- Obscure gastrointestinal bleeding.
  - Most sources located in small bowel.
  - Ideally during/in the first 24–72 h after the bleeding onset to have a higher chance of identifying the source.
- Occult gastrointestinal bleeding.
- Unexplained iron-deficiency anemia.
  - Performed after no source has been identified by upper and lower gastrointestinal endoscopy.

- Malabsorption syndrome.
- Evaluation of chronic diarrhea.
- Surveillance of gastrointestinal polyposis syndromes.
  - Particularly in familial adenomatous polyposis and Peutz–Jeghers syndrome.
- Diagnosis of suspected small bowel Crohn's disease.
  - Recommended as the initial diagnostic method in the absence of obstructive symptoms or previously known stenosis [3].
  - CT/MRI enterography are the first diagnostic modalities if obstructive symptoms are present or there is a previously known stenosis.
- Evaluation of the location/extent/flare of a previously diagnosed small bowel Crohn's disease.
  - Indicated only when CT/MRI enterography results are inconclusive and only if it impacts management.
  - Should be preceded by administration of a patency capsule to ensure safe passage of the capsule endoscopy.

5.4   Advantages and Disadvantages

- Advantages
  - Noninvasive technique.
  - No need for patient sedation.
  - No need for hospital admission (usually performed as an outpatient procedure).
- Disadvantages

- Does not allow tissue sampling and therapeutic maneuvers.
- Impossibility of exact lesion localization.
- Low-quality image in case of poor bowel preparation because it lacks possibility of aspiration and lavage.
- Expensive

5.5 Complications

- Tracheobronchial aspiration
  - Extremely rare.
  - In patients with impaired deglutition.
  - The capsule can be introduced with the endoscope into the duodenum.
- Intestinal perforation
- Capsule retention
  - Most important complication (1.4%) [4].
  - Increased risk in patients with small bowel obstruction (stenosing Crohn's disease, small bowel tumors, history of abdominal or pelvic radiotherapy).
  - Suspected if the capsule is not eliminated in stool after 14 days.
  - In case of prolonged retention or presence of obstructive symptoms, endoscopic or surgical retrieval is necessary.
  - Patency capsules can be used in cases of suspected obstruction to minimize the risk of retention.
    Traceable capsule that dissolves itself if not eliminated in a certain time limit.

References

1. Hale MF, Sidhu R, McAlindon ME. Capsule endoscopy: current practice and future directions. World J Gastroenterol. 2014;20(24):7752–9. https://doi.org/10.3748/wjg.v20.i24.7752.
2. Rondonotti E, Spada C, Adler S, May A, Despott EJ, Koulaouzidis A, Panter S, Domagk D, Fernandez-Urien I, Rahmi G, Riccioni ME, van Hooft JE, Hassan C, Pennazio M. Small-bowel capsule endoscopy and

device-assisted enteroscopy for diagnosis and treatment of small-bowel disorders: European Society of Gastrointestinal Endoscopy (ESGE) Technical Review. Endoscopy. 2018;50(4):423–46. https://doi.org/10.1055/a-0576-0566.

3. Akpunonu B, Hummell J, Akpunonu JD, Ud DS. Capsule endoscopy in gastrointestinal disease: Evaluation, diagnosis, and treatment. Cleve Clin J Med. 2022;89(4):200–11. https://doi.org/10.3949/ccjm.89a.20061.

4. Wang YC, Pan J, Liu YW, Sun FY, Qian YY, Jiang X, Zou WB, Xia J, Jiang B, Ru N, Zhu JH, Linghu EQ, Li ZS, Liao Z. Adverse events of video capsule endoscopy over the past two decades: a systematic review and proportion meta-analysis. BMC Gastroenterol. 2020;20(1):364. https://doi.org/10.1186/s12876-020-01491-w.

Part III

Examination Techniques

Preparation Before Endoscopy

6

Irina F. Cherciu Harbiyeli
and Mihaela Calița

6.1 General Preparation [1, 2]

- Patients history (allergies, heart/lung disease).
- The treatment for chronic diseases (heart, etc.) will not be interrupted, will be administered in the morning with a small amount of fluid.
  - Exceptions: anticoagulants and antiplatelets drugs will be discontinued according to the recommendations, in case of procedures with risk of bleeding (see Chap. 11).
- For patients with diabetes:
  - Oral antidiabetic medication will not be administered pre-procedurally.
  - The insulin will be administered as follows: half of the morning dose at the usual time and the other half together with the first post-procedural meal.
- Submitting all medical documents that could guide the diagnosis and further therapy.

I. F. Cherciu Harbiyeli (✉) · M. Calița
Research Center of Gastroenterology and Hepatology Craiova,
University of Medicine and Pharmacy Craiova,
Craiova, Romania

A. Săftoiu (ed.), *Pocket Guide to Advanced Endoscopy in Gastroenterology*, https://doi.org/10.1007/978-3-031-42076-4_6

- Informed consent is essential!
  - Provides information on the nature of a proposed procedure or specific treatment for which the procedure is suggested, with risks, benefits, possible complications, and reasonable alternatives.
  - Must be obtained within a predefined time and in a favorable environment.
  - It is necessary for the document to cover the separate endoscopic procedure, respectively, the sedation.
    The endoscopist will document in the final result the preprocedural consent.
  - The recognized exceptions to the informed consent process include the following:
    Emergency.
    The possibility that the information may harm the patient.
    Legal waiver and power of attorney.
  - All informed refusals must be documented!
- Creating the venous approach by mounting a catheter in a peripheral vein in patients undergoing deep sedation investigation (see Chaps. 13, 14, and 15).

6.2 Special Preparation for the Upper Digestive Tract [3]

- Fasting 6–8 h before the procedure + liquid rest for at least 2 h.
  - Exceptions: patients with diabetes and gastrointestinal stenosis, in whom rest may be prolonged.
- Removal of denture prosthesis to prevent migration into the trachea!
- When biliary obstruction is suspected, appropriate antibiotic therapy is recommended prior to ERCP procedures (see Chap. 12).
- Corticosteroid prophylaxis may be considered in patients with a history of anaphylactic reactions to the contrast agent, prior to the EUS procedure.

6.3   Special Preparation for the Lower Digestive Tract [4, 5]

- Instructions regarding the preparation for colonoscopy.
  - As detailed as possible (provided verbally and in writing), increasing the degree of adherence of patients proportionally.
- Dietary changes.
  - On the day before preparation, a diet low in vegetable fiber is recommended (Table 6.1).
- Additional medication changes:
  - Iron medication should be stopped 7 days before the colonoscopic examination.
  - It is recommended to avoid agents with constipating effect, medicinal charcoal, laxative oils, etc.
  - Oral simethicone can be added to the colonoscopy preparation scheme.
  - The use of prokinetic agents is not recommended.
- Required before performing colonoscopy:
  - Preparation of the intestine by ingesting a purgative solution in order to eliminate the intestinal contents.
  - The most commonly used purgative solution in RO is the electrolytic solution with polyethylene glycol (PEG):
      The first dose will be administered in the afternoon of the day before the investigation.
      The second dose will be completed approximately 2–3 h before the investigation (split dose).

Table 6.1 Recommendations regarding the low-fiber diet

Category	Allowed foods	Foods to avoid
Type of food	Dairy products, white bread, white rice, chicken, turkey, fish, eggs, fruit juice without pulp, strained soups, fruits without peel and seeds (apples, cantaloupe melons, peaches), vegetables (carrots, mushrooms, potatoes, asparagus) thermally prepared	Fresh or dehydrated fruits and vegetables, any whole grain, red meat, nuts, seeds, granola, etc.

- The characteristics of the purgative solutions are summarized in Table 6.2.
- Not recommended.
  - Osmotic laxatives with nonabsorbable carbohydrates (mannitol, lactulose, sorbitol)/oral sodium phosphate.
- Preparation in particular cases:
  - Patients with constipation do not require any specific preparation.
  - Pregnant/lactating women: if colonoscopy is absolutely necessary, PEG-based protocols may be considered. For sigmoidoscopy, water enemas are preferred.
  - Patients with inflammatory bowel disease: PEG-based protocols will be used.

Table 6.2 Validated purgative solutions for colonoscopy/enteroscopy preparation

Product	Characteristics	Not recommended for patients with:
PEG	Izo-osmotic agent Safe and effective The 4 L of liquid can be difficult to ingest, even in two doses	Congestive heart failure (NYHA class III or IV)
Low volume PEG and adjuvants	Hypo-osmotic agent Similar to PEG regarding safety and efficacy 2 L PEG plus ascorbate/ascorbic acid/citrate/bisacodil administered in two doses	Severe renal impairment (creatinine clearance <30 mL/min) Congestive heart failure (NYHA class III or IV) Unstable angina Acute myocardial infarction Phenylketonuria Glucose-6-phosphate dehydrogenase deficiency
Magnesium salts (Mg citrate and picosulfate)	Hyper-osmotic agent Similar to PEG regarding safety and efficacy 2 L of liquid administered in two doses	Congestive heart failure Severe renal failure Hypermagnesemia Rhabdomyolysis
Trisulfate solutions (Na, Mg, and K sulphate)	Hyper-osmotic agent Similar to PEG regarding safety and efficacy 2.5 L liquid administered in two doses	Congestive heart failure Severe renal failure Ascites

- Inadequate preparation:
  - Makes colonoscopic screening inefficient.
      Decreases the detection rate of polyps and adenomas.
      Cecal intubation failure.
  - Requires to repeat colonoscopy in maximum 1 year.
  - Colonoscopy can be rescheduled on the same day or the next day, after additional preparation (with laxative or enema), individualized according to the possible reasons for the initial failure.

References

1. Haycock A, Cohen J, Saunders BP, Cotton PB, Williams CB. Cotton and Williams' practical gastrointestinal endoscopy: the fundamentals, vol. 3. 7th ed. Chichester: Wiley Blackwell; 2014. p. 19–32.
2. Zuckerman MJ, Shen B, Harrison ME, Baron TH, Adler DG, Davila RE, et al. Informed consent for GI endoscopy. Gastrointest Endosc. 2007;66:213–8.
3. Standards of Practice Committee, Faigel DO, Eisen GM, Baron TH, Dominitz JA, Goldstein JL, et al. Preparation of patients for GI endoscopy. Gastrointest Endosc. 2003;57:446–50.
4. Hassan C, East J, Radaelli F, Spada C, Benamouzig R, Bisschops R, et al. Bowel preparation for colonoscopy: European Society of Gastrointestinal Endoscopy (ESGE) Guideline—Update 2019. Endoscopy. 2019;51: 775–94.
5. ASGE Standards of Practice Committee, Saltzman JR, Cash BD, Pasha SF, Early DS, Muthusamy VR, Khashab MA, et al. Bowel preparation before colonoscopy. Gastrointest Endosc. 2015;81:781–94.

Enhanced Imaging

7

Maria Monalisa Filip
and Daniela Ștefănescu

7.1 Definition

Advanced imaging techniques improve the examinations quality through enhancement of fine structural mucosal visualization and microvascular detail (pit pattern and vessel pattern).

7.2 High-Definition Endoscopy (HD)

- Resolutions from 850,000 to more than 1 million pixels.
  - Discriminates details on mucosal surface.
  - HD video imaging can be displayed on computer monitor formats (Fig. 7.1).

M. M. Filip (✉) · D. Ștefănescu
Research Center of Gastroenterology and Hepatology, University of Medicine and Pharmacy Craiova, Craiova, Romania

© The Author(s), under exclusive license to Springer Nature Switzerland AG 2023

A. Săftoiu (ed.), *Pocket Guide to Advanced Endoscopy in Gastroenterology*, https://doi.org/10.1007/978-3-031-42076-4_7

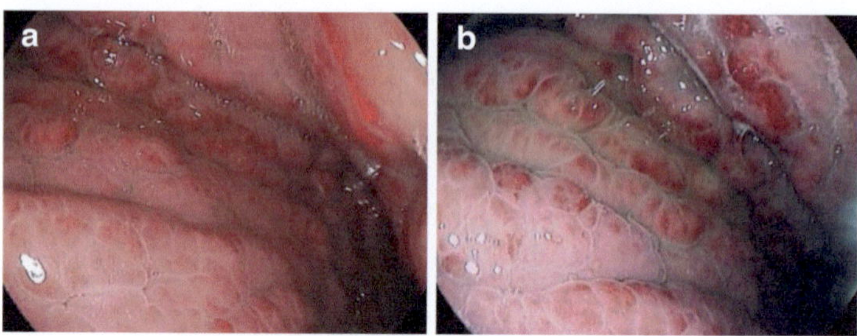

Fig. 7.1 High-definition (HD) endoscopy in white light mode (**a**) and enhanced visualization (I-scan 2) (**b**): portal-hypertensive gastropathy

7.3 Magnification Endoscopy

- Enlarge the image by performing optical zoom.
  - Images can be optically zoomed up to 150 times without losing image quality.

7.3.1 Magnification Chromoendoscopy

- Uses dye agents to visualize mucosal surface (absorptive, contrast, or reactive staining agents).
  - The dyes may be applied on the whole surface or on a small area.
  - Enhance mucosal visualization (i.e., microvascular networks).
  - Can distinguish among different types of epithelium.
  - Abnormal mucosa may stain positively or negatively.
  - Chromoendoscopy with magnification allows a detailed mucosal surface analysis (Fig. 7.2).

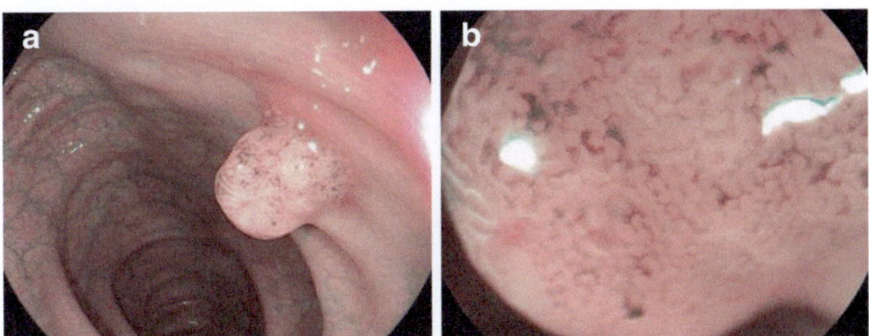

Fig. 7.2 "Virtual" chromoendoscopy (**a**), with magnification (**b**), both in optical enhancement (OE) mode: tubular adenomatous colonic polyp

7.4   Narrowed-Spectrum Technologies

- Image enhancement techniques rely on using only a narrowed part of the available spectral bandwidth, mainly corresponding to "blue light"
  - It is accomplished through optical or digital filtering, being termed "virtual chromoendoscopy".
  - It improves the visualization of the mucosal pattern and the mucosal and submucosal vessels, by using the characteristics of the light spectrum.

7.4.1   Narrow Band Imaging (NBI)

- Uses narrow band optical filters that illuminate the tissue with blue (415 nm) and green (540 nm) light (Olympus Medical Systems, Tokyo, Japan) (Fig. 7.3)
  - The longer the wavelength of light used, the deeper the penetration into tissue.
  - Superficial blood vessels appear brown.
  - Blood vessels from deep mucosa and submucosa appear cyan.

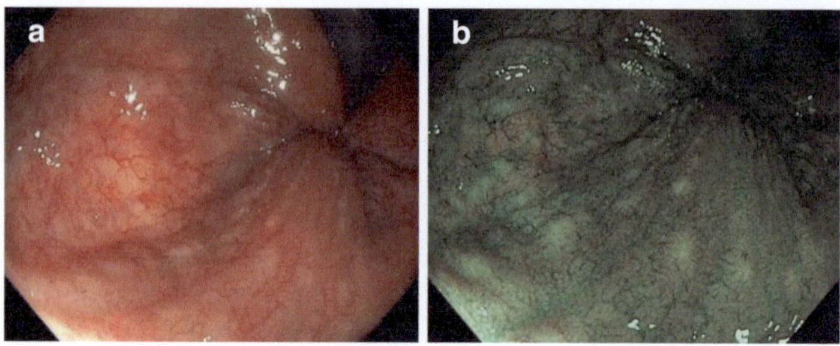

Fig. 7.3 White light endoscopy (**a**) and narrow band imaging (**b**): normal appearance of anorectal microvascularity

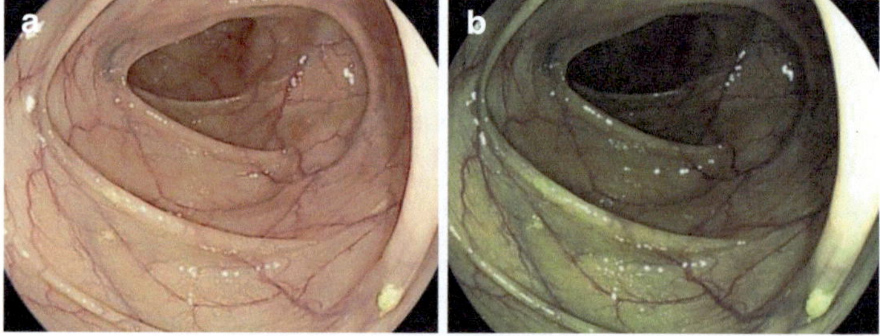

Fig. 7.4 Digital "virtual" chromoendoscopy in I-scan 1 mode (**a**) and I-scan 2 mode (**b**): normal appearance of colonic microvascularity

7.4.2 I-Scan Digital Contrast

- A post-processing algorithm functioning as a digital filter is applied on images obtained with WLE, thus resulting a virtual image (Pentax, Tokyo, Japan) (Fig. 7.4)
  - Mucosal surface and capillary patterns are enhanced on the virtual image.
  - Three digital filters are used to perform: surface, contrast, and tone enhancement.

7.4.3 Flexible Spectral Imaging Color Enhancement (FICE)

- Uses different wavelengths of red, green, and blue to process the light reflected from a surface (Fujifilm, Tokyo, Japan)
  - The color intensity spectrum for each pixel of the white-light image is analyzed in a "spectral estimation" circuit in the video processor.
  - Shorter wavelengths are used to analyze surface structures and longer wavelengths are used to visualize blood vessels.

7.5 Autofluorescence Imaging (AFI)

- Certain endogenous substances from the tissue emit fluorescence light when illuminated with short wavelength (Fig. 7.5)
  - Blood volume, fluorophore concentration, and tissue metabolic activity influence AF.
  - Normal mucosa is colored green, while blood vessels are dark green.
  - Inflamed mucosa and mucosal lesions are coloured differently from the normal tissue (magenta) [1–3].

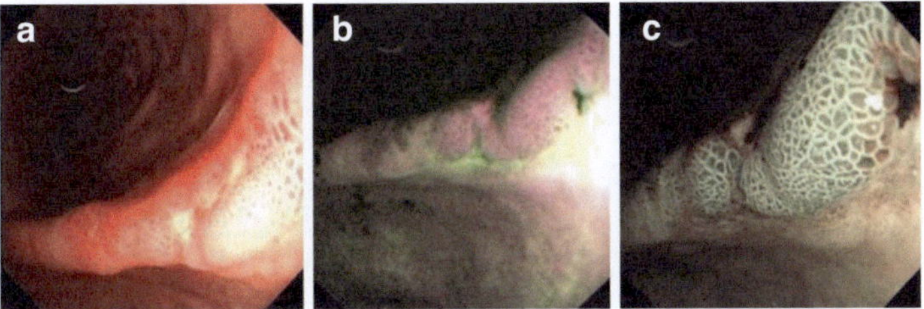

Fig. 7.5 Upper GI endoscopy using white light (**a**), autofluorescence (**b**), and narrow band imaging (**c**): early gastric adenocarcinoma

7.6 Endoscopic Ultrasound (EUS)

- Combines endoscopy with ultrasound, through placement of a miniaturized ultrasound transducer in the end of the endoscope.
  - Visualizes GI tract wall and structures nearby.
  - Useful in guiding fine-needle aspiration biopsy.

7.6.1 Contrast-Enhanced EUS

- Combines CEUS performance with the high resolution of EUS (Fig. 7.6).
  - It is performed after the injection of a microbubble contrast agent (Sonovue, Bracco, Italy).
  - Advantages: real-time intervention guidance, microvascularity and microperfusion imaging, good detail resolution [4].

7.6.2 EUS Elastography

- Visualizes and evaluates tissue elasticity.
  - (a) Strain (Fig. 7.7) and (b) shear wave (SWE)
- Elastography facilitates the differential diagnosis of focal pancreatic lesions.
  - Benign lesions have high strain (soft).
  - Malignant lesions have low strain (hard) [5].

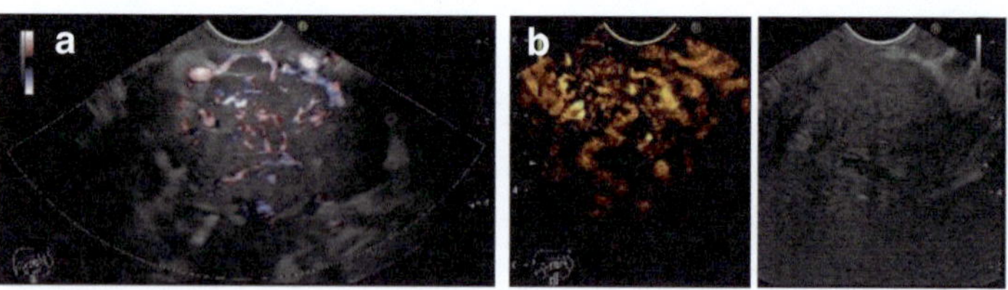

Fig. 7.6 Contrast-enhanced EUS, in color Doppler mode (**a**) and low mechanical index (**b**): pancreatic neuroendocrine neoplasm

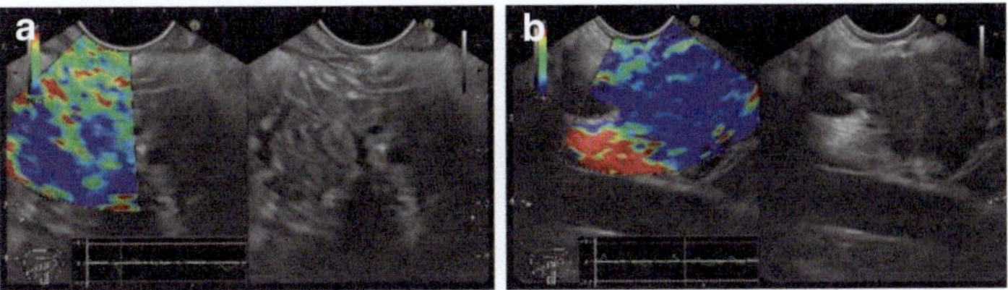

Fig. 7.7 EUS elastography, with mixed (**a**) and hard appearance, that is, low strain (**b**): chronic pseudotumoral pancreatitis and pancreatic adenocarcinoma

7.7 Optical Coherence Tomography

- Obtains 2D anatomical images, in transverse section, corresponding to the digestive tract structures.
  - Uses a catheter placed through the biopsy channel of a conventional endoscope.
  - Light source has low coherence (superluminescent diode), usually near-infrared (NIR) light.
  - Penetration of OCT scanning is 1–2 mm.

7.8 Confocal Laser Endomicroscopy

- Real-time alternative for histology, performed during endoscopy (Fig. 7.8).
  - In vivo microscopic analysis of mucosa, with depth up to 250 μm.
  - Uses a blue light laser: → tissues reflect back a fluorescent signal converted into gray-scale images.
  - Needs contrast agents: topical (acriflavine)/intravenous (fluoresceine).
  - Two types: eCLE (Pentax, Tokyo, Japan)—integrated in the endoscope/pCLE (Mauna Kea Technology, Paris, France) with miniprobes passing through the working channel of a conventional endoscope [6].

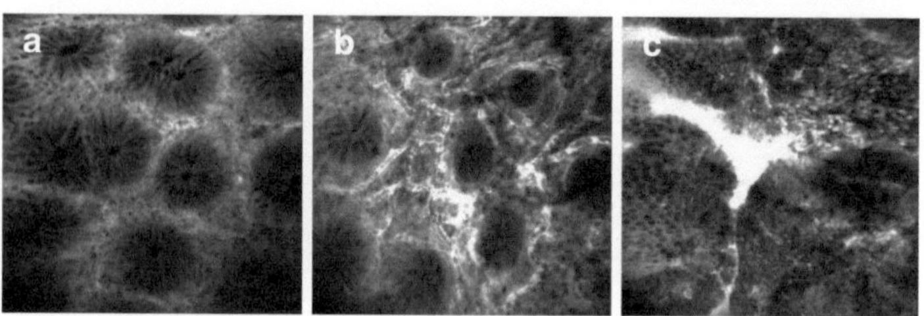

Fig. 7.8 Confocal laser endomicroscopy with i.v. fluoresceine: superficial (**a**) and profound (**b**) appearance of the normal colonic mucosa, in contrast with the distorted architecture and fluorescein leakage in the lumen characteristic of a colonic adenocarcinoma (**c**)

References

1. East JE, Vleugels JL, Roelandt P, et al. Advanced endoscopic imaging: European Society of Gastrointestinal Endoscopy (ESGE) technology review. Endoscopy. 2016;48:1029–45.
2. ASGE Technology Committee. High-definition and high-magnification endoscopes. Gastrointest Endosc. 2014;80:919–27.
3. Wang TD, Van Dam J. Optical biopsy: a new frontier in endoscopic detection and diagnosis. Clin Gastroenterol Hepatol. 2004;2:744–53.
4. Dietrich CF, Sharma M, Hocke M. Contrast-enhanced endoscopic ultrasound. Endosc Ultrasound. 2012;1:130–6.
5. Săftoiu A, Vilman P. Endoscopic ultrasound elastography—a new imaging technique for the visualization of tissue elasticity distribution. J Gastrointestin Liver Dis. 2006;15:161–5.
6. Gheonea DI, Cârţână T, Ciurea T, Popescu C, Bădărău A, Săftoiu A. Confocal laser endomicroscopy and immunoendoscopy for real-time assessment of vascularization in gastrointestinal malignancies. World J Gastroenterol. 2011;17:21–7.

Interventional Endoscopy Techniques

8

Sergiu Cazacu and Adrian Săftoiu

8.1 Definition and Methods

Interventional endoscopy includes a series of minimally invasive techniques with significant clinical impact, low morbidity and mortality, as well as an improved cost-efficiency ratio [1].

- Complex therapeutic procedures have benefited from the introduction of sedation, thus increasing the comfort of patients, but also the quality of examinations and therapeutic interventions.
- Moreover, a constant evolution of endoscopic devices and accessories that are more reliable and ergonomic, enabled the rapid and safe performance of interventional endoscopic procedures [2, 3].

S. Cazacu
Department of Gastroenterology and Hepatology, Emergency County Clinical Hospital, University of Medicine and Pharmacy Craiova, Craiova, Romania

A. Săftoiu (✉)
Department of Gastroenterology and Hepatology, Elias Emergency University Hospital, Carol Davila University of Medicine and Pharmacy, Bucharest, Romania

A. Săftoiu (ed.), *Pocket Guide to Advanced Endoscopy in Gastroenterology*, https://doi.org/10.1007/978-3-031-42076-4_8

8.2 Endoscopic Hemostasis (See Also Chaps. 27 and 36)

- Injection
  - Adrenaline 1:10,000 diluted in saline.
  - Sclerosing agents/fibrin.
  - Polymers (cyanoacrylate).
- Thermal treatments
  - Bipolar coagulation.
  - Monopolar coagulation.
  - Argon plasma jet coagulation (APC).
  - Coagrasper.
- Mechanical methods.
  - Metal clips (Fig. 8.1a, b).
  - Elastic ligatures/nylon bands.
  - Endoscopic sutures.
  - "Over-the-scope" clips (OTSC).
- Other methods
  - Hemostatic powders/ els.

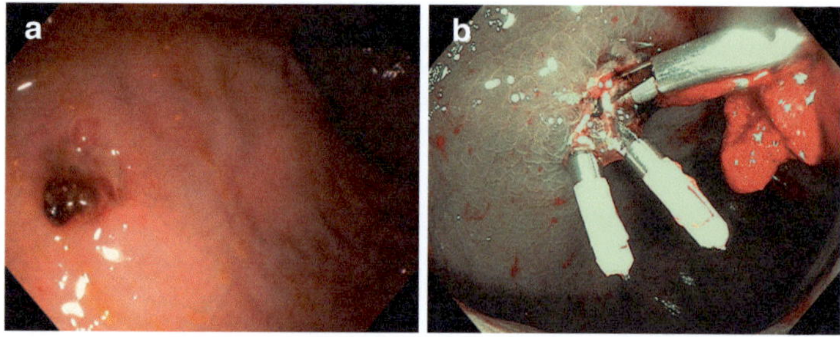

Fig. 8.1 Solitary rectal ulcer with visible vessel (**a**), with hemostasis by placement of metal clips, visualized in narrow band imaging (NBI) (**b**)

8.3   Conventional Polypectomy (See Also Chap. 34)

- Principles of electrosurgery [4]
  - Generates heat > vessel coagulation > transection.
  - Does not generate pain due to the high frequency.
    Modern pacemakers are not affected.
    Defibrillators must be temporarily disabled.
  - Types of electrical current.
    Coagulation current (deep, high power).
    Cutting current (superficial, low power).
    Mixed current (blended).
- Pedunculated polyps
  - Pedicle <10 mm and polyp <20 mm (Fig. 8.2a, b).
    Hot snare polypectomy.
  - Pedicle ≥10 mm and polyp ≥20 mm.
    Prophylactic pedicle hemostasis:
      1. Injection.
      2. Clips.
      3. Nylon bands (Fig. 8.3a, b).
    Hot snare polypectomy.
- Sessile polyps
  - Diminutive (≤5 mm) and small (6–9 mm) polyps.
    Cold snare polypectomy (CSP) (Fig 8.4a, b).
    Suction retrieval of the polyps.

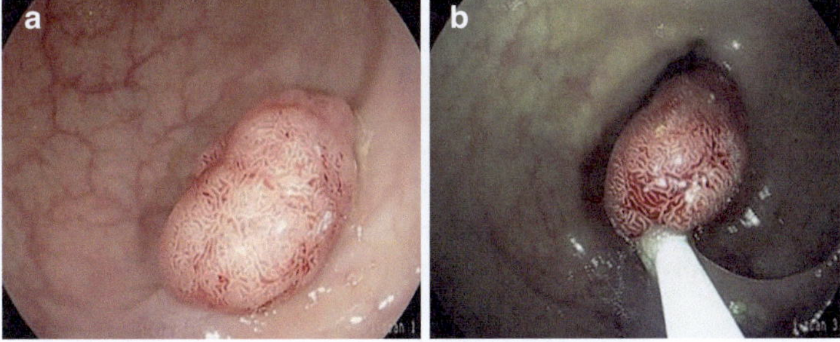

Fig. 8.2 Pedunculated polyp with short thin pedicle visualized in white light (**a**) with simple polypectomy after examination in iSCAN mode (**b**)

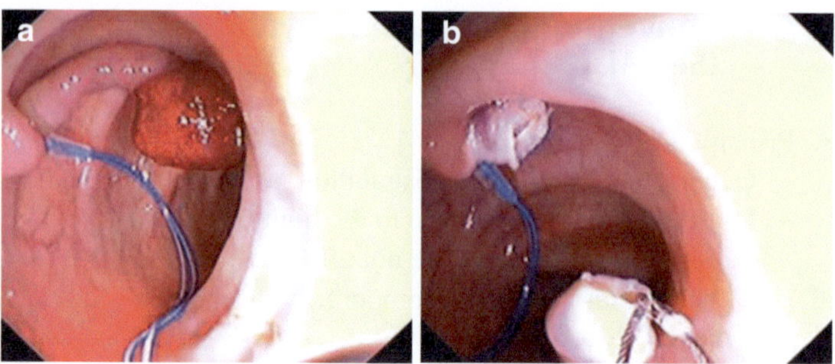

Fig. 8.3 Pedunculated polyp, viewed under white light (**a**), with hot snare polypectomy after placement of EndoLoop at the base of the pedicle (**b**)

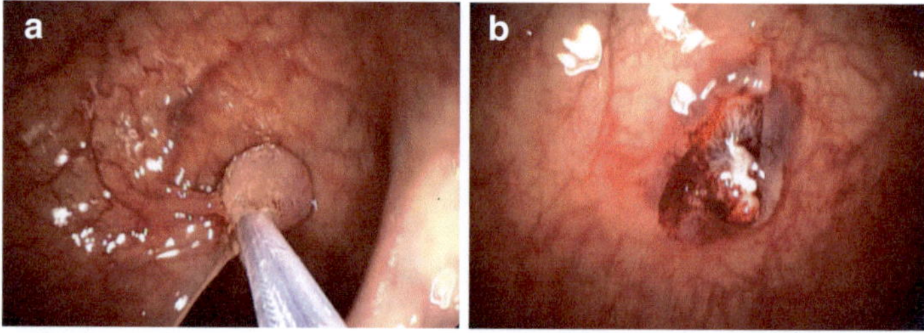

Fig. 8.4 Diminutive sessile polyp (3 mm), visualized under white light (**a**), with cold snare polypectomy, with visualization of the submucosa, with no immediate complications (**b**)

- Intermediate sessile polyps (10–19 mm).
    Advanced imaging (NBI/iSCAN/FICE).
    NICE (NBI International Colorectal Endoscopic classification) + Kudo classifications.
       1. Noninvasive sessile/flat lesions
       >En bloc mucosal resection (Fig. 8.5).
       >Piecemeal mucosal resection (Fig. 8.6).
    After elevation by injection of adrenaline 1:10,000 dissolved in saline/Gelofusine.

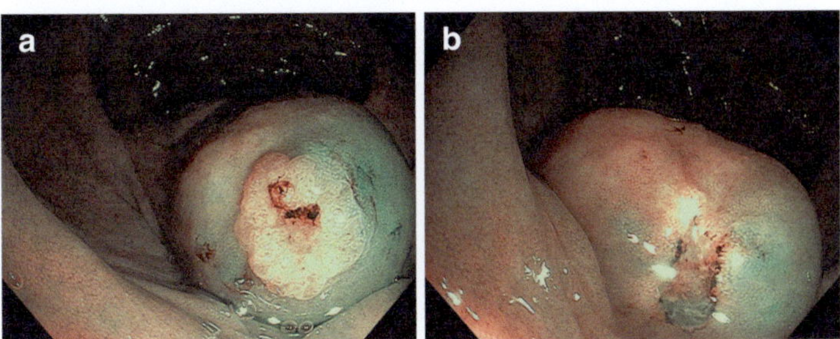

Fig. 8.5 Sessile polyp (10 mm), visualized under white light after adrenaline injection 1:10,000 dissolved in saline (**a**), with en bloc hot snare polypectomy, with no immediate complications (**b**)

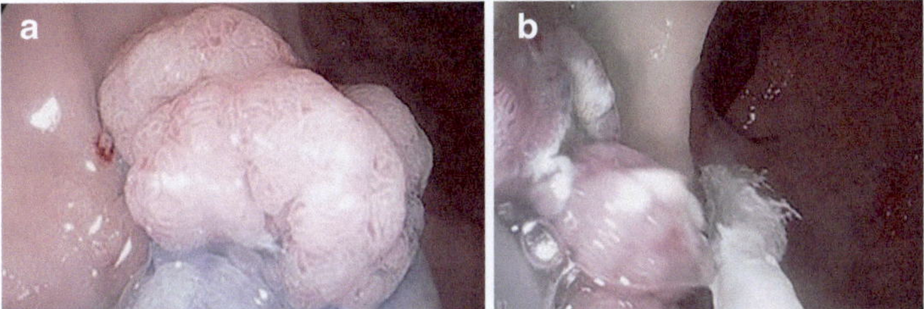

Fig. 8.6 Sessile sigmoid polyp (15 mm), visualized in white light, with piecemeal hot snare polypectomy (HSP), after injection of 1:10,000 adrenaline (**a**), with fragments recovered with a mesh snare (**b**)

- Difficult sessile polyps ≥20 mm.
    Advanced imaging (NBI/iSCAN/FICE).
    NICE (NBI International Colorectal Endoscopic classification) + Kudo classification.
    1. Noninvasive sessile/flat lesions
        >Piecemeal mucosal resection (Fig. 8.7).
    2. Invasive lesions (Fig. 8.8) > proximal and distal tattoo (at approximately 2–3 cm) > submucosal dissection/laparoscopic surgery.

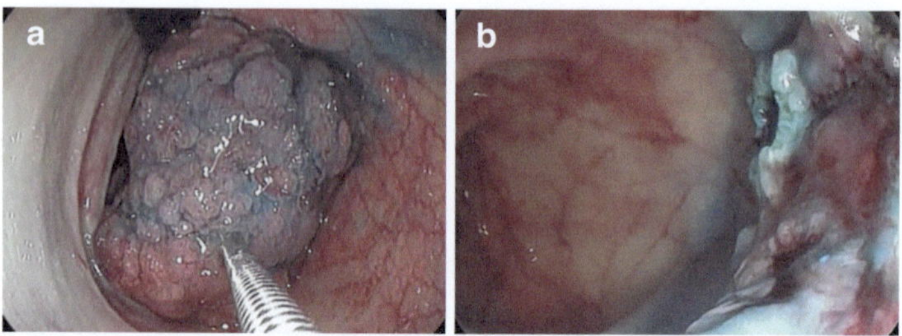

Fig. 8.7 Sigmoid villous sessile polyp (>40 mm), visualized in white light (**a**) with NICE 2A/Kudo IIIL appearance, resected by piecemeal polypectomy after injection of 1:10,000 adrenaline (**b**)

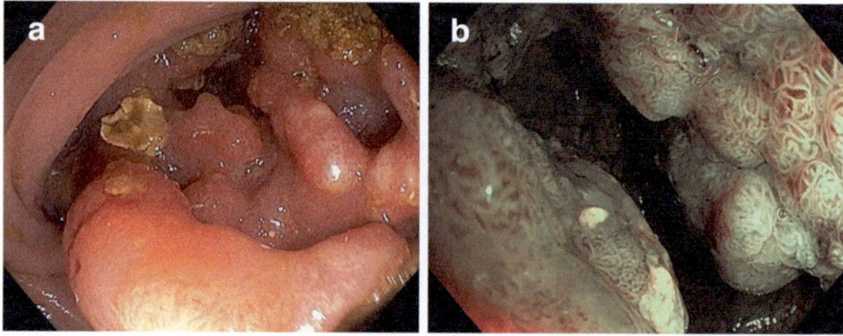

Fig. 8.8 Rectal sessile villous polyp (>50 mm), viewed under white light (**a**) and narrow band light (NBI), with NICE 2B/Kudo Vi (**b**) appearance, referred for laparoscopic resection

8.4 Endoscopic Mucosal Resection

- Implies injection into the submucosal space.
  - Saline/macromolecular agents (succinylated gelatin) + adrenaline 1:10,000 + methylene blue.
  - Proximal > distal injection.
    En bloc/piecemeal resection (Fig. 8.9).
  - Procedural complications.
    Coagrasper coagulation.
    Clips for defect closure (Fig. 8.10).

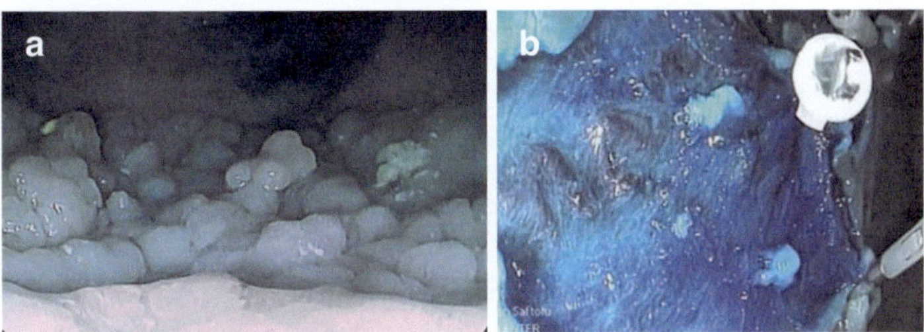

Fig. 8.9 Flat rectal polyp (>30 mm) LST-G type (granular laterally spreading tumor), visualized in iSCAN mode (**a**) with NICE 2A/Kudo IIIL appearance, resected by piecemeal polypectomy after injection of adrenaline 1:10,000 dissolved in Gelofusine + methylene blue (**b**)

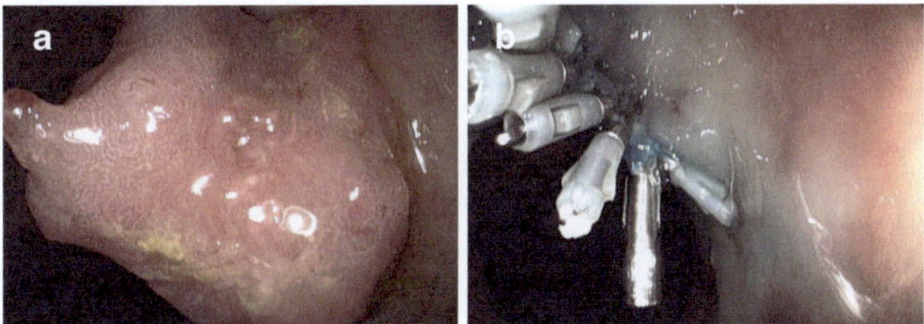

Fig. 8.10 Malignant pedunculated sigmoid polyp (aprox. 15 mm), resected by endoscopic mucosal resection (**a**), with mucosal defect closed with clips (**b**)

8.5   Endoscopic Submucosal Dissection

- Implies en bloc resection
  - Saline/macromolecular agents (succinylated gelatin) + adrenaline 1:10,000 + methylene blue.
  - Proximal > distal injection
    Dissection in the submucosal space.
    En bloc resection.
  - Procedural complications
    Coagrasper coagulation.
    Clips for defect closure.

8.6   Transmural Resections

- Usually performed with laparoscopic control
  - Endoscopic procedures combined with laparoscopic procedures—CELS (combined endoscopic laparoscopic surgery).
  - Defect closure with OTSC clips/endoscopic sutures.

8.7   Dilations

- Digestive stenoses require dilatation under endoscopic + radiological control.
  - Mechanical (bougie dilators)—radial + linear force.
  - Pneumatic (with balloon)—radial force.
    Guide wire
    TS balloons ("through-the-scope").
    Variable diameter depending on pressure.

8.8   Extraction of Foreign Bodies

- They cause problems for children, elderly people with missing teeth, alcoholics, or people with mental disabilities [5, 6].
  - -Foreign bodies represent emergencies if:
    Patients complain of complete dysphagia.
    Foreign bodies are sharp/impacted.
    Batteries cause local damage.
  - Overtube is used, preferably with deeply sedated and intubated patients for respiratory protection.

8.9   Endoscopic Stenting

- Self-expanding metallic (Fig. 8.11) or plastic stents are used [7–9].
- Indicated in malignant or less often benign stenoses, extrinsic compressions, digestive fistulas, exceptionally in achalasia or bleeding from esophageal varices.
- Under radiological or endoscopic guidance, on guide wire or transendoscopic.

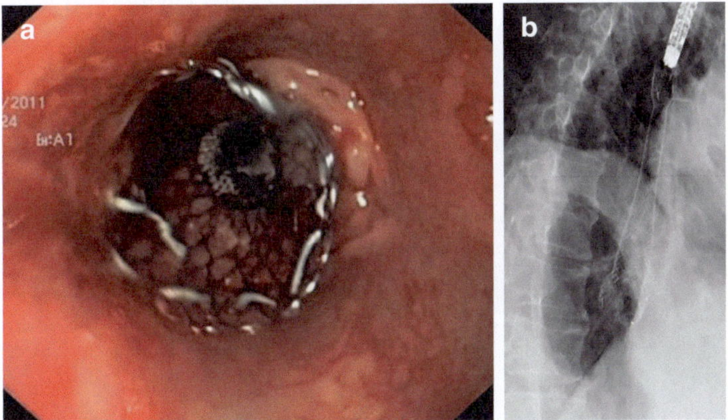

Fig. 8.11 Endoscopically placed expandable metal stent for palliation of an esophageal tumor (**a**), with radiological appearance (**b**)

8.10 Percutaneous Endoscopic Gastrostomy/ Jejunostomy (PEG/PEJ)

- Useful for eating disorders secondary to neurological pathology, oro-maxillofacial or esophageal obstructive pathology, for decompression in small intestine obstructions.
- Involves the penetration of the stomach with the endoscope, followed by the transillumination of the abdominal wall with the identification of the puncture site, the introduction of a guide wire through the puncture site with the help of which the gastrostomy tube is pulled through the oral cavity (pull technique) (Fig. 8.12).

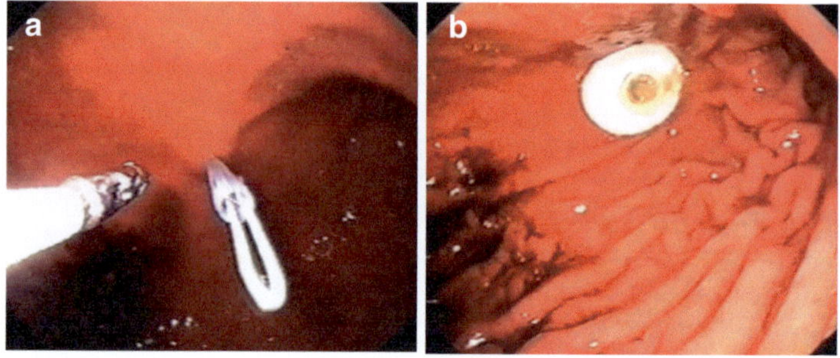

Fig. 8.12 Endoscopic gastrostomy: trocar visible on anterior gastric surface (**a**), inner end of gastrostomy visible (**b**)

8.11   Other Ablative Therapeutic Procedures

- Useful for Barrett's esophagus or digestive cancers.
  - Radiofrequency ablation.
  - Photodynamic therapy.

8.12   POEM (Per-Oral Esophageal Myotomy)

- Technique derived from submucosal dissection [10].
- Useful in achalasia.
- Implies making a tunnel in the esophageal and gastric submucosa, followed by sectioning the circular muscle layer and closing the tunnel opening area.

References

1. Haycock A, Cohen J, Saunders BP, Cotton PB, Williams CB. Cotton and Williams' practical gastrointestinal endoscopy: the fundamentals, vol. 7. 7th ed. Chichester: Wiley Blackwell; 2014. p. 153–79.
2. Ferlitsch M, Moss A, Hassan C, et al. Colorectal polypectomy and endoscopic mucosal resection (EMR): European Society of Gastrointestinal Endoscopy (ESGE) clinical guideline. Endoscopy. 2017;49:270–97.
3. Dumoulin FL, Hildenbrand R. Endoscopic resection techniques for colorectal neoplasia: current developments. World J Gastroenterol. 2019;25:300–7.
4. Gutta A, Gromski MA. Endoscopic management of post-polypectomy bleeding. Clin Endosc. 2020;53:302–10.
5. Chirica M, Kelly MD, Siboni S, Aiolfi A, Riva CG, Asti E, et al. Esophageal emergencies: WSES guidelines. World J Emerg Surg. 2019;14:26.
6. Cologne KG, Ault GT. Rectal foreign bodies: what is the current standard? Clin Colon Rectal Surg. 2012;25:214–8.
7. Spaander MC, Baron TH, Siersema PD, Fuccio L, Schumacher B, Escorsell À, et al. Esophageal stenting for benign and malignant disease: European Society of Gastrointestinal Endoscopy (ESGE) clinical guideline. Endoscopy. 2016;48(939–48.

8. Kim EJ, Kim YJ. Stents for colorectal obstruction: past, present, and future. World J Gastroenterol. 2016;22:842–52.
9. Arvanitakis M, Gkolfakis P, Despott EJ, Ballarin A, Beyna T, Boeykens K, et al. Endoscopic management of enteral tubes in adult patients—Part 1: definitions and indications. European Society of Gastrointestinal Endoscopy (ESGE) guideline. Endoscopy. 2021;53:81–92.
10. Lundell L. Current and future treatment options in primary achalasia. The role of POEM. J Gastrointestin Liver Dis. 2020;29:289–93.

Advanced Endoscopy (EUS and ERCP)

9

Adrian Săftoiu

9.1 Therapeutic Endoscopic Ultrasound

- Fine-needle aspiration biopsy [1–3].
  - Refrain from eating 6–8 h beforehand.
  - Preferably with deep sedation (propofol).
  - Procedure variable depending on the indications:
    FNA (Fig. 9.1)—aspiration, with smears and cell block (formalin) for cytological and microhistological examination.
    FNB (Fig. 9.2)—microbiopsy, with standard microhistological examination by formalin fixation, followed by immunohistochemical/molecular techniques.
  - Variable puncture technique.
    Various needles: 19G vs. 22G (frequently) vs. 25G.
    Use suction (yes/no) or fanning technique.
    Multiple passages.
    1. Minimum three for pancreatic formations.
    2. 1–2 for adenopathies/mediastinal tumors.

A. Săftoiu (✉)
Department of Gastroenterology and Hepatology, Elias Emergency University Hospital, Carol Davila University of Medicine and Pharmacy, Bucharest, Romania

A. Săftoiu (ed.), *Pocket Guide to Advanced Endoscopy in Gastroenterology*, https://doi.org/10.1007/978-3-031-42076-4_9

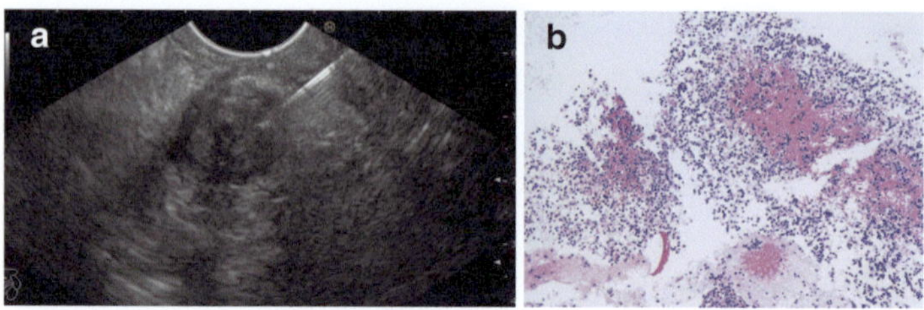

Fig. 9.1 Hypoechoic pancreatic tumor for which EUS-FNA was performed with a 22G needle (**a**), with a cytological appearance suggestive of a neuroendocrine tumor (**b**)

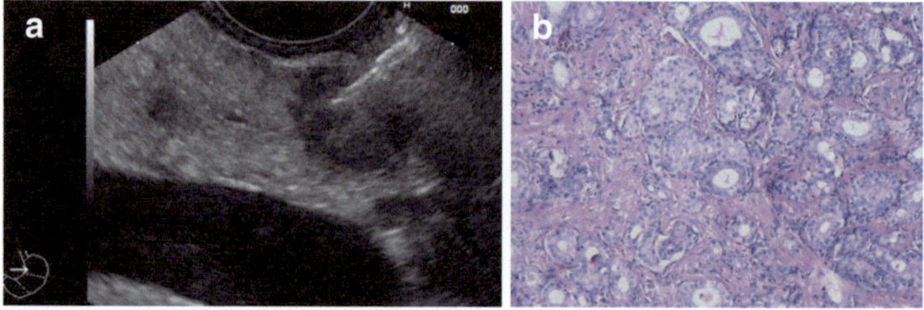

Fig. 9.2 Hypoechoic pancreatic tumor, for which an EUS-FNB was performed, with a 22G "histological" needle (**a**), with a histological appearance suggestive of a neuroendocrine tumor (**b**)

Evaluation of the aspirated sample.
1. ROSE (rapid on-site evaluation of cytological samples), with cytologist present.
2. MOSE (macroscopic on-site quality evaluation), for FNB.
- Indications include (Table 9.1):
- Contraindications include (Table 9.2):
- Variable accuracy dependent on multiple factors.
    Location of the punctured tumor.
    Type of needle used (FNA vs FNB).
    Endoscopist/cytopathologist experience.

Table 9.1 EUS-FNA/FNB indications

Region	Indication
Posterior mediastinum	Positive diagnosis of primary tumors/adenopathies (lymphomas, sarcoidosis, tuberculosis, etc.) Lung cancer staging
Subepithelial tumors	Leiomyoma GIST tumors
Hypertrophic gastric folds	Ménétrier disease Gastric lymphoma Linitis plastica
Pancreatico-biliary tumors	Solid pancreatic tumors Cystic pancreatic tumors Cholangiocarcinomas
Liver tumors	Metastases Primary tumors (HCC/CCC)
Adrenal tumors	Primary/secondary

Table 9.2 EUS-FNA/FNB contraindications

Type	Condition
Endoscopy contraindications	Heart/respiratory failure Acute abdomen Improper preparation
Coagulation disorders/risk of bleeding	Antiplatelet treatment (e.g., clopidogrel) Anticoagulant treatment (INR > 1.5) Thrombocytopenia ($<50{,}000/mm^3$)
Inaccessible tumors	Incomplete visualization Interposition of large vessels/tumor tissue
Absence of clinical impact	The procedure (and outcome) will not influence clinical management

   Number of passages.
   1. Sensitivity >90% (FNA) and > 98% (FNB).
   2. Specificity and NPV ~100%.
 − Minor and self-limited complications (1–2%).
   Minor intra−/extra-luminal bleeding.
   Intracystic bleeding.
   Mild acute pancreatitis.
   Infectious risk in cystic/mediastinal tumors.
   Needle tract seeding (exceptional).

- Celiac plexus neurolysis [4].
  - Transgastric approach to the celiac plexus (Fig. 9.3).
  - Procedure performed with EUS guidance in real time, using conventional / dedicated 22G needles.
  - Indications include:

    Pancreatic cancer—neurolysis (dehydrated alcohol).

    Chronic pancreatitis—block (triamcinolone).
  - The technique is different.

    Color Doppler visualization of the celiac trunk.

    1. Central approach—injection into celiac axis.

    2. Bilateral technique—injection in both sides.

    Aspiration (10 s).

    Bupivacaine injection (10 mL).

    Dehydrated alcohol injection (10 mL).
  - The results consist in reducing the need for opiates (including side effects).

    Pain reduction in 80% of patients (pancreatic cancer), respectively 60% (chronic pancreatitis).

    The effect is transient.
  - Complications/side effects.

    Postprocedural hypotension.

    Diffuse abdominal pain/diarrhea.

    Bleeding/abscesses/abdominal ischemia (exceptional).

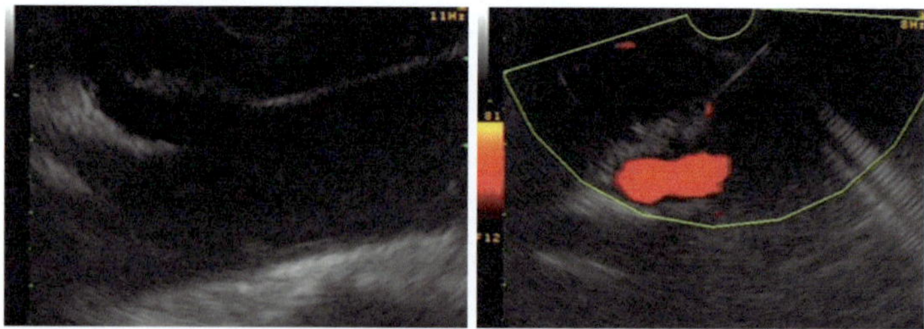

Fig. 9.3 Celiac plexus neurolysis with a central approach, with the 22G needle placed near the emergence of the celiac trunk from the aorta

- Drainage of pancreatic fluid collections [5–7].
  - Indication for EUS-guided drainage is based on the Atlanta classification of pancreatic fluid collections:
    Acute peripancreatic fluid collections (AFC).
    Pancreatic pseudocysts (PPC).
    Acute necrotic collections (ANC).
    Walled off necrotic collections (WON).
  - PPC and WON require a minimum of 4–6 weeks for the formation of its own wall.
  - Drainage is indicated in symptomatic patients.
    EUS guided drainage is preferred to percutaneous/surgical drainage.
    Reviewed before drainage:
    1. History, clinical examination, laboratory tests.
    2. Imaging studies (CT, MR, preferably EUS).
    3. Antiaggregant/anticoagulant treatment (INR < 1.5, platelets <50,000/mm3).
    4. Broad spectrum antibiotics.
    5. Multidisciplinary team (gastroenterologist, surgeon, anesthetist, interventional radiologist).
  - Pancreatic pseudocyst drainage technique (PPC).
    PPC puncture with a 19G needle (aspiration: bacteriological, biochemical, cytological examination).
    Placement of hydrophilic guide wire.
    Tract dilation (cystotome, ERCP cannula, TTS dilation balloon).
    Plastic "pigtail" stent placement (1–2 stents 7 Fr, 5–7 cm) (Fig. 9.4).
    Lumen-apposing covered self-expandable metal stents (LAMS) can be used (Fig. 9.5), with significant costs.
  - Necrotic collection drainage technique (WON).
    The initial stages of drainage are similar, LAMS type stents being preferred (Fig. 9.6).
    "Multi-gate" technique > creation of multiple tracts (rare in PPC, frequent in WON)
    Irrigation of the necrotic cavity (naso-cystic/percutaneous drain) = dual drainage.
    Endoscopic necrosectomy (Fig. 9.7) ~50%:

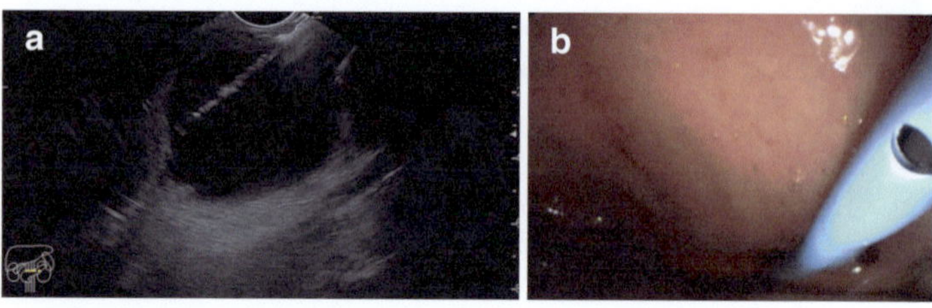

Fig. 9.4 EUS-guided drainage of a pancreatic pseudocyst using 19G needle +6 Fr cystotome (**a**) + 7Fr 7 cm pigtail stent placement (**b**)

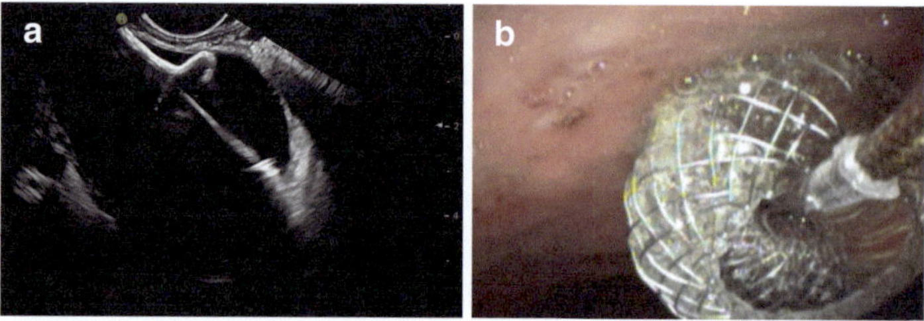

Fig. 9.5 EUS-guided drainage of a pancreatic pseudocyst using freehand LAMS stent placement, with EUS visualization of the distal end (in PPC) (**a**) and proximal end (in stomach) respectively (**b**)

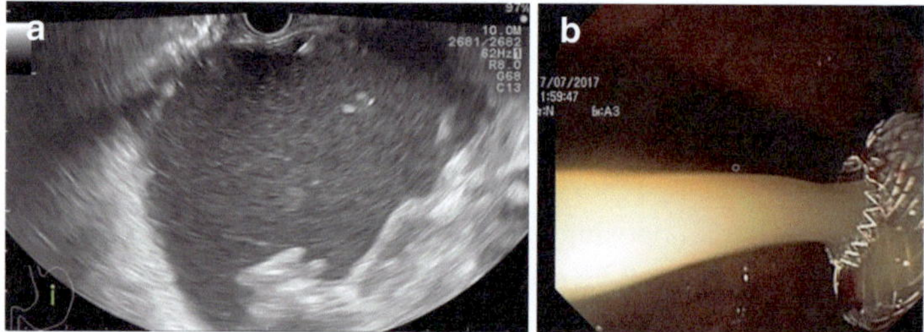

Fig. 9.6 EUS-guided drainage of a walled-off necrotic collection (WON) (**a**) using 19G needle approach + guidewire + LAMS stent placement, with visualization of the proximal end (into the stomach) and effective drainage (**b**)

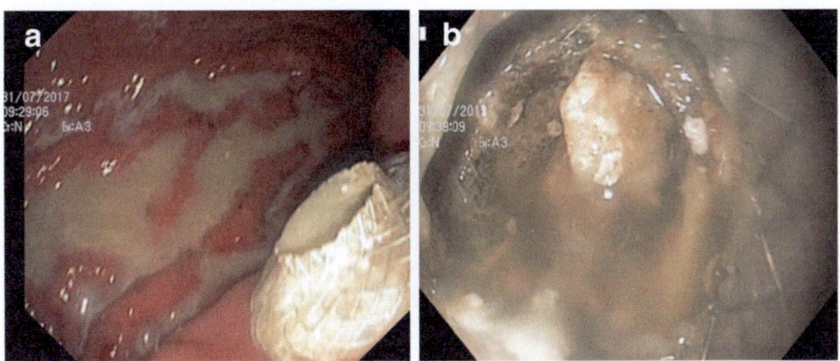

Fig. 9.7 Endoscopic necrosectomy after EUS-guided drainage of a walled-off necrotic collection (WON) with visualization of the proximal end (in the stomach) (**a**) and retrieval of solid necroses via stent (**b**)

1. Patients unresponsive to dual/multi-gate drainage.
2. Persistent symptoms: SIRS, sepsis, organ failure.
3. Continue until elimination of solid necrosis.

- Complications/side effects.
  Infection.
  Bleeding (more often for LAMS).
  1. Minor > endoscopic hemostasis.
  2. Major > interventional radiology / surgery.
  Perforation.
  Stent migration / obstruction (exceptional).
- Follow-up.
  CT scan at 6 weeks for plastic stent > maintained at least 6 months.
  CT scan at 3–4 weeks for LAMS > extraction (bleeding risk).

- EUS-guided drainage of the bile ducts.
  - Alternative for patients in whom ERCP cannot be performed (altered anatomy/obstructive tumors).
    Option for percutaneous/surgical drainage.
  - Types of procedures.
    Rendezvous: EUS allows the placement of a transpapillary guide wire, followed by ERCP.
    Transluminal drainage: choledocho-duodenostomy (CDS) and hepatico-gastrostomy (HGS).
    Anterograde drainage.

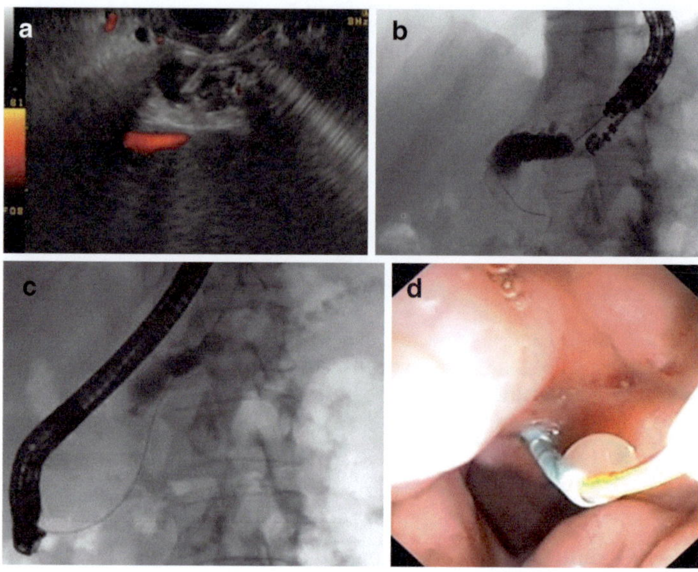

Fig. 9.8 EUS-guided transgastric puncture (**a**) of the dilated Wirsung duct, followed by guidewire passage through papilla (**b**), with EUS scope exchange to duodenoscope (**c**) with stent placement (**d**)

- – Clinical success rate up to 80–100% (lower in CDS).
- – Complications up to 10–20% (higher in HGS).
    - Bleeding/bile fistulas/leakage.
    - Cholangitis/biliary peritonitis/sepsis.
- EUS-guided drainage of the pancreatic duct.
  - – Generally used in patients with Wirsung's stenosis.
      - Rendezvous: EUS allows placement of a transpapillary guidewire, followed by ERCP (Fig. 9.8).
      - Transmural drainage (transgastric/transduodenal).
  - – Technical success rate 80–100%.
  - – Complications up to 25%.
      - Stent dysfunction > pancreatitis.
      - Peripancreatic fistulas/abscesses.

- EUS-guided drainage of the cholecyst.
  - Currently, indications in patients with acute cholecystitis and contraindication to surgical intervention.
    Avoids percutaneous drainage of the gallbladder.
    Cholecystogastric/duodenal communication.
  - Technical and clinical success rate of 90–98%.
  - Complications up to 20%.
    Bleeding.
    Recurrent cholecystitis/biliary peritonitis/sepsis.
- Perspectives [8].
  - Molecular analysis of FNA/FNB samples.
    DNA/RNA analysis of EUS-FNAB samples is feasible and allows molecular characterization (KRAS/GNAS/VHL mutations, etc.)
  - Intratumoral treatment.
    Phase 1/2 studies for intratumoral injection of oncolytic viruses/oligonucleotides/dendritic cells/anti-KRAS agents.
  - Endovascular treatment.
    Used especially in gastric varices.
    Involves injection of cyanoacrylate and/or coils (to minimize embolic risk).
  - Tumoral ablation.
    Various ablative methods used:
    1. Radiofrequency (especially in neuroendocrine/cystic tumors with a contraindication to surgical intervention, respectively in locally advanced adenocarcinoma of the pancreas).
    2. Cryothermia/microwaves.
  - Placement of markers for radiotherapy.
    Recommended for patients selected for stereotactic radiotherapy.
    EUS is the modality of choice for placement in pancreatic/esophageal/rectal cancer.
  - Digestive anastomoses.
    EUS-guided gastroentero-anastomoses can be performed by placing expandable LAMS stents.
    The method can avoid open/laparoscopic surgical anastomoses.

9.2   Endoscopic Retrograde Cholangiopancreatography

Strictly therapeutic procedure, combination of endoscopy and fluoroscopy, with access to the biliary tract and pancreatic duct, transpapillary from the level of the second duodenum. Retrograde injection of radiopaque contrast allows visualization of the biliopancreatic system with the possibility of therapeutic interventions.

- Choledocholithiasis [9].
    - ERCP with endoscopic sphincterotomy and stone extraction (Fig. 9.9) is the procedure of choice.
        Clearance rate of calculi up to 95%. Failure of ERCP:
        1. Inability of selective biliary cannulation.
        2. Altered anatomy (Billroth 2 gastrectomies, Roux-en gastrojejunal anastomoses, etc.)
        3. Diverticula/duodenal strictures.
    - Procedures used for "difficult" calculi.
        Balloon dilation (sphincteroplasty).
        Temporary insertion of stents (Fig. 9.10).
        Mechanical lithotripsy.
        Direct cholangioscopy with electrohydraulic/laser lithotripsy.
        1. "Single-operator mother-daughter" (spyglass)
        2. Per-oral cholangioscopy.
    - Complications.
        Post-sphincterotomy bleeding.
        Perforation.
        Acute post-ERCP pancreatitis.
        Acute cholangitis.
- Stenosis of bile ducts [10].
    - Complex evaluation.
        EUS-FNA and/or ERCP with biopsy + brushing.
        Cholangioscopy with direct biopsies.

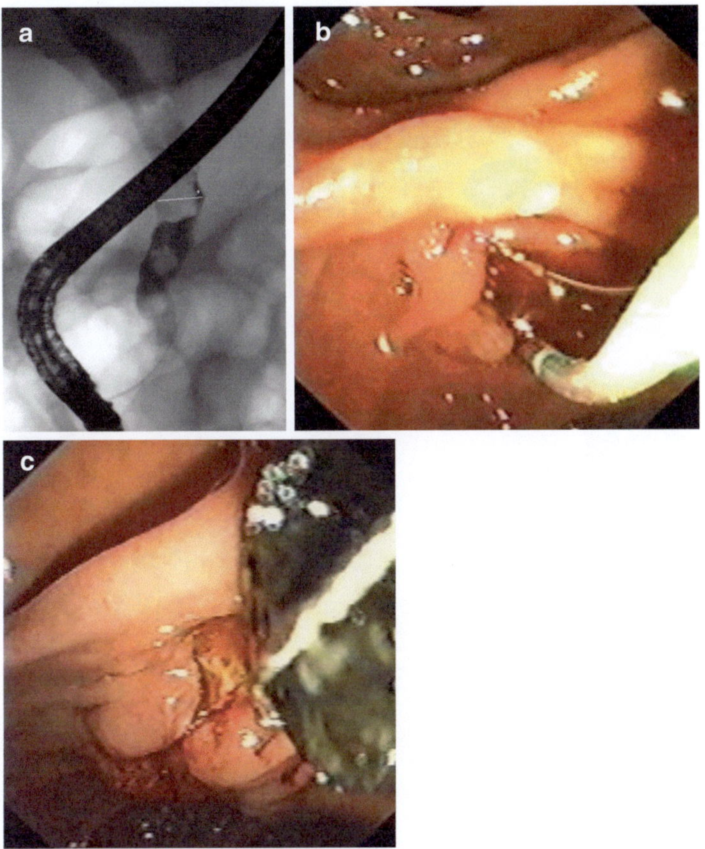

Fig. 9.9 ERCP with injection of contrast material (**a**), with sphincterotomy (**b**) and stone extraction (**c**)

- Benign stenoses.

     Causes: postoperative (especially after cholecystectomy/ orthotopic liver transplantation), chronic pancreatitis, primary/secondary sclerosing cholangitis (Fig. 9.11), IgG4 cholangiopathy, post-sphincterotomy.

     Dilatation with a single/multiple plastic stents, long-term (12 months, with replacement every 3 months)/ metallic covered stents.

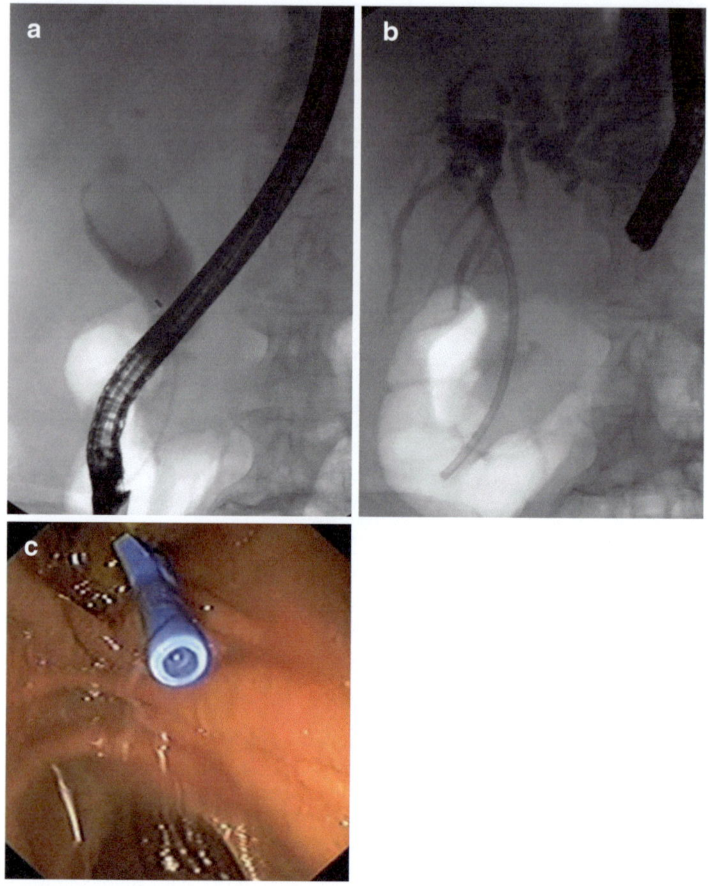

Fig. 9.10 ERCP with contrast injection, with visualization of a radiopaque choledochal calculus of approx. 35 × 25 mm (**a**), with placement of a transpapillary biliary stent (**b, c**)

- Malignant stenoses.
    ERCP = the method of choice for bile duct drainage in pancreatico-biliary cancers.
    Causes: peri-ampullary tumors, cholangiocarcinoma, pancreatic adenocarcinoma, gallbladder carcinoma, hilum tumors (Klatskin), etc.

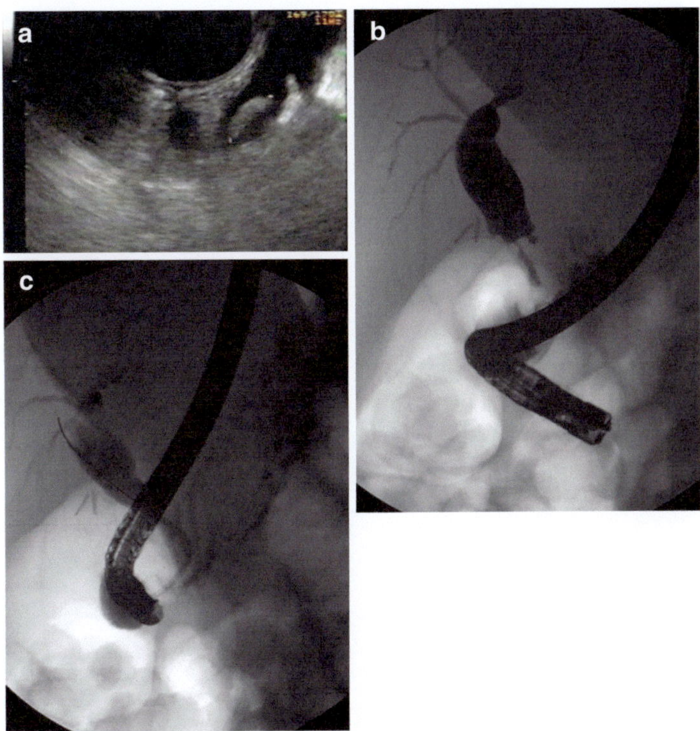

Fig. 9.11 EUS with visualization of dilated PBC, with a calculus image above the area of stenosis (**a**). ERCP allows the visualization of a tight post-cholecystectomy stenosis (**b**) and placement of a plastic stent (**c**)

>   Drainage with biliary stents (frequently 10 Fr, maximum 3 months) (Fig. 9.12)/expandable stents.
> – Complications.
>   Post-sphincterotomy bleeding.
>   Perforation.
>   Acute post-ERCP pancreatitis.
>   Acute cholangitis/recurrent biliary obstruction.
• Pancreatic diseases.
> – Stenoses of the pancreatic duct.
>   Causes: acute/chronic pancreatitis/tumors.
>   Placement of plastic stents (Fig. 9.13).
>   Cholangioscopy + lithotripsy.

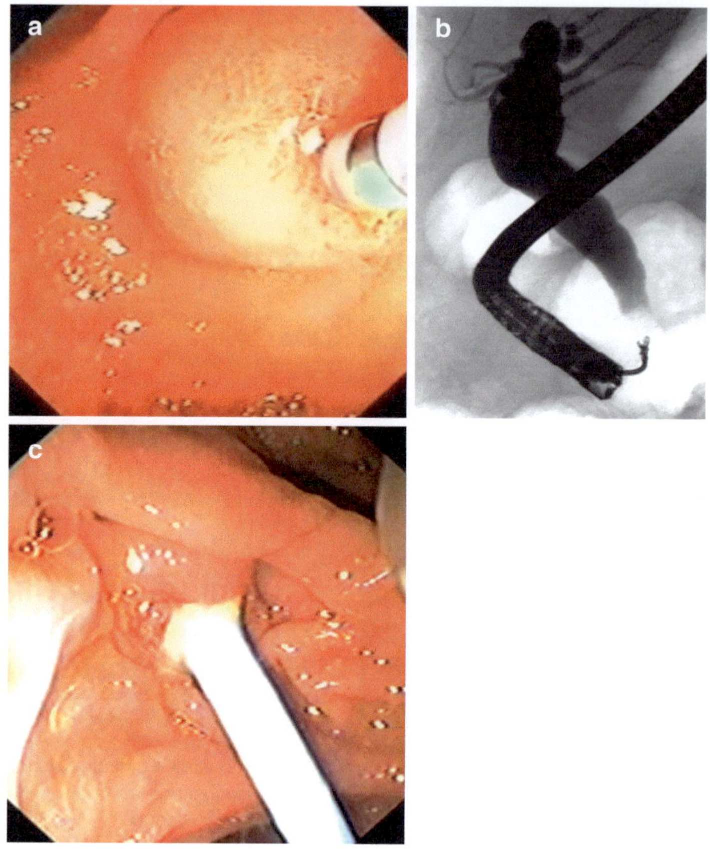

Fig. 9.12 ERCP in an intramural ampulalry cancer (**a**) with biopsies taken under radiological guidance (**b**) and placement of a plastic stent (**c**)

- Pancreatic fistulas.

    Causes: acute/chronic pancreatitis/pancreatic trauma/post-operative.

    Placement of plastic stents (Fig. 9.14) ± pancreatic sphincterotomy.

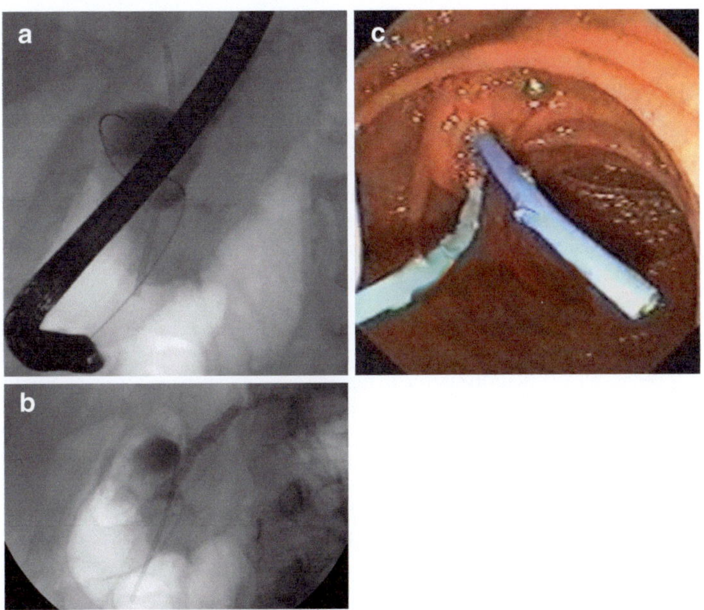

Fig. 9.13 ERCP with sequential transpapillary drainage of the CBD (compressed by a pancreatic head pseudocyst) (**a**) and pancreatic duct (**b**, **c**)

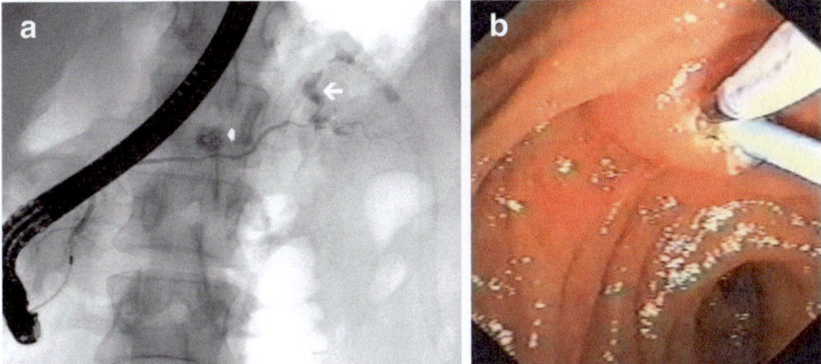

Fig. 9.14 ERCP in a patient with chronic pancreatitis, pseudocyst of the body of the pancreas, and fistula of the tail of the pancreas (**a**) in whom a plastic pancreatic stent was inserted, followed by pancreatic sphincterotomy over the stent (**b**)

References

1. Rimbas M, Larghi A. Techniques for endoscopic ultrasound-guided biopsy. In: Hawes R, Fockens P, Varadarajulu S, editors. Endosonography, vol. 21. 4th ed. Elsevier; 2019. p. 261–71.
2. Costache MI, Iordache S, Karstensen JG, Săftoiu A, Vilmann P. Endoscopic ultrasound-guided fine needle aspiration: from the past to the future. Endosc Ultrasound. 2013;2:77–85.
3. Guo J, Sahai AV, Teoh A, et al. An international, multi-institution survey on performing EUS-FNA and fine needle biopsy. Endosc Ultrasound. 2020;9:319–28.
4. Kaufman M, Singh G, Das S, Concha-Parra R, Erber J, Micames C, Gress F. Efficacy of endoscopic ultrasound-guided celiac plexus block and celiac plexus neurolysis for managing abdominal pain associated with chronic pancreatitis and pancreatic cancer. J Clin Gastroenterol. 2010;44:127–34.
5. Ang TL, Teoh AYB. Endoscopic ultrasonography-guided drainage of pancreatic fluid collections. Dig Endosc. 2017;29:463–71.
6. Singhal S, Rotman SR, Gaidhane M, Kahaleh M. Pancreatic fluid collection drainage by endoscopic ultrasound: an update. Clin Endosc. 2013;46:506–14.
7. Bang JY, Varadarajulu S. Endoscopic ultrasound-guided drainage of pancreatic fluid collections. In: Hawes R, Fockens P, Varadarajulu S, editors. Endosonography, vol. 23. 4th ed. Elsevier; 2019. p. 291–301.
8. Cazacu IM, Singh BS, Săftoiu A, Bhutani MS. Endoscopic ultrasound-guided treatment of pancreatic cancer. Curr Gastroenterol Rep. 2020;22:27.
9. Wilson P, Webster G. Endoscopic management of biliary stone disease. Frontline Gastroenterol. 2017;8:129–32.
10. Mangiavillano B, Pagano N, Baron TH, Luigiano C. Outcome of stenting in biliary and pancreatic benign and malignant diseases: a comprehensive review. World J Gastroenterol. 2015;21:9038–54.

Alina Constantin

10.1 Quality and Safety Indicators for Endoscopy Department [1–3]

Componence	Task
Leadership and organization	• Sharing responsibilities • Annual operational plan
Equipment and facilities	• Review of equipment and facilities • Program of maintenance, inspection, and calibration • Equipment and facilities deficiencies addressed • Compliance with national decontamination guidelines
Quality	• System to capture procedural indicators • Measurement of performance indicators and feedback to doctors • Action taken for persistent underperformance • Granting privileges

A. Constantin (✉)
Ponderas Academic Hospital, Bucharest, Romania

A. Săftoiu (ed.), *Pocket Guide to Advanced Endoscopy in
Gastroenterology*, https://doi.org/10.1007/978-3-031-42076-4_10

Componence	Task
Safety	• Procedures in place to mitigate risks well known
	• Known adverse events captured
	• The cause analysis of adverse events
	• STOP procedures where risks outweigh benefits
Appropriateness	• Guidelines for all procedures
	• Compliance with guidelines assessed periodically
Information, consent, further care	• Informed consent according to national requirements
	• Patient information regarding all procedures
	• Discharge recommendations given to patients
Comfort, dignity, privacy	• Patient feedback regarding comfort during procedures
	• Action taken in order to improve patient comfort
	• Proper environment for maintaining patient privacy
Staffing	• Review of staffing in relation to activity
	• New staff induction period
	• Specific training for each role in endoscopy department
Patient involvement	• Patient feedback collected
	• Negative feedbacks reviewed
	• Action taken accordingly

10.2   Quality Indicators for Upper Endoscopy [4]

Componence	Task
Pre-procedure	• Proportion of patients with proper indications for fasting (more than 95%)
Completeness of procedure	• Proportion of reports containing procedure time (more than 90%)
	• Proportion with accurate photodocumentation (more than 90%)

Componence	Task
Identification of pathology	• Proportion of reports with standardized terminology (more than 95%)
Management of pathology	• Proportion using Seattle biopsy protocol in Barrett surveillance (more than 90%)
Complications	• Proportion of complication recorded and documented after therapeutic procedures (more than 95%)
Number of procedures	• No current standard
Patient experience	• No current standard
Post-procedure	• No key indicator defined

10.3   Quality Indicators for Lower Endoscopy [5]

Componence	Task
Pre-procedure	• Proportion of patients who received instructions regarding bowel preparation (>90%)
Completeness of procedure	• Cecal intubation rate (more than 90%)
Identification of pathology	• Adenoma detection rate (more than 25%) and polyp detection rate (more than 40%)
	• Withdrawal time (7 min)
Management of pathology	• Standardized polypectomy technique (above 80%)
Complications	• Complication rate
Patient experience	• Patient feedback collected
	• Negative feedbacks reviewed
Post-procedure	• Post-polypectomy surveillance according to guidelines

10.4   Quality Indicators for ERCP [6]

Componence	Task
Pre-procedure	• Adequate antibiotic prophylaxis before ERCP (*more than 90%*) (incomplete biliary drainage, sclerosing cholangitis, hilar tumors, immunocompromised patients)
Completeness of procedure	• Bile duct cannulation rate (more than 90%)
Management of pathology	• Clearance of common bile duct stones (more than 90%)
	• Stent placement regarding biliary obstruction (more than 95%)
Safety of ERCP	• Post-ERCP (<10%) pancreatitis
Patient experience	• Patient feedback collected
	• Negative feedbacks reviewed
Post-procedure	• No key indicator defined

10.5   Quality Indicators for Endoscopic Ultrasound (EUS) [6]

Componence	Task
Pre-procedure	• Adequate antibiotic prophylaxis before EUS (cystic lesions) more than 95%
Identification of pathology	• Tissue sampling during EUS-FNA and FNB (more than 85%)
	• Documentation of EUS landmarks (more than 90%)
Patient experience	• Patient feedback collected
	• Negative feedbacks reviewed
Post-procedure	• No key indicator defined

10.6 Indicators That Should Be Evaluated in the Future in Order to Improve Quality in ERCP and EUS

- The role of NSAIDS for prevention of post ERCP pancreatitis.
- Documentation of EUS landmarks according to each pathology.
- Completeness of ERCP video and radiological documentation Accuracy of T and N staging for cancer.
- Radiation exposure and protection.

References

1. Valori R, Cortas G, de Lange T, et al. Performance measures for endoscopy services: a European Society of Gastrointestinal Endoscopy (ESGE) Quality Improvement Initiative. Endoscopy. 2018;50:1186–204.
2. Day LW, Cohen J, Greenwald D, et al. Quality indicators for gastrointestinal endoscopy units. VideoGIE. 2017;2:119–40.
3. Armstrong D, Barkun A, Bridges R, et al. Canadian Association of Gastroenterology consensus guidelines on safety and quality indicators in endoscopy. Can J Gastroenterol. 2012;26:17–31.
4. Bisschops R, Areia M, Coron E, et al. Performance measures for upper gastrointestinal endoscopy: a European Society of Gastrointestinal Endoscopy (ESGE) Quality Improvement Initiative. Endoscopy. 2016;48:843–64.
5. Kaminski MF, Thomas-Gibson S, Bugajski M, et al. Performance measures for lower gastrointestinal endoscopy: a European Society of Gastrointestinal Endoscopy (ESGE) Quality Improvement Initiative. Endoscopy. 2017;49:378–97.
6. Domagk D, Oppong KW, Aabakken L, et al. Performance measures for ERCP and endoscopic ultrasound: a European Society of Gastrointestinal Endoscopy (ESGE) Quality Improvement Initiative. Endoscopy. 2018;6:1448–60.

Antiplatelet and Anticoagulant Therapy in Endoscopy

11

Alina Constantin

11.1 Stratification of Endoscopic Procedures as Stated by International Guidelines (Table 11.1) [1–4]

A. Constantin (✉)
Ponderas Academic Hospital, Bucharest, Romania

Table 11.1 Stratification of endoscopic procedures as stated by international guidelines

Practice guidelines			
Thrombotic risk group	ASGE	ESGE/BSG	APAGE/APSDE
Low risk	Diagnostic upper endoscopy and lower endoscopy including mucosal biopsy, ERCP with stent placement or papillary balloon dilation without sphincterotomy, diagnostic enteroscopy, capsule endoscopy, enteral stent placement (controversial), EUS without FNA, argon plasma coagulation, Barrett esophagus ablation	Diagnostic upper endoscopy and lower endoscopy including mucosal biopsy, ERCP with stent placement, EUS without FNA, diagnostic enteroscopy	Diagnostic upper endoscopy and lower endoscopy including mucosal biopsy, ERCP with stent placement, EUS without FNA, diagnostic enteroscopy, capsule endoscopy, enteral stent placement (colonic, esophageal), plasma argon coagulation
High-risk and ultrahigh-risk	Polypectomy ERCP with sphincterotomy varices PEG/PEJ placement; therapeutic enteroscopy; EUS with FNA; endoscopic hemoastasis; tumor ablation; cyst-gastrostomy ampullectomy EMR, ESD, pneumatic or bougie dilation	Polypectomy; ERCP with sphincterotomyampullectomy EMR, ESD dilatation of strictures Varices PEG EUS with FNA Oesophageal, enteral, or colonic stenting	Polypectomy; ERCP with sphincterotomy ± ballon sphincteroplasty dilatation of strictures; injection or banding of varices; PEG/PEJ placement; EUS with FNA, Ampullectomy ESD, EMR of polyps bigger than 2 cm

ASGE American society for gastrointestinal endoscopy, *ESGE/BSG* European society of gastrointestinal endoscopy and British society of gastroenterology, *APAGE/APSDE* Asian Pacific association of gastroenterology and Asian Pacific society for digestive endoscopy, *EUS* endoscopic ultrasound, *FNA* fine-needle aspiration, *ERCP* endoscopic retrograde cholangiopancreatography, *PEG* percutaneous endoscopic gastrostomy, *PEJ* percutaneous endoscopic jejunostomy, *EMR* endoscopic mucosal resection, *ESD* endoscopic submucosal dissection

11.2   Stratification of Thrombotic Risk Stated by International Guidelines (Table 11.2) [1–4]

Table 11.2 Stratification of thrombotic risk

Practice guidelines		
Risk group	ASGE	ESGE/BSG	APAGE/APSDE
Low/ moderate risk	*Anticoagulant therapy* Bileaflet aortic valve prosthesis with no CVA risk factors or AF VTE more than 12 months previous and no other risk factor for CVA 3. AF + CHA2DS2-VASc score < 2 Bileaflet aortic valve prosthesis and one or more risk factors—AF, prior CVA or TIA, diabetes, hypertension, congestive heart failure, age more than 75 year 2. VTE within the past 3–12 months + thrombophilia (heterozygous factor V Leiden or prothrombin gene mutation Recurrent VTE active cancer	*Anticoagulant therapy* Prosthetic metal heart valve in aortic position Xenograft heart valve AF with no valvular disease More than 3 months after VTE Thrombophilia syndrome *Antithrombotic therapy* Ischaemic heart disease without coronary stent cerebrovascular disease Peripheral vascular disease	*Anticoagulant therapy* Nonvalvular AF + CHA2DS2-VASc score ≤ 5 Prosthetic valve with no AF More than 3 months after VTE *Antithrombotic therapy* 1. Acute coronary syndrome / coronarography more than 6 months ago 2. Stable coronary artery disease

High risk/ ultrahigh risk	*Anticoagulant therapy*	*Anticoagulant therapy*	*Anticoagulant therapy*
	Any mitral valve prosthesis Any caged-ball or tilting disk aortic valve prothesis Recent (last 6 months) TIA or CVA AF + CHA2DS2-VASc score > 2	Prosthetic metal heart valve in mitral position Prosthetic heart valve + AF AF + mitral stenosis Less than 3 months after VTE *Antithrombotic therapy* Drug eluting coronary artery stents within 12 months of placement Bare metal coronary artery stents within 1 month of placement	AF with no valvular disease + CHA2DS2-VASc score > 5 Metallic mitral valve Prosthetic valve with AF Less than 3 months after VTE Severe thrombophilia (protein C or protein S deficiency) Antiphospholipidic syndrome) *Antithrombotic therapy* Acute coronary syndrome or coronarography 6 weeks to 6 months *Antithrombotic therapy* Acute coronary syndrome or coronarography less than 6 weeks

ASGE American society for gastrointestinal endoscopy, *ESGE/BSG* European society of gastrointestinal endoscopy and British society of gastroenterology, *APAGE/APSDE* Asian Pacific association of gastroenterology and Asian Pacific society for digestive endoscopy, *EUS* endoscopic ultrasound, *FNA* fine-needle aspiration, *ERCP* endoscopic retrograde cholangiopancreatography, *PEG* percutaneous endoscopic gastrostomy, *PEJ* percutaneous endoscopic jejunostomy, *EMR* endoscopic mucosal resection, *ESD* endoscopic submucosal dissection, AF atrial fibrillation, CVA cerebrovascular accident, VTE venous thromboembolism, TIA transient ischemic attack

11.3 Management of Aspirin and NSAID Drugs in Elective Endoscopic Procedures as Stated by International Guidelines (Table 11.3) [1–4]

Table 11.3 Management of aspirin and NSAID drugs in elective endoscopic procedures

Aspirin/AINS			
Risk group	ASGE	ESGE/BSG	APAGE/APSDE
Low-risk procedures	Continue low doses of aspirin and NSAIDS	Continue aspirin	Continue aspirin
High–/ ultrahigh risk procedures	Continue low doses of aspirin and NSAIDS	Discontination of aspirin in patients scheduled for ampullectomy, ESD, EMR for upper gastrointestinal lesions and colonic lesions more than 2 cm	Discontinuation of aspirin in patients scheduled for ESD and EMR of polyps larger than 2 cm

NSAID nonsteroidal antiinflammatory drugs, *ASGE* American society for gastrointestinal endoscopy, *ESGE/BSG* European society of gastrointestinal endoscopy and British society of gastroenterology, *APAGE/APSDE* Asian Pacific association of gastroenterology and Asian Pacific society for digestive endoscopy, *EUS* endoscopic ultrasound, *EMR* endoscopic mucosal resection, *ESD* endoscopic submucosal dissection

11.4 Antiplatelet Drugs: Thienopyridines (Clopidogrel, Prasugrel, Ticlopidine) + Ticagrelor: In Elective Endoscopic Procedures as Stated by International Guidelines (Table 11.4) [1–4]

Table 11.4 Antiplatelet drugs—thienopyridines (clopidogrel, prasugrel, ticlopidine) + ticagrelor—in elective endoscopic procedures

Practice guidelines			
	ASGE	ESGE/BSG	APAGE/APSDE
Low-risk procedures	Continue therapy	Continue therapy as single or dual antiplatelet therapy	Continue therapy
High–/ultrahigh-risk procedures	*Low cardiovascular risk* Stop therapy before procedure In the case of dual antiplatelet therapy, continue aspirin *High cardiovascular risk* Stop therapy at least 5 days before the procedure or switch to aspirin In the case of dual antiplatelet therapy, continue aspirin	*Low cardiovascular risk* Stop therapy before procedure In the case of dual antiplatelet therapy, continue aspirin *High cardiovascular risk* Stop therapy at least 5 days before the procedure or switch to aspirin In the case of dual antiplatelet therapy, continue aspirin	Stop therapy at least 5 days before the procedure In the case of dual antiplatelet therapy, with aspirin and clopidogrel, in patients with coronary stents, continue aspirin and stop clopidogrel Ultrahigh-risk procedures may need stopping dual antiplatelet therapy

ASGE American society for gastrointestinal endoscopy, *ESGE/BSG* European society of gastrointestinal endoscopy and British society of gastroenterology, *APAGE/APSDE* Asian Pacific association of gastroenterology and Asian Pacific society for digestive endoscopy

11.4.1 Warfarin: In Elective Endoscopic Procedures as Stated by International Guidelines (Table 11.5)

Table 11.5 Warfarin in elective endoscopic procedures

Practice guidelines			
	ASGE	ESGE/BSG	APAGE/APSDE
Low-risk procedures	Continue therapy	Continue therapy Check the INR the week before endoscopy (it should be in therapeutic range)	Continue therapy Check the INR the week before endoscopy (it should be in therapeutic range)
High–/ ultrahigh-risk procedures	*Low cardiovascular risk*	*Low cardiovascular risk*	*Low cardiovascular risk*
	Stop warfarin/ acenocumarol	Stop warfarin 5 days before the procedure and check INR (it should be less than 1.5)	Stop warfarin 5 days before the procedure and check INR (it should be less than 2)
	High cardiovascular risk	*High cardiovascular risk*	*High cardiovascular risk*
	Stop warfarin and bridge with LMWH	Stop warfarin 5 days before the procedure Stop therapy at least 5 days before the procedure and bridge with LMWH. Stop LMWH more than 24 h before endoscopy	Stop warfarin 5 days before the procedure and bridge with LMWH When INR is less than 2

ASGE American society for gastrointestinal endoscopy, *ESGE/BSG* European society of gastrointestinal endoscopy and British society of gastroenterology, *APAGE/APSDE* Asian pacific association of gastroenterology and Asian Pacific society for digestive endoscopy, *INR:* international normalized ratio, *LMWH* low-molecular-weight heparin

11.5   DOACs: In Elective Endoscopic Procedures as Stated by International Guidelines (Table 11.6) [1–4]

Table 11.6 DOACs—in elective endoscopic procedures

DOACs			
	ASGE	ESGE/BSG	APAGE/APSDE
Low-risk procedures	Continue therapy	Continue therapy and omit the dose the morning of procedure	Continue therapy
High–/ ultrahigh-risk procedures	Stop therapy before procedure for the appropriate drug-specific interval	Stop therapy before procedure for the appropriate drug-specific interval Take last dose of DOAC ≥48 h before procedure	Stop therapy before procedure for the appropriate drug-specific interval Take last dose of DOAC ≥48 h before procedure

ASGE American society for gastrointestinal endoscopy, *ESGE/BSG* European society of gastrointestinal endoscopy and British society of gastroenterology, *APAGE/APSDE* Asian Pacific association of gastroenterology and Asian Pacific society for digestive endoscopy, *INR* international normalized ratio, *DOAC* direct anticoagulant

References

1. Maida M, Sferrazza S, Maida C, Morreale GC, Vitello A, Longo G, et al. Management of antiplatelet or anticoagulant therapy in endoscopy. World J Gastrointest Endosc. 2020;12:172–97.
2. Veitch AM, Vanbiervliet G, Gershlick AH, Boustiere C, Baglin TP, Smith LA, et al. Endoscopy in patients on antiplatelet or anticoagulant therapy, including direct oral anticoagulants: British Society of Gastroenterology (BSG) and European Society of Gastrointestinal Endoscopy (ESGE) guidelines. Endoscopy. 2016;48:1–18.
3. ASGE Standards of Practice Committe, Acosta RD, Abraham NS, Chandrasekhara V, Chathadi KV, Early DS, Eloubeidi MA, et al. The management of antithrombotic agents for patients undergoing GI endoscopy. *Gastrointest.* Endoscopy. 2016;83:3–16.
4. Chan FKL, Goh KL, Reddy N, Fujimoto K, Ho KY, Hokimoto S, et al. Management of patients on antithrombotic agents undergoing emergency and elective endoscopy. Joint Asian Pacific Association of Gastroenterology (APAGE) and Asian Pacific Society for Digestive Endoscopy (APSDE) practice guidelines. Gut. 2018;67:405–17.

Antibiotic Use in Endoscopy

12

Irina F. Cherciu Harbiyeli

12.1 Subsequent to Endoscopic Procedures, Infections Can Occur Due to [1]

- Bacterial translocation or bacteremia.
  - The pathogen transfers to the blood flow as a result of mucosal trauma.
- Invasive procedures.
  - The use of contaminated endoscopes and/or accessories into a previously known sterile cavity determines translocation of gut flora during procedures such as drainage, aspiration, or pathological sampling.

12.2 Transient Bacteremia [2]

- Often occurs even during routine day-to-day activity, frequently at rates surpassing those associated with endoscopic procedures.

I. F. Cherciu Harbiyeli (✉)
Research Center of Gastroenterology and Hepatology Craiova,
University of Medicine and Pharmacy Craiova, Craiova, Romania

© The Author(s), under exclusive license to Springer Nature Switzerland AG 2023
A. Săftoiu (ed.), *Pocket Guide to Advanced Endoscopy in Gastroenterology*, https://doi.org/10.1007/978-3-031-42076-4_12

- Tooth brushing and flossing (20–68%), toothpicks use (20–40%), ingesting chewable foods (7–51%) carry a risk of temporary bacteremia.
  - These findings provide a solid foundation against routine administration of antibiotic for infective endocarditis (IE) prophylaxis prior to endoscopic procedures.

12.3 Bacteremia [2]

- Can occur after endoscopic procedures.
- Has been endorsed as a surrogate marker for IE risk, but clinically significant infections are extremely rare.
- The prophylactic use of antibiotics, exclusively to prevent IE, is no longer recommended for patients undergoing endoscopic procedures.

12.4 Questions to be Answered when Assessing the Patients Need for Antibiotic Prophylaxis

- Which endoscopic procedure is planned to be performed?
- Does the planned procedure pose a risk of a new infection or bacteremia?
- What are the patient-dependent risk factors in terms of infectious complications?
- Which antibiotics should be used, in which doses, is it given before or after the procedure?

12.5 Endoscopic Procedures Associated with a High Risk of Bacteremia [1, 3]

- Esophageal dilation, sclerotherapy of varices, instrumentation of obstructed bile ducts.
- The rate of bacteremia associated to ERCP in patients with non-obstructed bile ducts is as low as 6.4%, and the incidence reaches 18% in the case of biliary obstruction due to stones/strictures.

12.6 Endoscopic Procedures with High Risk for Infection Independent of Bacteremia [4]

- EUS-guided fine-needle aspiration (EUS-FNA).
- Gastrostomy-PEG/jejunostomy-PEJ.

12.7 Procedures Associated with a Low Risk for Infection and Bacteremia [2, 4]

- Diagnostic gastroscopy, colonoscopy, flexible rectosigmoidoscopy, polypectomy.
- Rates of bacteremia associated to gastroscopy with/without biopsy go up to 8%, with a mean of 4.4%.
- Rates of colonoscopy associated bacteremia varies between 0% and 25%, with a mean of 4.4%.
- Bacteremia associated with therapeutic procedures of the colon (e.g., colonic stent insertion) is unusual (6.3%).
- The rate of flexible sigmoidoscopy-associated bacteremia is 1%.
- No data are available regarding the risk of bacteremia related with enteroscopy, but it is probable minor and comparable to the risk of routine upper/lower endoscopic procedures.

12.8 Practical Aspects Regarding Antibiotic Therapy [4–6]

- Antibioprophylaxis in routine endoscopy is no longer indicated for the prevention of IE, septic arthritis, or graft/device infection.
- Antibiotic prophylaxis is presently recommended in invasive procedures: the placement of PEG/PEJ, EUS-FNA of cystic lesions, ERCP with incomplete biliary drainage (see Table 12.1).

I. F. Cherciu Harbiyeli

Table 12.1 Types of patients and procedures requiring antibiotic drug prophylaxis in endoscopy

Endoscopic procedures	Patient condition	Periprocedural antibioprophylaxis
ERCP with incomplete drainage	– Cholangitis – Biliary obstruction (hilar stenosis, biliary conditions after liver transplantation, etc.)	– Ciprofloxacin 500 mg oral within 60 min before the procedure alternatives: – Ciprofloxacină 400 mg i.v. infused over 60 min, beginning within 120 min before the procedure – Augumentin 2 g oral – Ampicillin-sulbactam 3 g i.v. – Ampicillin 2 g + gentamicin 5 mg/kg i.v. – Antibiotics should be continued until effective biliary drainage
ERCP with complete drainage	– Bile duct obstruction In absence of cholangitis	– Not recommended
EUS-FNA	– Solid lesion in upper/lower GI tract	– Not recommended
	– Drainage of pancreatic/peripancreatic/mediastinal cysts – Sampling of pancreatic masses with cystic component – Walled-off pancreatic necrosis (WOPN)	– Ciprofloxacin 500 mg oral within 60 min before the procedure Or – Ciprofloxacin 400 mg i.v. infused over 60 min, within 120 min before the procedure – Antibiotherapy should be continued 3 days post-procedural
ESD/EMR/POEM	*All patients*	– Same as the suggested regimens for EUS-FNA

PEG/PEJ	*All patients*	– Cefazolin within 60 min before the procedure 2 g i.v. < 120 kg 3 g i.v. ≥ 120 kg If penicillin allergy: – Clindamycin 900 mg i.v. If MRSA risk: – Vancomycin 15 mg/kg (max 2 g) i.v. infused over 60–90 min, beginning within 120 min before the procedure
Colonoscopy or polipectomy	– Peritoneal dialysis	– Ampicillin 2 g + gentamicin 5 mg/kg i.v., max: 120 mg pre-procedure
High-risk endoscopic procedures	*Immunocompromised patients:* – Severe neutropenia (absolute neutrophil count <500 cells/mL) – Advanced hematologic malignancy	– Antibioprophylaxis in these scenarios must be individualized after discussing it with the hematologist/infectionist – Amoxicillin 2 g oral, within 60 min before the procedure or – Ampicillin 2 g i.v./i.m. within 60 min before the procedure If penicillin allergy: – Clindamycin 900 mg i.v.
	– Cirrhosis with variceal bleeding	– Third-generation cephalosporin: – Ceftriaxone 1–2 g i.v. IV once per day or – Cefuroxime – Cefotaxime

(continued)

Table 12.1 (continued)

Endoscopic procedures	Patient condition	Periprocedural antibioprophylaxis
Any endoscopic procedure	– Synthetic vascular graft; other nonvalvular cardiovascular devices – Prosthetic joints	– Not recommended
	Cardiac conditions associated with highest risk of IE: – History of IE – Prosthetic cardiac valve – Cardiac transplant recipients who develop cardiac valvulopathy – Patients with congenital heart disease (CHD)	– Recommended for IE prevention: Either antimicrobial agent active against enterococci: – Penicillin – Ampicillin – Piperacillin – Vancomycin
	All cardiac conditions, except the ones above	– Not recommended

- *The haphazardous use of antibiotics* can be correlated with the development of antibiotic resistance, unnecessary expense, *C. difficile* colitis, drug toxicity.
- Numerous *GI-related infections* are due to gram-negative or anaerobic bacteria. The choice of antibiotics is wide, and only a frequently used selection in GI practice is mentioned in Sect. 12.9 of this chapter.

12.9   Agents Used for Antibioprophylaxis in Endoscopy [4, 6, 7]

- Cephalosporins.
  - Indications:
    - Esophageal rupture.
    - Cholangitis.
    - Intra-abdominal sepsis.
    - Variceal hemorrhage.
    - Often used in combination with metronidazole.
    - Prevention of sepsis after ERCP.
  - Mode of action:
    - Bactericidal B-lactam antibiotic with a broad spectrum of activity.
    - Active against gram-negative and gram-positive bacteria (a slighter coverage).
  - Examples and dose:
    - Cefuroxime 750 mg i.v. every 8 h.
    - Cefotaxime 1–2 g i.v. every 12 h.
    - Ceftriaxonă 1–2 g i.v. once per day.
  - Contraindications:
    - Penicillin hypersensitivity.
    - History of urticaria/angioedema.
    - Porphyria.
    - Caution in renal insufficiency.

- Side effects:
  - Nausea and vomiting.
  - Headache.
  - Rash.
  - Pseudomembranous colitis.
  - Fever and arthralgia.
  - Abnormal liver function tests (cholestasis).
  - Large-scale use of cephalosporins has been correlated with outbreaks of *C. difficile* infection.
- Quinolonnes.
  - Indications:
    - Prevention of infective complications following ERCP (gram-negative sepsis).
  - Mode of action:
    - Active against gram-negative microorganisms.
    - Less effective against gram-positive bacteria, hence insufficient for the prevention of IE.
  - Examples and dose:
    - Ciprofloxacin: 400 mg i.v. every 12 h/500 mg oral every 12 h.
  - Contraindications:
    - Epilepsy.
    - Stroke or preexisting CNS lesions/inflammation.
    - QT prolongation.
    - To be avoided in athletes.
  - Side effects:
    - Dyspepsia, nausea, vomiting.
    - Insomnia, dizziness, neuralgy, phototoxicity.
    - Cartilage damage.
- Aminoglicosides.
  - Indications:
    - Suitable for use in neutropenic patients.
  - Mode of action:
  - Enhance the bactericidal power of ampicillin or amoxicillin against drug-resistant germs (gram-negative Pseudomonas, Proteus, Serratia, or gram-positive Staphylococci).

- Examples and dose:
    Gentamicin 3–6 mg/kg i.v./i.m. once daily.
- Contraindications:
- Myasthenia gravis.
- Dose adjustment in renal impairment patients.
- Side effects:
    Even though associated with significant neuro/nephro-toxicity/ototoxicity, a single dose of gentamicine is safe.
- Metronidazole.
    - Indications:
        Can be added to the prophylaxis regimen in all neutropenic patients.
    - Mode of action:
        Offers cover against anaerobic organisms.
        Doze: 7.5 mg/kg i.v., maximum 4 g.
    - Contraindications:
        Meningitis.
        Seizure.
        Peripheral neuropathy.
        Alcoholism.
        Prolonged QT interval.
        Chronic kidney disease stage 5.
        Severe liver disease.
        Cockayne syndrome.
    - Side effects:
        Nausea, vomiting, loss of appetite, dyspepsia.
        Metallic taste.
        Diarrhea, constipation.
        Headache.
        Rash and itching.
        Mouth sores.
- Glycopeptides.
    - Indications:
        Prophylaxis of IE in patients who are allergic to penicillins or received penicillin/ampicillin/amoxicillin during last month.

- Mode of action:

  A very broad spectrum of activity against gram-positive bacteria.

  Occasionally it can be used in prophylaxis against MRSA infection.
- Examples and dose:

  Vancomycin 15 mg/kg (max. 2 g) i.v. over 60 min.
- Teicoplanin is easier and quicker to administer, more sustained blood levels occur after a single dose.
- Contraindications:

  Mastocytosis.

  Neutrophilia.

  Kidney diseases.

  Ototoxicity.
- Side effects:

  Bitter taste.

  Nausea and vomiting.

  Red man syndrome.

  Fever.

  Eosinophilia.

- Ampicillin and amoxicillin.
  - Indications:

    Prevention of IE: ampicillin or amoxicillin are preferred to penicillin in prophylaxis of enterococcal bacteremia after instrumentation of the lower GI tract.

    Augumentin (amoxycillin + clavulanic acid) seems to be suitable in the prophylaxis of cholangitis after ERCP.
  - Mode of action:

    Active against gram-positive bacteria, especially streptococci and enterococci.
  - Dose:

    Ampicillin 2 g i.v., amoxicilin 1 g i.m.
  - Contraindications:

    Infectious mononucleosis.

    Preceding allergic reactions to any antibiotics.
  - Side effects:

    Might determine hypersensitivity reactions.

- Pipperacillin.
  - Indications:
    Together with tazobactam is effective in preventing post-ERCP cholangitis.
  - Mode of action:
    Broad spectrum agent.
    Limited activity against most strains of staphylococci.
  - Dose:
    4 g i.v. administered over 30 min
  - Contraindications:
    Patients with history of allergic reactions to any of the penicillins, β-lactamase inhibitors, cephalosporins.
  - Side effects:
    Dyspepsia, nausea, vomiting, diarrhea.
    Phlebitis, thrombophlebitis.
    Erythema, rash, pruritus.
    It might induce pseudomembranous colitis, while the risk to cause *C. difficile* might be smaller than other antibiotics.

References

1. Khashab MA, Chithadi KV, Acosta RD, Bruining DH, Chandrasekhara V, et al. Antibiotic prophylaxis for GI endoscopy. Gastrointest Endosc. 2015;81:81–9.
2. Koksal AR, Ramazani-Necessary C. Antibiotic prophylaxis in gastrointestinal system endoscopy. J Gastroenterol Hepatol. 2019;4:025.
3. Domagk D, Oppong KW, Aabakken L, Czako L, Gyokeres T, et al. Performance measures for endoscopic retrograde cholangiopancreatography and endoscopic ultrasound: a European Society of Gastrointestinal Endoscopy (ESGE) quality improvement initiative. United European Gastroenterol J. 2018;6:1448–60.
4. Allison MC, Sandoe JAT, Tighe R, et al. Antibiotic prophylaxis in gastrointestinal endoscopy. Gut. 2009;58:869–80.
5. Gorospe EC, et al. Preprocedural considerations in gastrointestinal endoscopy. Mayo Clin Proc. 2013;88:1010–6.

6. Wilson W, Taubert KA, Gewitz M, Lockhart PB, Baddour LM, et al. Prevention of infective endocarditis: guidelines from the American Heart Association: a guideline from the American Heart Association Rheumatic Fever, Endocarditis, and Kawasaki Disease Committee, Council on Cardiovascular Disease in the Young, and the Council on Clinical Cardiology, Council on Cardiovascular Surgery and Anesthesia, and the Quality of Care and Outcomes Research Interdisciplinary Working Group. Circulation. 2007;116:1736–54.
7. Rey JR, Axon A, Budzynska A, Kruse A, Nowak A. Guidelines of the European Society of Gastrointestinal Endoscopy (E.S.G.E.) antibiotic prophylaxis for gastrointestinal endoscopy. European Society of Gastrointestinal Endoscopy. Endoscopy. 1998 Mar;30(3):318–24.

Part IV

Sedation and Monitoring

Superficial ("Conscious") Sedation

13

Andreea Stănculescu
and Alice Drăgoescu

13.1 Definition

Pharmacological depression of the state of consciousness with the aim of reducing patient anxiety and discomfort for a better endoscopic examination, while providing procedure amnesia [1–6].

13.2 Sedation Levels

- Minimal sedation (anxiolysis).
  - The patient reacts to verbal stimuli by performing commands, spontaneous breathing is not affected.
- Moderate sedation (conscious).
  - The patient is drowsy, but reacts to wider verbal stimuli, spontaneous breathing is adequate and no support is needed.

A. Stănculescu · A. Drăgoescu (✉)
University of Medicine and Pharmacy Craiova, Craiova, Romania

A. Săftoiu (ed.), *Pocket Guide to Advanced Endoscopy in Gastroenterology*, https://doi.org/10.1007/978-3-031-42076-4_13

13.3   Indications

- Simple endoscopic procedures, gastroscopy or colonoscopy.

13.4   Medical Team

- Anesthesiologist with or without nurse anesthetist.

13.5   Preoperative Assessment

- Patients are assessed using the ASA scale (American society of anesthesiologists) [7] and the Mallampati score [8].

13.5.1 ASA Scale

  I Healthy patient.
  II Patient with minor systemic diseases, for example, arterial hypertension or diabetes mellitus controlled therapeutically.
  III Patient with severe systemic diseases, for example, stable angina or diabetes mellitus with systemic impact.
  IV Patient with severe systemic diseases (life threatening), for example, congestive heart failure or end-stage chronic kidney disease.
  V Patient with death risk in the next 24 h (without surgery).
  VI Patient which is declared brain-dead.

13.5.2 Mallampati Score

It is performed by visualizing the oral cavity and is useful for the assessment of difficult tracheal intubation and/or ventilation.

  I The soft palate, uvula, pillars are visualized.
 II The soft palate, part of the uvula is visualized.
III The soft palate, the base of the uvula is visualized.
 IV The hard palate only is visualized.

13.6 Patient Preparation

- Obtaining the written informed consent of the patient or his/her legal representative.
- Mandatory venous access setup.
- Administration of supplemental oxygen.
- Establishing the optimal patient positioning during the procedure.

13.7 Drugs Used

- Benzodiazepines.
  - Midazolam or diazepam.
  - Midazolam is preferred, in doses of 1–2 mg intravenous, due to its short action time.
- Opioids.
  - Fentanyl, sufentanil, or alfentanil.
- Propofol.
  - Administered intermittently as boluses—monotherapy or in combination with other drugs: benzodiazepines, opioids, or ketamine—balanced therapy.
- Nonpharmacological measures.
  - Music therapy reduces the need for administered drugs, offering superior sedation.

13.8 Patients Monitoring

- Pulse oximetry.
- Electrocardiography (D2 lead).
- Noninvasive, automatic, intermittent measurement of blood pressure by plethysmography at 3–5-min intervals.
- Capnography if deepening of sedation is required.

13.9   Assessment of Sedation

Visual assessment of respiratory chest movements, use of sedation scales such as the RASS scale (Richmond agitation-sedation scale) [9].

13.9.1 Richmond Agitation-Sedation Scale: RASS

+4—combative patient
+3—very agitated patient
+2—agitated patient
+1—restless patient
0—patient calm, quiet
−1—dizzy patient, stays awake for more than 10 s after verbal stimulation
−2—lightly sedated patient, stays awake for less than 10 s when verbally stimulated
−3—moderately sedated patient, opens eyes and moves to verbal stimulation
−4—deeply sedated patient, opens eyes and moves only on painful stimulation
−5—unresponsive patient, does not respond to painful stimulation.

13.10 Waking-up Patients

Spontaneous or following administration of the antagonists' drugs, flumazenil and/or naloxone.

13.11 Complications and Side Effects

- Pain at the propofol injection site. Lidocaine can be associated to reduce discomfort.
- Unwanted deepening of sedation.

- Apnea, hypoxemia.
- Cardiac complications:
  - Arterial hypotension.
  - Arrhythmias.
  - Bradycardia.

13.12 Discharge Criteria

- Performing the modified Aldrete scores [10] and the post-anesthetic discharge scoring system (PADSS), which include the following evaluation criteria:
  - Motor activity.
  - Breath.
  - Blood pressure.
  - State of consciousness.
  - Skin appearance.
  - The patient must have stable vital functions for at least 1 h, be conscious, cooperative, time and space oriented, have no pain, bleeding, nausea or vomiting, be able to walk alone/supported [11].

13.13 Advices After Discharge

- The patient must leave accompanied by a responsible adult, is not allowed to drive a car, sign official/legal documents for 24 h and must provide a contact phone number.
- These recommendations are provided to the patient verbally and in writing prior to the sedation (as part of the written informed consent procedure).

References

1. Early DS, Vargo JJ, Chandrasekhara V, et al. Guidelines for sedation and anesthesia in GI endoscopy. Gastrointest Endosc. 2018;87:327–37.
2. Külling D, Orlandi M, Inauen W. Propofol sedation during endoscopic procedures: how much staff and monitoring are necessary? Gastrointest Endosc. 2007;66:443–9.
3. Baudet JS, Borque P, Borja E, et al. Use of sedation in gastrointestinal endoscopy: a nationwide survey in Spain. Eur J Gastroenterol Hepatol. 2009;21:882–8.
4. Radaelli F, Meucci G, Sgroi G, Minoli G, Italian Association of Hospital Gastroenterologists (AIGO). Technical performance of colonoscopy: the key role of sedation/analgesia and other quality indicators. Am J Gastroenterol. 2008;103:1122–30.
5. McQuaid KR, Laine L. A systematic review and meta-analysis of randomized, controlled trials of moderate sedation for routine endoscopic procedures. Gastrointest Endosc. 2008;67:910–23.
6. Qadeer MA, Vargo JJ, Khandwala F, et al. Propofol versus traditional sedative agents for gastrointestinal endoscopy: a meta-analysis. Clin Gastroenterol Hepatol. 2005;3:1049–56.
7. ASA. Physical Status Classification System. www.asahq.org/clinical/physicalstatus.htm; Accessed Oct 15, 2014.
8. Mallampati SR, Gatt SP, Gugino LD, et al. A clinical sign to predict difficult tracheal intubation: a prospective study. Can Anaesth Soc J. 1985;32:429–34.
9. Ely EW, Truman B, Shintani A, et al. Monitoring sedation status over time in ICU patients: reliability and validity of the Richmond Agitation-Sedation Scale (RASS). JAMA. 2003;289:2983–91.
10. Aldrete JA. Modifications to the postanesthesia score for use in ambulatory surgery. J Perianesth Nurs. 1998;13:148–55.
11. Dumonceau JM, Riphaus A, Aparicio JR, Beilenhoff U, et al. European Society of Gastrointestinal Endoscopy, European Society of Gastroenterology and Endoscopy Nurses and Associates, and the European Society of Anaesthesiology Guideline: non-anesthesiologist administration of propofol for GI endoscopy. Endoscopy. 2010; 42:960–74.

Deep Sedation

14

Daniela Burtea and Anca Dimitriu

14.1 Definition

Endoscopic procedures (diagnostic/therapeutic) are frequently performed with deep sedation in most tertiary centers because the sedation:

- Increases the number and complexity of procedures.
- Reduces patient's anxiety and discomfort.
- Increases the degree of addressability to gastroenterologists.

Sedation has a big role in increasing endoscopist satisfaction because it

D. Burtea (✉)
Endoscopy Department, Research Center of Gastroenterology and Hepatology, University of Medicine and Pharmacy Craiova, Craiova, Romania

A. Dimitriu
Intensive Care Anesthesia Department, County Hospital Craiova, Craiova, Romania

A. Săftoiu (ed.), *Pocket Guide to Advanced Endoscopy in Gastroenterology*, https://doi.org/10.1007/978-3-031-42076-4_14

- Improves the quality of endoscopic examination.
  - Increases rate of complete intubation to cecum.
  - Increases the detection of polyps/adenomas.
- Improves the results of therapeutic interventions [1–3]

14.2 Methodology

14.2.1 Procedure Type

- Diagnostic endoscopic examinations can be performed safely without sedation, with adequate pre-procedural psychological preparation.
- Therapeutic interventions require a longer time and higher doses of sedation [4]:
  - Endoscopic mucosal/submucosal resections (EMR sau ESD).
  - Ultrasound endoscopy (EUS).
  - Retrograde endoscopic cholangiopancreatography (ERCP).
  - Enteroscopy.

14.2.2 Sedation Type

Depends on a variety of factors [5]:

- Patient characteristics.
  - Age.
  - Comorbidities.
  - Personal option.
- Type of procedure.
  - Diagnostic.
  - Interventional/therapeutic.

14.2.3 Level of Sedation

It is variable, from minimal and moderate sedation to deep sedation and general anesthesia [1–3]:

- Conscious sedation.
  - Involves the i.v. administration of pharmacological agents that reduce the level of consciousness to a state of drowsiness, relaxation, but the patient remains awake throughout the procedure.
  - Maintains open airways and spontaneuous breathing (patients do not need intubation or mechanical ventilation).
  - Normal cardiac output.
  - There is the possible of communicate with the medical team and to respond to the verbal commands.
- Deep sedation.
  - The pain is tolerable.
  - Decreases anxiety and discomfort.
  - The patient does not remember the negative emotions.
  - Facilitates the performance of the endoscopist.

14.2.4 Advantages of Propofol

- Current guidelines support the use only the propofol vs benzodiazepines and/or opioides [6, 7].
  - Provides security and satisfaction.
  - Reduces the time allocated to the procedure.
  - It is easy to administer.
  - Prompt awakening with fast recovery.
  - Is antiemetic and anticonvulsivant being preferred for ambulatory endoscopy.

- Rate of cardiovascular, respiratory, or cerebral adverse effects.

  Cardiovascular side effects: decreased BP (high doses, fast injection, old age), decreased heart rate + cardiac output (up to asystole for old age, combination of beta-blockers, vagal reflex in long procedures).

  Respiratory side effects: respiratory depression (up to apneea).

  Cerebral side effects: decreases blood flow and intracranial pressure.

  The induction can sometimes be accompanied by excitatory phenomena: muscle spasms, opisthotonus or hiccups.

- *Administration dose*: The American Society of Anesthesiology (ASA) has published definitions for different levels of sedation, depending on the duration and type of endoscopic examination:

  - "Light sedation"—anxiolysis.
  - "Moderate sedation"—ventilatory and cardiovascular function is maintained and the patient is able to respond to verbal or tactile stimules.
  - "Deep sedation"—patients can not be easily awakened but are still able to respond to persistent stimulation.
  - "General anesthesia" with intubation of the patient and the use of other anesthetic agents (ketamine) depending on the particularities of the patient or the difficulty of the procedure.

- *Complications and risks*.

  - The most common complications of propofol and midazolam sedation are apneic episodes, bradycardia and hypotension.

    In the event of an apneic episode, the infusion of propofol should be stopped immediately and basic airways maneuvers should be initiated, including head extension, mandibular and/or chin traction, respectively high-flow oxygena provided via a mask.

In the absence of the effectiveness of these measures an urgent anesthetic examination is required.

Bradycardia should be treated with atropine bolus (0.4 mg to a total dose of 2 mg).

Hypotension should be treated by simultaneously discontinuing propofol, placing the patient in the Trendelenburg position and i.v fluids.

- *Administration of sedation*: the introduction of anesthetic agents into current endoscopy practice has also raised the question "Who should administer these agents?"
  - The use of i.v. sedation has increased the demand for qualified medical personnel.

    The pro-propofol arguments and its utility in endoscopy indicate that it can be administered not only by anesthesiologist but also by trained assistants or endoscopists/gastroenterologists.
  - Administration of propofol by another team member, "Non-anesthesiologist administered propofol sedation" (NAAPS), it is a viable option in many countries.

    However, the use of NAAPS is controversial due to ethical and medicolegal aspects but also due to divergent clinical guidelines.

    In România, the National Medicines Agency requires that propofol be administered only in hospitals/outpatient day hospitalization units and exclusively by doctors specialized in anesthesia.
  - The protocol of propofol requires:

    Constant monitoring of circulatory and respiratory functions (BP, ECG, O_2 saturation).

    The equipment to support the patency of the airways or necessary for artificial ventilation + other resuscitation devices must be available.

References

1. Ferreira AO, Cravo M. Sedation in gastrointestinal endoscopy: where are we at in 2014? World J Gastrointest Endosc. 2015;7:102–9.
2. Müller M, Wehrmann T. How best to approach endoscopic sedation? Nat Rev Gastroenterol Hepatol. 2011;8:481–90.
3. McQuaid KR, Laine L. A systematic review and meta-analysis of randomized, controlled trials of moderate sedation for routine endoscopic procedures. Gastrointest Endosc. 2008;67:910–23.
4. Cheriyan DG, Byrne MF. Propofol use in endoscopic retrograde cholangiopancreatography and endoscopic ultrasound. World J Gastroenterol. 2014;20:5171–6.
5. Igea F, Casellas JA, González-Huix F, Gómez-Oliva C, Baudet JS, Cacho G, Simón MA, De la Morena E, Lucendo A, Vida F. Sedation for gastrointestinal endoscopy. Endoscopy. 2014;46:720–31.
6. Sethi S, Wadhwa V, Thaker A, Chuttani R, Pleskow DK, Barnett SR, Leffler DA, Berzin TM, Sethi N, Sawhney MS. Propofol versus traditional sedative agents for advanced endoscopic procedures: a meta-analysis. Dig Endosc. 2014;26:515–24.
7. Vargo JJ, Zuccaro G, Dumot JA, Shermock KM, Morrow JB, Conwell DL, Trolli PA, Maurer WG. Gastroenterologist-administered propofol versus meperidine and midazolam for advanced upper endoscopy: a prospective, randomized trial. Gastroenterology. 2002;123:8–16.

General Anesthesia

15

Maria Stoica

15.1 Definition

In recent years, the complexity of endoscopic procedures (especially advanced ones) has required their practice in patients under deep sedation/general anesthesia (GA) [1–4].

- GA is an alternative to sedation used in endoscopic procedures, indicated in:
  - Prolonged therapeutic procedures (polypectomies, mucosectomies, EUS, ERCP, enteroscopy, etc.).
  - Procedures that require absolute immobilization of the patient.
  - Emergency endoscopic procedures (gastrointestinal bleeding).
  - Procedures performed on patients who are at high risk.
- Patient-related risk factors:
  - Children (especially under 7 years old).
  - ASA risk III/IV.
  - Patients with suspected difficult airway (Mallampati score).

M. Stoica (✉)
Anesthesiology Department, Emergency County Clinical Hospital Craiova, University of Medicine and Pharmacy Craiova, Craiova, Romania

A. Săftoiu (ed.), *Pocket Guide to Advanced Endoscopy in Gastroenterology*, https://doi.org/10.1007/978-3-031-42076-4_15

- Increased obesity
- Elderly patients (>70 years).
- Associated severe heart/pulmonary diseases.
- Chronic kidney disease (low creatinine clearance),
- Decompensated liver cirrhosis.

15.2 Methodology

- GA must be performed in the OR, by specialized personnel (anesthesiologist and nurse anesthetist).
- At the preanesthetic assessment (carried out at least 24–48 h before the procedure), the anesthesiologist will specify the duration of fasting, any premedication, guidance regarding the treatment of other comorbidities, and the correction of any fluid and electrolyte disturbances.

The Minimum Equipment Required
- Anesthesia machine, facial masks, laryngoscope and endotracheal tubes, laryngeal masks – depending on the patient's age.
- Secretion aspirator.
- Monitor—pulse oximetry, BP, HR, ECG, capnography, anesthetic gases.
- Emergency kit for cardiopulmonary resuscitation (including defibrillator and resuscitation drugs – adrenaline, atropine, etc.)

Pharmacological Agents
- The choice of anesthetics for induction and maintenance depends on the particularities of the patient and the type of intervention.
    - Benzodiazepines (midazolam, diazepam).
        Midazolam – residual amnesia, good systemic tolerance, large interindividual variations.
- Hypnotics (propofol, etomidate).
        Propofol—rapid action, short duration, anxiolytic and amnesic effect comparable to midazolam, good general tolerance in slow administration, pain on injection.

- Central analgesics (opioids, ketamine).
    Opioids (fentanyl, remifentanil)—analgesic effect, weak sedative effect, with possible side effects: respiratory ++++, hemodynamic +/−.
    Ketamine.
- Inhalation anesthetics (sevoflurane, nitrous oxide).
    Sevoflurane—ensures rapid induction and awakening, with minimal cardiovascular effects, does not irritate the airways, ideal for maintaining anesthesia, but increases the risk of POVN (postoperative nausea and vomiting).
- Non-depolarizing neuromuscular blockers.
    Rocuronium.
    Cisatracurium.
- Antagonists.
    Flumazenil.
    Naloxone.

Methods of Administration

- Iterative boluses adapted to intervention times.
    - Combining several drugs with a synergistic effect allows the reduction of individual doses and limits the side effects.
- IV continuous administration is possible with automated infusion pumps.

Postoperative Care

- After the intervention, patients are transferred to the "recovery room" or to intensive care (in serious cases), the decision belonging to the anesthesiologist.
- The Aldrette score quantifies the patient's awakening.
- Pharmacological agents indicated immediately post-intervention.
    - Analgesics/NSAIDs (paracetamol, tramadol, dexketoprofen, etc.).
    - Multimodal analgesia reduces side effects and postoperative opioid consumption (in complex cases).

- Antiemetics.

    5-HT antagonists, i.v. dexamethasone

    Cyclizine, im prochlorpromazine.
- In general, in patients at risk (female, nonsmoker, history of motion sickness, postoperative opioid use), antiemetics should be administered pre- or intraoperatively for good efficiency.
- Adequate analgesia and hydration can prevent POVN.

References

1. Obara K, Haruma K, Irisawa A, et al. Guidelines for sedation in gastroenterological endoscopy. Dig Endosc. 2015;27:435–49.
2. Sidhu R, Turnbul D, Newton M, et al. Deep sedation and anaesthesia in complex gastrointestinal endoscopy: a joint position statement endorsed by the British Society of Gastroenterology (BSG), Joint Advisory Group (JAG) and Royal College of Anaesthesics (RCoA). Frontline Gastroenterol. 2019;10:141–7.
3. ASGE Standards of Practice Committee, Early DS, Lightdale JR, Vargo JJ 2nd, et al. Guidelines for sedation and anaesthesia in GI endoscopy. Gastrointest Endosc. 2018;87:327–37.
4. Hinkelbein J, Lamperti M, Santos J, et al. European Society of Anaesthesiology and European Board of Anaesthesiology guidelines for procedural sedation and analgesia in adults. Eur J Anaesthesiol. 2018;35:6–24.

Part V

Clinical Impact of Endoscopy

Clinical Impact of Endoscopy: Gastroenterology

16

Dan Ionut Gheonea and Ion Rogoveanu

16.1 Endoscopy in Current Practice

- Over time, it became the diagnostic standard for the majority of diseases of the digestive tract as well as bile ducts [1–3]:
- The accumulated knowledge currently allows:
  - Understanding the associated etiopathogenic mechanisms of gastroenterological diseases.
  - Reorganization of digestive tract conditions.
  - The introduction of innovative noninvasive treatments.
- It has become a widely used method, being relatively easily accepted by patients, due to the following [4, 5]:
  - Permanent modernization of equipment and endoscopic accessories.
  - Continuous improvement of the team that uses them.
  - The possibility of sedation.
- It has brought several benefits in dealing with patients:
  - Implementation of screening programs with consequences directly on the reduction of morbidity and mortality.

D. I. Gheonea (✉) · I. Rogoveanu
Gastroenterology Department, University of Medicine and Pharmacy Craiova, Craiova, Romania

A. Săftoiu (ed.), *Pocket Guide to Advanced Endoscopy in Gastroenterology*, https://doi.org/10.1007/978-3-031-42076-4_16

- Some procedures (polypectomies, use of stents in biliary and pancreatic pathology, drainage, dilations of stenoses, endoscopic hemostasis, PEGs) have radically changed their attitude toward patient management.
- Major advantages that gastroenterology has gained for the patient through endoscopy [4]:
  - Increasing periprocedural comfort.
  - Improved the quality of life of patients.
  - Reduction of mortality, complications, period of post-intervention hospitalization.
  - The existence of a favorable balance of the time cost-effectiveness.

16.2 Implications of Endoscopy in Gastroenterology

- The use of endoscopy in the pathology of the bile ducts and the pancreas which for a long time represented the prerogative of surgery [6]:
  - The introduction of endoscopic retrograde cholangio-pancreatography (ERCP) with associated techniques has improved considerably patient morbidity and mortality.
- The use of endoscopy in the field of pathological anatomy:
  - Made the transition in many cases from the analysis of evidence postsurgical intervention to those obtained by harvesting biopsies.
  - This aspect was reflected in the benefit of patient's quality of life who improved significantly.
- The discovery of Helicobacter pylori and the macroscopic consequences of the mucosal changes revealed by endoscopy.
- All endoscopic procedures, with a diagnostic or therapeutic role, are widely used in medical practice replacing to a large extent or even totally the old techniques of approach (plain abdominal X-ray, irrigography, enteroclysis, defecography, laparoscopy, arteriography, etc.).

16.3   Therapeutic Role and Clinical Impact

- Mechanical or thermal endoscopic hemostasis by using different techniques such as hemostatic clips, coagulation with argon plasma, bipolar probe, elastic ligatures, injection of other substances.
- Polypectomy, endoscopic submucosal dissection, as well as endoscopic mucosal resection are techniques that allow resection of preneoplastic lesions as well as T1 cancers and have intervened in decreasing the incidence of esophageal, gastric and colorectal cancer.
- Dilation or fitting of stents in case of certain pathologies which causes stenoses in the digestive tube or the biliary tract.
- Peroral endoscopic myotomy (POEM) in the treatment of motility esophageal disorders, esophageal diverticula.
- Different endoscopic suturing techniques in the treatment of obesity.
- Endoscopic drainage of pseudocysts, walled-off pancreatic necrosis (WOPN), abscesses, or even anastomoses between different organs as in endoscopic gastrojejunostomy.

References

1. Trifan A, Gheorghe C, Dumitrascu D, Diculescu M, Gheorghe L, Sporea L, Tantau M, Ciurea T, editors. Gastroenterologie si Hepatologie clinica București. Medicală; 2018. p. 852–920.
2. Patel N, Darzi A, Teare J. The endoscopy evolution: 'the superscope era'. Frontline Gastroenterol. 2015;6:101–7.
3. Brill JV, Chapman FJ, Dahl J. The practice of gastroenterology: evolution versus intelligent design. Gastrointest Endosc Clin N Am. 2006;16: 623–41.
4. Classen M, Tytgat GNJ, Lightdale CJ. Gastroenterological endoscopy. 2nd ed. Thieme; 2010.
5. Fatima H, Rex DK. General approach to endoscopy: sedation, monitoring, and preparation. In: Podolsky DK, editor. Yamada's textbook of gastroenterology. 6th ed. Wiley; 2015. p. 2535–42.
6. Stockland AH, Baron TH. Endoscopic and radiologic treatment of biliary disease. In: Qayed E, Shahnavaz N, Srinivasan S, editors. Sleisenger and Fordtran's gastrointestinal and liver disease. 10th ed. Elsevier; 2016. p. 1201–13.

Clinical Impact of Endoscopy: Hepatology

Larisa Săndulescu
and Elena Codruța Gheorghe

The rapid expansion of endoscopic techniques and continuous clinical research has expanded the potential clinical utility of interventional procedures in the field of hepatology, being commonly used for the diagnosis and evaluation of:

- Portal hypertension.
- Liver lesions.
- Biliary pathology.

17.1 Portal Hypertension

- Upper gastrointestinal endoscopy (UGE) is the most sensitive method for the diagnosis and evaluation of esophageal and gastric varices.
- The endoscopic appearance of varices is found in most prognostic scores for predicting the individual bleeding risk.

L. Săndulescu
Department of Gastroenterology, Research Center of Gastroenterology and Hepatology, University of Medicine and Pharmacy Craiova, Craiova, Romania

E. C. Gheorghe (✉)
University of Medicine and Pharmacy of Craiova, Craiova, Romania

A. Săftoiu (ed.), *Pocket Guide to Advanced Endoscopy in Gastroenterology*, https://doi.org/10.1007/978-3-031-42076-4_17

- UGE can be used for the management of esophageal varices:
  - Bleeding prophylaxis (ligation reduces the risk of bleeding by ~60% compared to propranolol and reduces bleeding related mortality).
  - Treatment of acute hemorrhages.
  - Prophylaxis of recurrent bleeding (the risk of rebleeding using ligation is lower than sclerotherapy).
- The management of gastric varices has the same objectives, for the prophylaxis and treatment of bleeding using, instead, cyanoacrylate glue injection with a higher success rate than band ligation [1].

17.2 Liver Lesions

- Endoscopic ultrasound (EUS) and endoscopic ultrasound-guided fine-needle aspiration (EUS-FNA) may be alternatives to classical imaging methods and liver biopsy, with a lower risk for adverse reactions.
- These techniques have been proven to be useful for:
  - Parenchymal disease of unclear etiology.
  - Imagistic unconclusive liver tumors [2].
- EUS is a feasible investigation for the preoperative staging of suspicious liver lesions as:
  - It can detect small lesions that can be missed by other imaging methods (e.g., CT scan).
  - EUS-FNA can confirm the diagnosis, can establish cancer stage, and thus change the clinical management [3].

17.3 Biliary Pathology

- EUS is a potential alternative to ERCP or it can be used as a complementary method to other imaging techniques for:
  - Identification of gallstones and assessment of biliary strictures.
  - Characterization of suspicious lesions and use FNA for a final diagnosis.
  - Identification of vascular and lymphatic structures that may facilitate the staging of cholangiocarcinoma.

- Regarding patient management, EUS has an impact on clinical decisions for patients suspected of cholangiocarcinoma.
  - It can reduce the rate of unnecessary surgery in healthy patients.
  - It can determine the resectability of tumors that can spare patients of additional invasive procedures [4].

References

1. Luigiano C, Iabichino G, Judica A, Virgilio C, Peta V, Abenavoli L. Role of endoscopy in management of gastrointestinal complications of portal hypertension. World J Gastrointest Endosc. 2015;7(1):1–12.
2. Lau GK, Ng M, Wu WH, Lam SK. The use of endoscopy in liver diseases. Hong Kong Med J. 1997;3(3):267–273.
3. Parekh PJ, Majithia R, Diehl DL, Baron TH. Endoscopic ultrasound-guided liver biopsy. Endosc Ultrasound. 2015;4(2):85–91.
4. Strongin A, Singh H, Eloubeidi MA, Siddiqui AA. Role of endoscopic ultrasonography in the evaluation of extrahepatic cholangiocarcinoma. Endosc Ultrasound. 2013;2(2):71–76.

Clinical Impact of Endoscopy: Surgery

18

Valeriu Surlin and Ştefan Pătraşcu

Endoscopy plays an important clinical role in surgery, and as we see it, the most evident clinical impact would be in three main areas:

- Diagnosis and treatment of postoperative intestinal bleedings.
- Diagnosis and treatment of postoperative anastomotic strictures.
- Treatment of postoperative anastomotic leakages.

18.1 Endoscopic Diagnosis and Treatment of Postoperative Gastrointestinal Bleedings

Postoperative bleeding is one of the most common complications after GI (gastrointestinal) tract surgery and in some situations may be life threatening.

V. Surlin (✉) · Ş. Pătraşcu
First Department of Surgery, University of Medicine and Pharmacy Craiova, Craiova, Romania

© The Author(s), under exclusive license to Springer Nature Switzerland AG 2023

135

A. Săftoiu (ed.), *Pocket Guide to Advanced Endoscopy in Gastroenterology*, https://doi.org/10.1007/978-3-031-42076-4_18

Causes (Sources) and Pathogenesis

- Mucosal damage.
- Suture line, from either handsewn or stapled.
- Inflammatory, infectious, or ischemic.
- Erosions from foreign materials around the GI tract—gastroplasty plastic rings, intraperitoneal meshes (abdominal wall, from hiatal hernia repairs), duodenal erosion of hemoclips placed on cystic duct, etc. [1].

Location

- More frequently from upper GI tract, representing more than 80% of causes, mortality can reach 30% and four times more postoperative deaths compared with cases without bleeding.
- Less common after colocolic, colorectal, ileocolonic, ileorectal, enteroenteral anastomosis. It is usually self-limiting.

Pathogenesis

- Mucosal damage may occur from:
  - Mechanical surgical trauma.
  - Iatrogenic trauma due to nasogastric tube pressure ulcers.
  - Excessive vomiting with Mallory–Weiss syndrome.
  - Exacerbated gastric of esophageal varices.
- Bleeding from anastomosis:
  - Occur more after sutures on the stomach.
    Timing:
    Immediate postoperative bleeding—stitch to tight, cutting into the tissues, poor hemostasis
    On the anastomotic line, the stitches are too rare or not enough tighten.
    Intermediate postoperative bleeding >5–6 days.
    Breakdown of the anastomotic line.
    Ischemia of one of the anastomotic partners.
    Late postoperative bleeding.
    After 2–3 weeks
    From the granulation tissue of the anastomosis.
    Peptic ulcer of the anastomosis.

- Inflammatory, infectious, or ischemic:
  - Healing process go through a face of exacerbated inflammation, more frequently after stapled anastomoses and the granulation tissue is responsible for bleeding.
  - Local inflammation of the stapling line and formation of microabscesses may lead to rupture and bleeding.
  - Ischemia is one of the anastomotic partners could lead to bleeding.

Diagnosis

- Endoscopy is the best diagnostic tool and can mandate immediate therapy if expertise of the endoscopist available.
- Angiography, also with possibility of treating the bleeding (but higher risk for necrosis).
- I.V. contrast enhanced CT scan with oral/enema contrast agent.

Treatment

- It is adapted to the source, localization, status of patient, time from surgery, suspicion of an associated anastomotic leakage.
- Most cases will be managed by conservative measures: fluid resuscitation, blood, red cell pack and fresh frozen plasma administration, hemostatics, vasopressin, propranolol.
- In upper GI tract bleeding, insertion of nasogastric tube, for monitoring and lavage with cold saline fluids, vasopressin, antacids (where indicated).
- Upper anastomotic GI bleedings respond less to conservative measures compared with the lower GI anastomotic bleeding, probably because of the richer vascularization of the stomach and duodenum.
- Endoscopy is the best therapeutic choice because we can identify very precisely the lesion and apply one of the standard therapeutic measures:
  - Monopolar and bipolar coagulation.
    Caution with extended and deep monopolar coagulation on recent staple line, use spray function.
    Bipolar coagulation of the surface of staple line is considered more safe, especially where three staple lines are present.

- Injection of epinephrine.
- Hemostatic clips.
- Plasma argon beam coagulation.
- Laser coagulation.
- Endoscopic suturing with different devices (Overstich™ Apollo endosurgery, Over the Scope Clips™, etc.)
- Precaution should be taken with insufflation is mandatory in the first postoperative days, not to hyperinflate and overstretch the anastomotic line, and after 5–6 days a leakage may be existent and the probable cause for the bleeding.
- After 2–3 weeks the bleeding is from granulation tissue and the anastomosis is considered to have gained enough resistance to withstand insufflation.

18.2 Endoscopic Diagnosis and Treatment of Anastomotic Stenosis

Stenosis of an anastomosis performed between segments of GI tract can occur at any level in the late postoperative period.

18.2.1 Upper GI Anastomotic Strictures

- Esojejunal anastomosis after esophageal resections, esogastrectomies for cancer or for peptic stenosis.
- Gastrojejunal anastomotic strictures after RYGB (Roux-en-Y gastric bypass) in bariatric surgery patients [2, 3].

Diagnosis
- Stricture of gastrojejunal anastomosis.
  - Dysphagia, vomiting, nutritional deficiencies, is a relatively common late complication of Roux-en-Y gastric bypass (RYGB) with an incidence of 3–12% [2, 3].
  - Definition: anastomotic orifice less than 10 mm, or the inability to allow passage of a standard upper endoscope.

Primary Treatment

- Endoscopic dilatation of stenosis through the scope balloon dilatation or wire-guided bougie dilatation is safe and highly effective.
- Majority of patients can be successfully treated with 1–2 sessions and surgical revision is rarely necessary.
- NB: An over dilatation should be avoided because it may impact on the long term on the weight loss outcomes.

18.2.2 Lower GI Anastomotic Strictures

- Anastomotic stricture is a complication after colorectal surgery, especially after low anterior rectal resections, for rectal cancer, with an incidence between 3 and 30%, although only 5% of patients become symptomatic.
- Definition: The inability to pass a proctoscope (12 mm diameter) or a larger rigid sigmoidoscope (19 mm diameter) through the stenosis.

Risk Factors

- General nutrition status.
- Obesity.
- Technique employed for the anastomosis.
- Tension in anastomosis.
- Type of anastomosis (end-to-end, side-to-end, etc.).
- Insufficient blood supply.
- Infection, perianastomotic abscess.
- Anastomotic leakage.
- Male patients (2.4 times greater the risk compared to women, due to narrow pelvis and technical difficulties).
- Not freeing the splenic flexure, not dividing the origin of IMA (inferior mesenteric artery) and IMV (inferior mesenteric vein).
- Stapled anastomosis (2/3 of cases).
- Incomplete "doughnuts".
- Occur more frequently after stapled anastomosis probably due to more inflammation in the period of healing.

Symptoms

- Abdominal distension and pain.
- Fractioned and frequent stool passage.
- Pelvic pain.
- Sensations of emergency.

Diagnosis

- Digital examination—stricture of anastomosis.
- Anuscopy, proctoscopy with visualization of stenosis.
- X-ray contrast enema.
- I.V. contrast-enhanced CT scan + contrast enema.
- Pelvic MRI.
- Endoscopy, reduction of lumen, punctiform stenosis, complete stenosis.

Techniques Employed

- Higher colorectal, colocolic or ileocolic strictures are managed by endoscopic +/− fluoroscopic approach
    - Endoscopic electrocision in complete or cvasicomplete strictures.
    - Endoscopic balloon dilatation.
    - Placement of plastic stents or self-expanding metallic stents, coated preferably for easier extraction.

Rate of Success

- The higher the expertise of the endoscopist, the higher the rate of success.
- The procedure may be repeated from one up to several times until a patency is maintained over a long period of time.

Lower anastomotic strictures, reachable by digital tact, could be dilated digitally upon regular postoperative checkup, or by using metal dilators with or without sedation or general anesthesia.

18.3   Endoscopic Diagnosis and Treatment of Anastomotic Leakages After GI Surgery

Anastomotic leakages are specific complication after major GI surgery, unavoidable, and sometimes with severe consequences until potentially life threatening. Are one of the worse surgeons's nightmare. They are associated with postoperative comorbidities, prolongation of hospital stay, hospitalization in ICU, increase over all medical costs, increase postoperative mortality, and worse oncologic outcome [4].

Leakage can occur up to 3 weeks after surgery, the highest incidence is days 3–5. An immediate leakage is testimony of a defect in the execution of the anastomosis, leakages after 5–6 day are due to the impairment of healing.

Risk Factors
- Insufficient blood supply.
- Tension in the anastomosis.
- Inadequate suture material.
- Hipoproteinemia.
- Anemia.
- Poor nutritional status.
- Intraoperative hypotension.
- Abscesses in the suture line, hematomas.
- Staple misfiring.
- Multiple staples firing.
- Blood loss during surgery.
- Long operative times.
- Postoperative hemorrhage, etc.

Diagnosis
- Fever, leukocytosis, pain, tachycardia, mental confusion, hypotension, ileus.
- High values for C-reactive proteins, procalcitonin.
- Increase value of liver enzymes.
- Increase of urea, creatinine.

- Gas, pus, food, bile, intestinal fluid, fecal discharge on the drains.
- Pneumonia, basal pleurisy, mediastinitis in leakages after GI surgery.
- Pelvic abscesses, intraabdominal abscesses, peritonitis in leakages after lower GI surgery.

Imagistic Diagnosis
- Oral administration of blue methylene (for upper GI leakages).
- Radiological examination using water-soluble contrast agent.
- I.V. contrast-enhanced CT scan + water-soluble oral contrast.
- MRI (when acute renal failure).
- Endoscopy—should be the method of choice in all cases.

Advantages of Endoscopy
- Possible application at bed side.
- Early precise diagnosis, can estimate the size of the dehiscence, the existence of a perianastomotic abscess.
- Option for therapy.
  - Can clean the perianastomotic abscess by debridement.

    In upper GI leakages, install a nasogastric tube in the abscess cavity for drainage and lavage or apply endoscopic vacuum-assisted closure therapy by Endosponge™.

    In leakages after low colorectal anastomoses same principle of endoscopic repeated debridement of the abscess cavity can be applied the same endoscopic vacuum-assisted closure therapy by Endosponge™.

    Sealing of the fistulous tract with fibrin glue. This method is successful in case of small leakages and residual fistulas, and it has to be repeated for many times.
  - Can bypass the leak by an endoprothesis, best coated, in order to ensure feeding for patient, limit the leakage outside the lumen, and calibrate healing of the anastomosis, to reduce secondary anastomotic stenosis.

- In lower GI leakages, the placement of a plastic stent or a self-expanding metallic stent, after cleaning of the abscess and development of granulation tissue, may help guide healing and calibrate the anastomosis.
- Attempt closure by suturing devices such as Overstich™ (Apollo endosurgery), or OTSC® system (Ovesco endoscopy AG). The method is more successful in cases when the leakage is very early, in the first few days after surgery, due to a technical imparity, because there is very little inflammation due to leakage of intestinal fluid outside the lumen. The more time passes, the less success rate because of inflammation that impairs healing.

References

1. Ghallab E. Post-operative bleeding and its management. Egypt J Hosp Med. 2018;70(9):1480–3.
2. de Palma GD, Forestieri P. Role of endoscopy in the bariatric surgery of patients. World J Gastroenterol. 2014;20(24):7777–84.
3. Kumar N, Thompson CC. Endoscopic management of complications after gastrointestinal weight loss surgery. Clin Gastroenterol Hepatol. 2013;11(4):343–53.
4. Kähler G. Anastomotic leakage after upper gastrotintestinal surgery: endoscopic treatment. Visc Med. 2017;33:202–6.

Endoscopic Bariatric Therapies

19

Alina Constantin and Cătălin Copăescu

19.1 Endoscopic Bariatric Interventions and Intragastric Devices

- Obesity is considered a global burden due to its worldwide spread and increasing incidence and prevalence [1]. Bariatric endoscopy has several advantages, being an efficient method used to treat obesity with loss of limited number of kilos and higher safety profile. Several endoscopic optios are available [2, 3]:
- Endoscopic sleeve gastroplasty.
    - Endoluminally free hand, full thickness suture between prepyloric antrum and gastroesophageal junction using Overstitch.
    - The stomach reduces along the great curvature such as a "sleeve" (Fig. 19.1a, b).
- Intragastric balloons.

Orbera
- Silicone made balloon filled with saline 500–700 ml.
- Inserted and retrieved endoscopically.
- Complications—nausea and vomiting, very rare gastric perforation.
- Extra weight loss 6 months (EWL 6 M) 38.4%.

A. Constantin (✉) · C. Copăescu
Ponderas Academic Hospital, Bucharest, Romania

A. Săftoiu (ed.), *Pocket Guide to Advanced Endoscopy in Gastroenterology*, https://doi.org/10.1007/978-3-031-42076-4_19

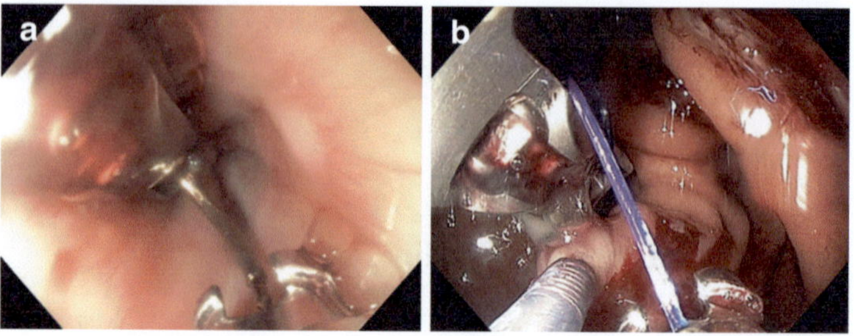

Fig. 19.1 Endoscopic gastroplasty using the Overstitch™ device, placed on a double-channel endoscope

Reshape Duo

- Two balloons interconnected by a flexible tube that is filled with saline 450 mL × 2.
- Each balloon has independent channel.
- Inserted and retrieved endoscopically.
- Complications—gastric erosions.
- EWL 6 M 25.1%.

Obalon

- Balloon ingested under fluoroscopy control and filled with air 250 mL.
- May be inserted up to three balloons at 4 weeks distance.
- Complications—gastric erosions.
- EWL 6 M 6.81%.

Transpiloric Shuttle

- Delays gastric emptying.
- Two silicon bulbs joined by a flexible transpyloric catheter which determines partial gastric obstruction.
- Complications – mucosal erosions.
- EWL 6 M 50% ± 26.4%.

"Full Sense" Device

- Fully covered gastroesophageal stent with a cylindrical esophageal component and a gastric disk.
- With the aim of increasing pressure on cardia in order to induce satiety.

"AspireAssist" Device

- Silicone tube that is inserted similar to a percutaneous endoscopic gastrostomy tube.
- After 2 weeks the external portion of the tube is connected to the AspireAssist device in order to allow aspiration of 30% of the meal at 20 min after ingestion.

19.2 Endoscopic Bariatric Procedures and Small Bowel Interventions [4]

- Duodenal mucosal resurfacing [5].
  - Radiofrequency ablation to the superficial duodenal mucosa after lifting it with saline injection into the submucosa in order to regenerate superficial layer.
  - Major benefits in improving glycemia.
- "Endobarrier" device.
  - Thin, flexible sleeve lined with teflon that is released in duodenal bulb extended 65 cm into the small bowel.
  - In order to create a mechanical barrier avoiding biliopancreatic secretions and absorption of food on this segment.
- Gastroduodenojejunal bypass sleeve.
  - 120 cm flexible sleeve used for gastroduodenojejunal bypass, that is secured all the GE junction and extended through the stomach, duodenum, proximal jejunum
- Self-assembling magnets for endoscopy.
  - Two endoscopes are used to access the small bowel.
  - Magnets are deployed from each endoscope.
  - The devices are connected in order to create a compression anastomosis.
  - Anastomosis has the role to bypass a portion of the small bowel.

References

1. Hales CM, Carroll MD, Fryar CD, et al. Prevalence of obesity among adults and youth: United States, 2015-2016. NCHS Data Brief. 2017;288:1–8.
2. Goyal D, Watson RR. Endoscopic Bariatric therapies. Curr Gastroenterol Rep. 2016;18:26.
3. ASGE Bariatric Endoscopy Task Force, ASGE Technology Committee, et al. Endoscopic bariatric therapies. Gastrointest Endosc. 2015;81:1073–86.
4. Štimac D, Klobučar Majanović S, Belančić A. Endoscopic treatment of obesity: from past to future. Dig Dis. 2020;6:1–13.
5. van Baar ACG, Holleman F, Crenier L, Haidry R, Magee C, Hopkins D, et al. Endoscopic duodenal mucosal resurfacing for the treatment of type 2 diabetes mellitus: one year results from the first international, open-label, prospective, multicentre study. Gut. 2020;69:295–303.

Part VI

Upper Gastrointestinal Tract

Motility Disorders

20

Sacerdoțianu Mihai

20.1 Definition and Classification

Gastrointestinal motility disorders are caused by primary or secondary abnormalities of the neuromuscular system of the oropharynx, esophagus, stomach, and intestine.

The disposition of the esophageal muscular system: striated muscle at the upper esophagus, smooth muscle for the lower esophagus, and mixed muscle type for the middle esophagus.

Classification of GI motility disorders:

- Upper oropharyngeal and esophageal motility disorders (skeletal muscle).
  - Pharyngeal paralysis.
  - Cricopharyngeal bar.
  - Globus pharyngeus.
  - Motility disorders encountered in other pathologies (Parkinson's disease, myasthenia gravis).

S. Mihai (✉)
Gastroenterology Department, University of Medicine and Pharmacy Craiova, Craiova, Romania

© The Author(s), under exclusive license to Springer Nature Switzerland AG 2023

A. Săftoiu (ed.), *Pocket Guide to Advanced Endoscopy in Gastroenterology*, https://doi.org/10.1007/978-3-031-42076-4_20

- Lower esophageal motility disorders (smooth muscle).
  - Achalasia.
  - Diffuse esophageal spasm (DES).
  - Hyperperistaltic esophagus.
  - Lower esophageal sphincter (LES) hypertension.
  - Gastroesophageal reflux disease (GERD).
  - Pseudoachalasia.
  - Chagas disease.
  - Presbyesophagus.
  - Motility disorders associated with collagen diseases (scleroderma).
  - Motility disorders associated with other pathologies (diabetes) [1, 2].

20.1.1 Achalasia

20.1.1.1 Definition

- Primary motor disorder of smooth muscle esophagus characterized by failure of the LES to relax and loss of esophageal peristalsis with swallowing, changes that cause progressive dilatation of the esophagus over time in the absence of appropriate treatment.

20.1.1.2 Epidemiology

- Achalasia usually appears:
  - Between 25 and 60 years.
  - Incidence around 1/100,000 per year.
  - Prevalence of 10/100,000.
  - Men = women.
- Known risk factors.
  - Viral (varicella zoster virus VVZ, HSV-1).
  - Autoimmune disorders (psoriasis, Sjogren syndrome).
  - Family aggregation HLA DKW1, DQA1 × 0103 and DQB1 × 0603.
  - Mutations in the AAAS gene that cause autonomic nervous system dysfunction.
  - Poor socioeconomic status.

20.1.1.3 Etiology and Pathogenesis

- Significant loss of ganglion cells within Auerbach myenteric plexus and degeneration of inhibitory neurons that release VIP and NO.
- The consequence is the imbalance between the excitatory and inhibitory neurons, with increasing LES pressure and loss of esophageal peristalsis.

20.1.1.4 Diagnosis

- Clinical signs.
  - Solid food and liquids dysphagia with insidious onset, progressive, sometimes paradoxical.
  - Chest pain, sometimes with irradiation in the shoulders, back, and mandible; may improve in advanced stages, with the dilatation of the esophagus; dominates the symptoms in vigorous variant.
  - Regurgitation of undigested food or saliva.
  - Heartburn gave by the low pH of lactic acid caused by the bacterial fermentation of retained food in the esophagus.
  - Weight loss (in advanced stages).
  - Respiratory symptoms (nocturnal cough, wheezing, feeling of suffocation due to regurgitation followed by aspiration).
  - Physical exam:
  - - No additional information in the absence of pulmonary complications.
- Laboratory studies.
  - No additional information.
- Barium swallow radiography.
  - Is the initial test; provide useful information regarding LES function, peristalsis, and bolus clearance through the EGJ.
  - Can describe various degrees of dilatation of the esophagus, with tortuous aspect—pseudosigmoid, aperistalsis; symmetrical narrowing of the LES (bird's beak); poor emptying of barium.

- Esophageal manometry.
  - Highlights the incipient motor changes of the disease; allows differential diagnosis with other esophageal motor disorders.
  - Classic manometry—basic exploration, divides achalasia into two variants (classical and vigorous); highlights insufficiency/absence of LES relaxation during swallowing and increased basal pressure, aperistaltic contractions in the lower two-third of the esophagus, with various amplitude depending on the form of achalasia, (can be performed mecholyl, bethanechol, or cholecystokinin tests).
  - High-resolution esophageal manometry with pressure topography (HRE-PT) divides achalasia into three distinct patterns (Chicago classification), with different treatment responses and prognosis; demonstrates the absence of LES relaxation by calculating the integrated relaxation pressure (IRP).

    Type I, IRP > 15 mmHg, absent peristalsis and esophageal pressurization.

    Type II, IRP > 15 mmHg, absence of esophageal body peristalsis and panesophageal pressurization >30 mmHg in more than 20% of swallows (the most common form with the best treatment response).

    Type III, IRP > 15 mmHg, premature contractions (DL < 4.5 s) in >20% of swallows.

20.1.1.5 Role of Endoscopy

- *EGD* (esophagogastroduodenoscopy) allows the assessment of the gastroesophageal junction and may rule out pseudoachalasia/mechanical obstruction.
  - Normal esophagus in initial stages; functional stenosis of LES—may have a pinpoint appearance and no relaxation with air insufflation, normal passage of the endoscope through it (strong resistance in pseudoachalasia).
  - In advanced disease—dilated esophagus with retained undigested food, liquid and saliva; inflammatory changes or ulcerations secondary to stasis, pill esophagitis, or Candida overgrowth.

- *EUS* (endoscopic ultrasound) excludes pseudoachalasia (in particular malignancy).
  - Thickened circular muscle layer (4) of the LES can be observed.
- Therapeutic role of EGD:
  - Pneumatic dilation (PD).
  - Per oral endoscopic myotomy (POEM).
  - Botulinum toxin injection (BTI).

20.1.1.6 Differential Diagnosis

- High suspicion of pseudoachalasia >>>.
  Endoscopic biopsies and CT/EUS
  - Pseudoachalasia caused by neoplasia—gastroesophageal junction adenocarcinoma, esophageal squamous-cell carcinoma, lymphoma, lung, pancreatic, hepatocellular, colonic, breast, and prostatic cancers (tumor infiltration/paraneoplastic syndrome).
  - Pseudoachalasia caused by benign disease—amyloidosis, sarcoidosis.
  - DES.
  - Chagas disease.

20.1.1.7 Treatment
There Is No Cure Treatment
- Aim: relieves patient's symptoms, and improves esophageal emptying.

Pharmacological Treatment
- Method with the lowest efficiency.
  Recommended for patients with no possibility of PD, myotomy, or BTI.
  - Nitrates (isosorbide dinitrate).
  - Calcium channel blockers (nifedipine).
  - Phosphodiesterase-5-inhibitors (sildenafil).

Endoscopic Treatment

- *Pneumatic dilation.*
  - With polyethylene balloons (30–35–40 mm).
  - With sedation; fluoroscopic/endoscopic guidance.
  - Most effective nonsurgical option.
  - Complications: perforation (Fig. 20.1) or hemorrhage.
- *POEM* (peroral endoscopic miotomy).
  - More than 6 cm above and 2 cm under cardia.
  - Longitudinal endoscopic dissection in the submucosal space, followed by cross-sectioning of the fibers and closure of the created tunnel.
- *Botulin toxin injection* at LES.
  - When endoscopic and laparoscopic methods are not possible.

Surgical Therapy

- *Heller laparoscopic myotomy with partial antireflux fundoplication antireflux.*
  - Anterior—Dor or posterior—Toupet.
  - Recommended as the first treatment option, like pneumatic dilation—similar results.
- *Esophagectomy* with gastric or colonic segment interposition, for advanced stages of achalasia [3–5].

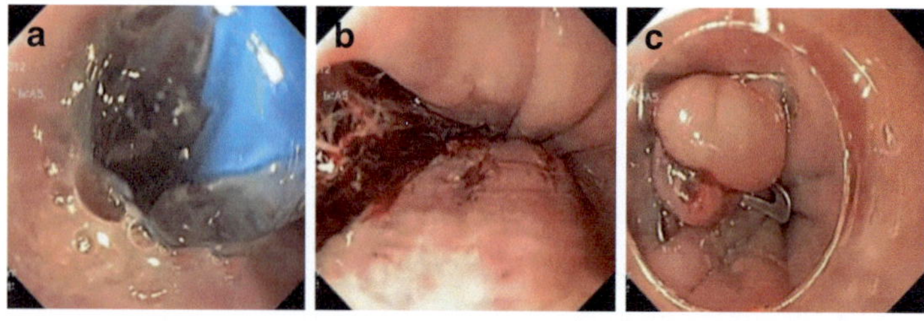

Fig. 20.1 Pneumatic dilation of LES with 30 mm balloon (**a**), under radiologic and endoscopic guidance followed by a 10 mm esophageal perforation (**b**). The OTSC (Osvesco) was applied (**c**)

20.1.2 Diffuse Esophageal Spasm (DES)

20.1.2.1 Definition
- Spastic motor disorder of the esophagus smooth muscle, manifested with retrosternal pain and dysphagia.
- It is characterized by uncoordinated, simultaneous contractions, with normal amplitude.

20.1.2.2 Epidemiology
- SED usually appears:
  - At 40 years old.
  - Incidence under 1/100,000 per year.
  - Women > men.
- Known risk factors:
  - Diseases like anxiety and depression.
  - Incidence increases with age.

20.1.2.3 Etiology and Pathogenesis
- Imbalance between the excitatory and inhibitory regulation of the esophageal smooth muscle in favor of excitation.
- Lower visceral pain threshold.

20.1.2.4 Diagnosis
- Clinical signs.
  - Dysphagia for solid and liquid food is usually intermittent, not progressive, suddenly installed, and sometimes related to swallowing extreme hot or cold liquids, stressful situations, or loud noises.
  - Chest pain, very similar to angina.
  - Regurgitation, heartburn—rare.
- Physical exam.
  - Normal.
- Laboratory studies.
  - No additional information.

- Barium swallow radiography.
  - Simultaneous, non-propulsive contractions or tertiary contractions in inferior two-third of the esophagus "corkscrew sign"; pseudo-diverticula.
- Esophageal manometry.
  - Classical manometry: aperistaltic contractions, simultaneous, repetitive, with multispike waves with increased duration and amplitude;
  - HRM (high-resolution manometry) is the accurate diagnostic modality—at least 20% of test swallows must have a short distal latency (<4.5 s).

20.1.2.5 Role of Endoscopy
- EGD—an important role in the differential diagnosis.
  - The appearance of layered esophageal rings (Fig. 20.2).

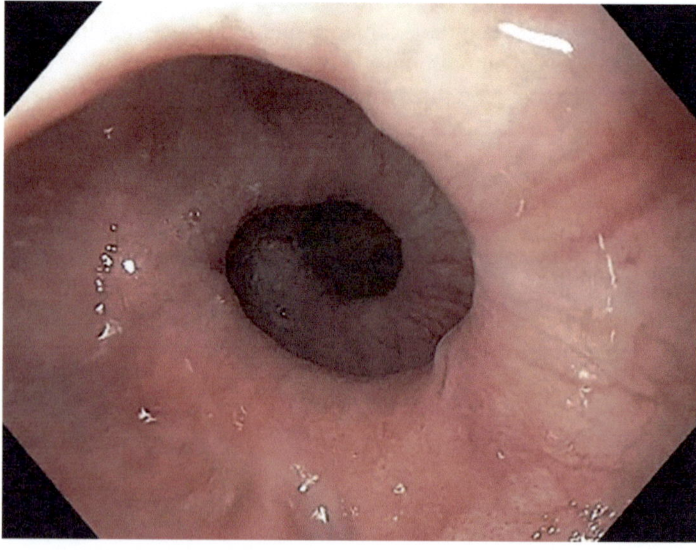

Fig. 20.2 Endoscopic image showing the presence of multiple narrowing in the lower esophagus, arranged in a spiral pattern, in a patient diagnosed with SED

20.1.2.6 Differential Diagnosis
- Achalasia (vigorous form).
- Esophageal cancer.
- Esophageal diverticula.
- Esophagitis/esophageal ulcer.
- Angina pectoris.
- Chagas disease.
- GERD.
- Hypertensive LES.

20.1.2.7 Treatment
- Aim: relieve patients symptoms.

Pharmacological Treatment
- Myorelaxants.
- Nitrates, calcium channel blockers, hydralazine, antidepressants, and anxiolytics.

Laparoscopic Treatment
- Heller myotomy + antireflux technique.
- Esophagectomy in severe cases.
  - If the pain becomes unbearable and cannot be improved medicinally with weight loss [3, 6, 7].

References

1. Schlottmann F, Herbella FA, Patti MG. Understanding the Chicago classification: from tracings to patients. J Neurogastroenterol Motil. 2017;23:487–94.
2. Rohof WOA, Bredenoord AJ. Chicago classification of esophageal motility disorders: lessons learned. Curr Gastroenterol Rep. 2017;19:37.
3. Roman S, Kahrilas PJ. Management of spastic disorders of the esophagus. Gastroenterol Clin N Am. 2013;42:27–43.
4. Zaninotto G, Bennett C, Boeckxstaens G, Constantini M, Ferguson MK, Pandolfino JE, et al. The 2018 ISDE achalasia guidelines. Dis Esophagus. 2018;31:doy071.
5. Vaezi MF, Pandolfino JE, Vela MF. ACG clinical guideline: diagnosis and management of achalasia. Am J Gastroenterol. 2013;108:1238–49.

 6. ASGE Standards of Practice Committee, Fukami N, Anderson MA, Khan K, Harrison ME, Appalaneni V, Ben-Menachem T, et al. The role of endoscopy in gastroduodenal obstruction and gastroparesis. Gastrointest Endosc. 2011;74:13–21.
 7. ASGE Standards of Practice Committee, Pasha SF, Acosta RD, Saltzman JR, Shergill AK, Cash B. The role of endoscopy in the evaluation and management of dysphagia. Gastrointest Endosc. 2014;79:191–201.

Gastroesophageal Reflux Disease and Esophagitis

Petrică Popa

21.1 Gastroesophageal Reflux Disease

21.1.1 Definition

- Gastroesophageal reflux disease (GERD) involves:
  - Symptomatology determined by the reflux of gastric contents into the esophagus.
  - The presence or absence of erosions.
- GERD is pathological when:
  - Episodes last more than 5 min.
  - More than 50 episodes/24 h.
  - Heartburn occurs more often than once a week.
  - Symptoms are present for at least 3 months.

21.1.2 Epidemiology

- GERD has a global reach.
- Increased frequency in developed countries.
- Varies between regions.

P. Popa (✉)
Gastroenterology Department, University of Medicine and Pharmacy Craiova, Craiova, Romania
e-mail: petrica.popa@umfcv.ro

© The Author(s), under exclusive license to Springer Nature Switzerland AG 2023
A. Săftoiu (ed.), *Pocket Guide to Advanced Endoscopy in Gastroenterology*, https://doi.org/10.1007/978-3-031-42076-4_21

- Risk factors:
  - Increased body mass index.
  - Increased fat intake.
  - Carbonated drinks.
  - Pregnancy.
  - Drugs (NSAIDs, anticholinergics, calcium blockers).
  - Smoking.
  - Alchol/coffee consumtion.

21.1.3 Etiology and Pathogenesis

- The direct cause is reflux of gastric contents into the esophagus.
- Predisposing causes can be:
  - Hiatal hernia.
  - Large abdominal tumors.
  - Voluminous ascites.
  - Surgical intervention (vagotomy, gastrectomy).
  - Scleroderma.
- GERD has a multifactorial pathogenesis:
  - Incompetent antireflux barriers.
  - Delayed gastric emptying.
  - Alteration of esophageal clearance [1].

21.1.4 Symptoms

- Typical symptoms.
  - Heartburn and regurgitation.
  - Non-cardiac chest pain.
- Atypical symptoms.
  - Retrosternal/epigastric pain.
  - Cough/dyspnea.
  - Early satiety.
  - Nausea and vomiting.
  - Belching.

- Alarm symptoms.
  - Weight loss.
  - Dysphagia and odynophagia.
  - Anemia.
  - Dysphonia.
  - Digestive bleeding.

21.1.5 Diagnostic

- Anamnesis.
  - Heartburn and/or regurgitation occuring two or more times a week are sugestive.
  - The initial assessment must include.
    The presence, severity, and frequency of heartburn and regurgitation.
    Alarm symptoms.
    Atypical symptoms.
    Assessment of risk factors.
    Evaluation of ameliorating factors.
- Clinical exam.
  - Anemia.
  - Weight loss.
  - Wheezing.
  - Minimal abdominal pain.
- Therapeutic test.
  - PPI, usually for 8 weeks is necessary to evaluate the response to the treatment [2].

21.1.6 Tests and Explorations

- **GIE:** high specificity for esophageal erosions.
  - It is not recommended in the presence of typical symptoms that yield to treatment.
  - Recommended for alarm symptoms [3].

- Los Angeles classification, the most used:

  Grade A: one/several erosions <5 mm.

  Grade B: at least one erosion >5 mm.

  Grade C: at least one extensive erosion between 3 and 4 mucosal folds, noncircumferential.

  Grade D: circumferential erosion [4].

- Endoscopically, sliding hiatal hernias (Figs. 21.1 and 21.2) or paraesophageal hernias can also be visualized.

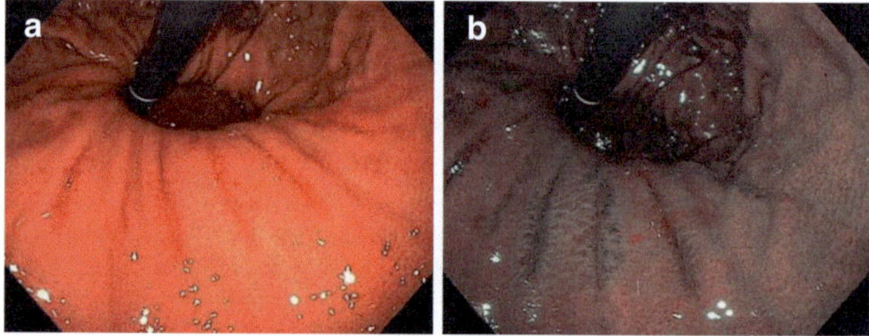

Fig. 21.1 Sliding hiatal hernia approximately 4 cm viewed in retroversion in white light mode (**a**) and narrow band imaging (**b**) mode, with longitudinal erosions in the subcardial region

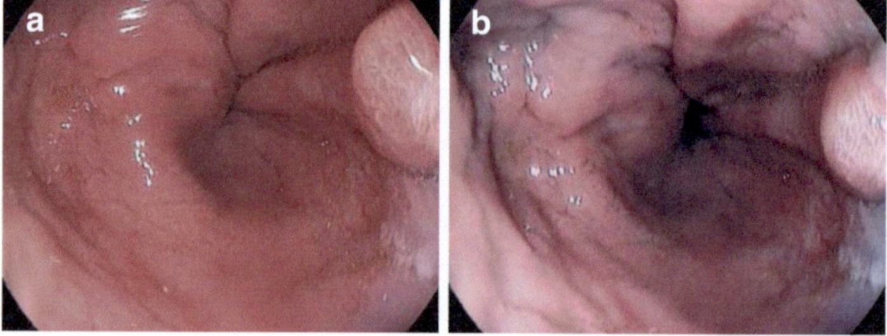

Fig. 21.2 Sliding hiatal hernia of approximately 3 cm visualized in direct view in white light mode (**a**) and I-scan "optical enhancement" mode (I-scan OE) (**b**), with a small "sentinel" polyp of approx 5 mm

- Taking biopsies by endoscopy.

    Esophageal biopsies confirm the presence of inflammation and exclude Barrett's esophagus.

    Gastric biopsies should be taken to diagnose *H. pylori* infection, atrophy, intestinal metaplasia, or dysplasia.

- Esophageal manometry is recommended:
  - For patients with persistent symptoms after appropriate treatment and normal endoscopy.
  - To rule out achalasia.
- **pH-metry** associated with intraluminal impedance.
  - Allows the evaluation of patients refractory to PPIs treatment.
  - The only test that can evaluate the association of reflux symptoms.
- Barium esophagram.
  - Used to evaluate a hiatal hernia or achalasia.
- *Helicobacter pylori* respiratory and fecal antigen test.
  - Recommended as noninvasive tests for the detection of active infection.

21.1.7 Differential Diagnosis

- Peptic ulcer.
- Achalasia.
- Gastric or duodenal ulcer.
- Ischemic cardiomyopathy.
- Functional hearburn.
- Angina pectoris.
- Diffuse esophageal spasm.
- Esophageal diverticulum.
- Eosinophilic esophagitis.

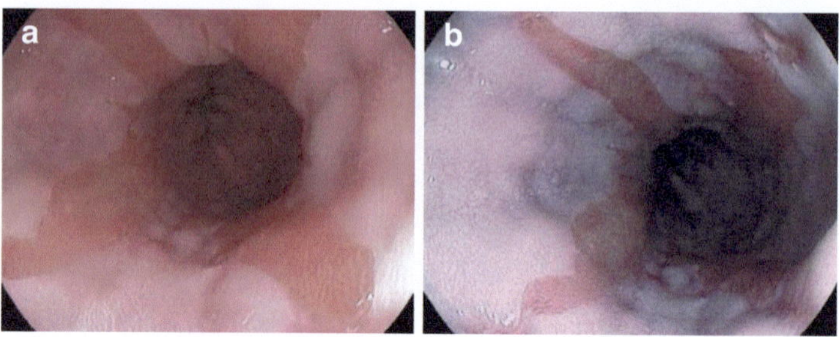

Fig. 21.3 Barrett's esophagus C30M33 (according to the Prague classification) viewed in white light (**a**) and I-scan (**b**) mode, with grade A esophagitis lesions superimposed

21.1.8 Complications

- Reflux esophagitis.
- Esophageal ulcer.
- Benign esophageal stenosis.
- Barrett's esophagus (Fig. 21.3a, b).
- Esophageal adenocarcinoma.

21.1.9 Treatment

21.1.9.1 General Measures

- Weight reduction in overweight/obese.
- Lifestyle:
  - Small lunches.
  - Avoiding late meals.
  - Avoiding precipitating factors:
    Alcohol and fats.
    Coffee and chocolate.
    Spices and citrus fruits.
- No smoking.

- Avoiding drugs that decrease lower esophageal sphincter pressure:
  - Nitrites.
  - Anticholinergics.
  - Progesterone.

21.1.9.2 Pharmaceutical Treatment

- Antacids.
  - Short-term therapy.
  - Simple antacids neutralize gastric acid.
  - Agents containing alginates: these include alginic acid with small doses of antacids.
- Histamin H2 blockers.
  - Short/medium term therapy.
  - Longer acting than antacids.
  - They cause tachyphylaxis.
    - Cimetidine.
    - Ranitidine.
    - Famotidine.
    - Nizatidine.
- Proton pump inhibitors (PPIs).
  - The most powerful inhibitors of gastric acid secretion.
  - Superior efficacy to H2 blockers,
  - Esophagitis cure rate of 90%.
  - They can be used in extraesophageal manifestations or in peptic esophageal stenosis.
  - Excellent clinical tolerance.
    - Omeprazole.
    - Rabeprazole.
    - Lansoprazole.
    - Pantoprazole.
    - Esomeprazole.

21.1.9.3 Therapeutic Strategy

- Lifestyle modification for mild symptoms.
- For average symptoms, with grade A/B esophagitis, standard dose H2 blockers or PPIs can be used.

- For severe symptoms and C/D esophagitis, PPIs are recommended in standard dose or double dose, 8 weeks.
  - Stepwise treatment includes two strategies:
      "**step-down**" in which PPIs are used in standard dose for 6–8 weeks, with subsequent dose reduction.
      "**step-up**" in which antacids or histamine H2 blockers are used, followed by PPIs if symptoms persist.
  - Step-down therapy is currently the most accepted one.

21.1.9.4 Surgical Treatment

- It is indicated for building an antireflux barrier.
- Complications are the major indication.
  - Stenosis.
  - Barrett's esophagus.
- Can also be used for:
  - Severe extradigestive manifestations.
  - Voluminous hiatal hernia.
  - Young people with severe symptoms.
- Laparoscopic technique is the gold standard.
  - Efficacy is high for symptoms.
  - Increases the quality of life.
- The disadvantage of surgery is the complications.
  - Postoperative dysphagia.
  - Denervation syndrome.

21.1.10 Evolution and Prognosis

- The evolution is favorable.
  - Symptoms may recur often, requiring long-term maintenance treatment.
- The prognosis remains good.
  - Mortality is low [5–8].

21.2 Esophagitis

21.2.1 Clasification

21.2.1.1 Reflux Esophagitis
- See Sect. 21.1.6 (Fig. 21.4a, b).

21.2.1.2 Drug-Induced Esophagitis
- NSAIDs.
- Antibiotics (doxycycline—Fig. 21.5a, b).
- Potassium chloride.
- Bisphosphonates.

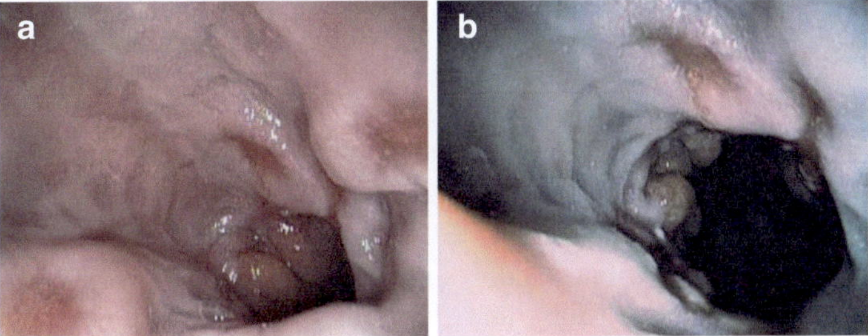

Fig. 21.4 Grade A (Los Angeles) reflux esophagitis viewed in white light (**a**) and I-scan mode (**b**)

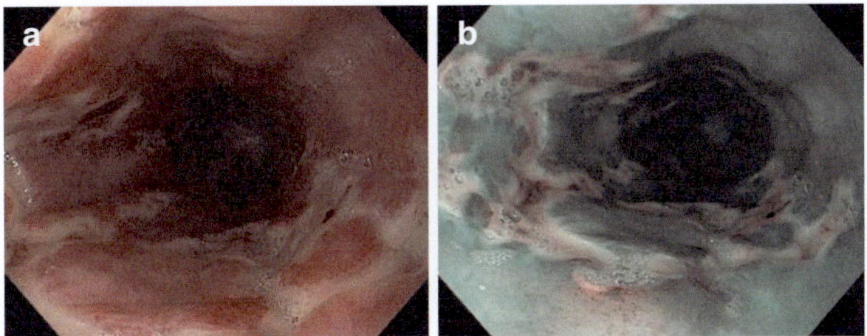

Fig. 21.5 Drug-induced esophagitis (doxycycline) viewed in white light mode (**a**) and NBI mode (**b**), with confluent ulcerations in one-third of the esophagus, associated with edema and hyperemia

21.2.1.3 Infectious Esophagitis

Infectious esophagitis especially in immunosuppressed patients (HIV/AIDS, cancer, etc.)

- Bacteria.
- Viral.
  - HSV: superficial ulcerations.
  - CMV: giant ulcers especially in HIV.
  - EBV.
- Mycotic (*Candida albicans*) (Fig. 21.6a, b).

21.2.1.4 Eosinophilic Esophagitis

- Inflammatory condition triggered by food antigens trough a TH2 immune-mediated mechanism.
- Patients have air allergen sensitivity and other atopic diseases: asthma, allergic rhinitis, eczema.
- The clinical presentation depends on the age of onset.
  - Children: vomiting, dysphagia.
  - Young people: dysphagia for solids, retrosternal pain, vomiting and regurgitation.
  - Adults: heartburn and dysphagia.
- **GIE**: circular rings and longitudinal bands ("furrows") (Fig. 21.7), papules and white deposits, strictures, and friability generated by the insertion of the scope.

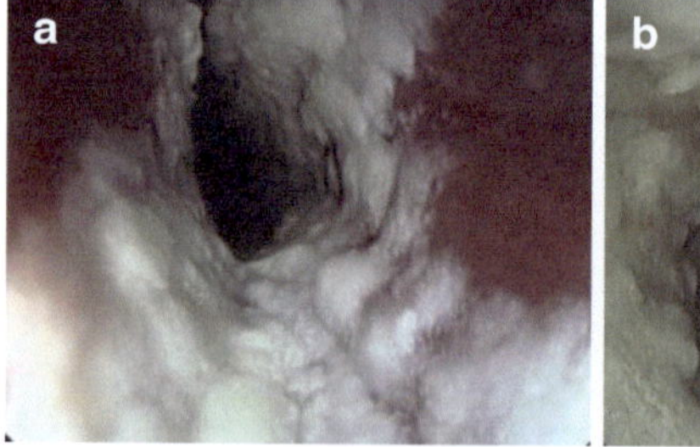
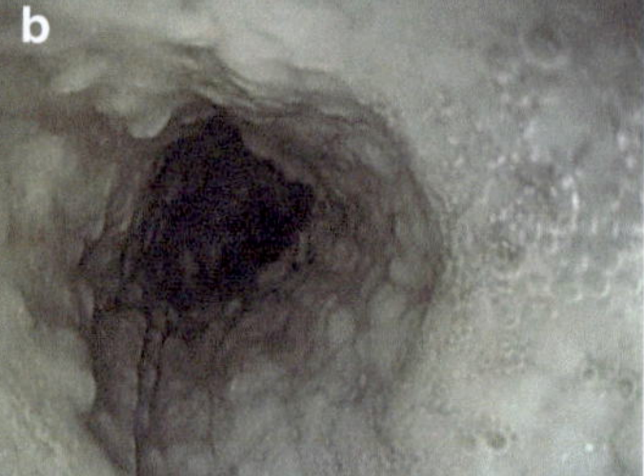

Fig. 21.6 Severe candidal esophagitis

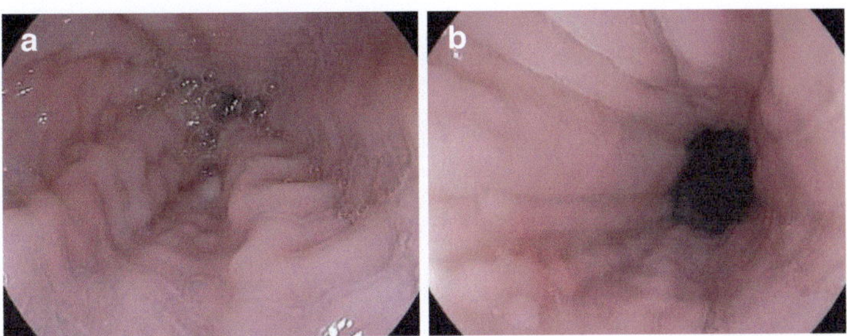

Fig. 21.7 Eosinophilic esophagitis with circular rings and longitudinal bands, with characteristic histological appearance

- For symptomatic patients the treatment includes:
  - PPI in high dose (20–40 mg × 2/day) 8 weeks > histologica remission >50%.
  - Topical corticosteroids (budesonide) 1 mg daily for 8 weeks > histological remission >90%.
  - The use of empiric elimination diets or based on antigen tests is useful.
  - In the presence of dilations/strictures, endoscopic dilations are required.
  - Experimental anti-IL, montelukast, immunomodulator or anti-TNF treatments have been used in clinical trials [9].

21.2.1.5 Esophagitis Dissecans Superficialis
- Has unknown pathogenesis.
- **GIE**: desquamation of the squamous epithelium (Fig. 21.8a, b).

21.2.1.6 Acute Necrotizing Esophagitis
- Also called "Black esophagus".
- Combination of ischemic damage, corrosive effect of gastric acid, and decreased mucoasal barrier function in malnourished or immunosuppressed patients.
  - Multiorgan dysfunction/hypoperfusion hypothermia/vasculopathy/sepsis.
  - Diabetic ketoacidosis/renal failure.
  - Intoxication/acute alcoholic hepatitis.

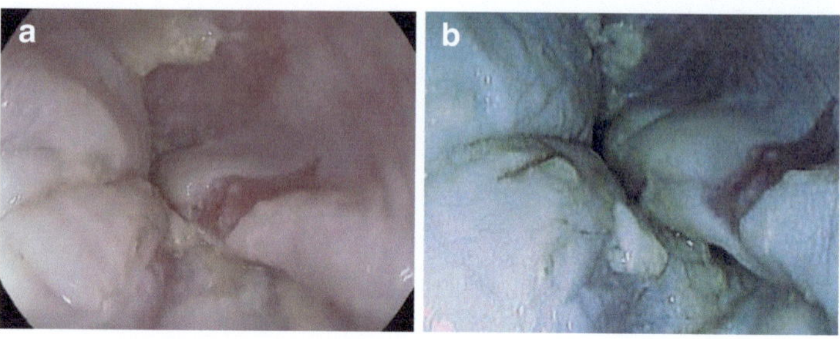

Fig. 21.8 Esophagitis dissecans superficialis viewed in white light mode (**a**) and I-scan mode (**b**)

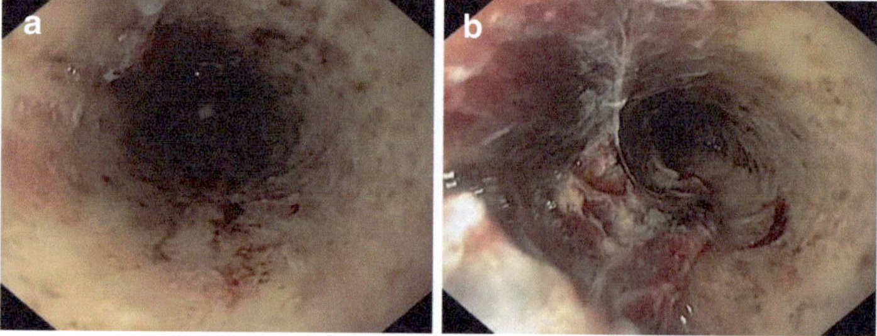

Fig. 21.9 Acute necrotizing esophagitis, with a white: black appearance of the esophagus, with a necrotic appearance

- – Nasogastric tube/gastric volvulus.
  – Pulmonary thromboembolism/aortic dissection.
  – Advanced cancer/severe infection (HSV, CMV, etc.)
- Clinical presentation.
  – Upper digestive bleeding.
  – Nausea/vomiting/epigastric pain.
  – Dysphagia.
- **GIE**: circumferential white / black discoloration (Fig. 21.9a, b).
  – Clearly defined at the level of the esogastric junction.

- Complications.
  - Perforation/mediastinitis/abscesses.
  - Esophageal strictures.
  - Death, especially in the presence of comorbidities.
- Treatment.
  - Supportive + high dose of PPI [10].

References

1. El-Serag H. The association between obesity and GERD: a review of the epidemiological evidence. Dig Dis Sci. 2008;53:2307–12.
2. Moayyedi P, Talley NJ. Gastro-oesophageal reflux disease. Lancet. 2006;367:2086–100.
3. Chen SL, Gwee KA, Lee JS, Miwa H, Suzuki H, Guo P, et al. Systematic review with metaanalysis: prompt endoscopy as the initial management strategy for uninvestigated dyspepsia in Asia. Aliment Pharmacol Ther. 2015;41:239–52.
4. Lundell LR, Dent J, Bennett JR, Blum AL, Armstrong D, Galmiche JP, et al. Endoscopic assessment of oesophagitis: clinical and functional correlates and further validation of the Los Angeles classification. Gut. 1999;45:172–80.
5. Person E, Rife C, Freeman J, Clark A, Castell DO. A novel sleep positioning device reduces gastroesophageal reflux: a randomized controlled trial. J Clin Gastroenterol. 2015;49:655–9.
6. Weijenborg PW, Cremonini F, Smout AJPM, Bredenoord AJ. PPI therapy is equally effective in well-defined non-erosive reflux disease and in reflux esophagitis: a meta-analysis. Neurogastroenterol Motil. 2012;24:747–57.
7. Katz PO, Gerson LB, Vela MF. Guidelines for the diagnosis and management of gastroesophageal reflux disease. Am J Gastroenterol. 2013;108:308–28.
8. Sandhu DS, Fass R. Current trends in the management of gastroesophageal reflux disease. Gut Liver. 2018;12:7–16.
9. Hirano I, Chan ES, Rank MA, Sharaf RN, Stollman NH, Stukus DR, et al. AGA Institute and the joint task force on allergy-immunology practice parameters clinical guidelines for the Management of Eosinophilic Esophagitis. Gastroenterology. 2020;158:1776–86.
10. Săftoiu A, Cazacu S, Kruse A, Georgescu C, Comănescu V, Ciurea T. Acute esophageal necrosis associated with alcoholic hepatitis: is it black or is it white? Endoscopy. 2005;37:268–71.

Gastritis and Gastropathies 22

Ana-Maria Barbu and Sevastița Iordache

22.1 Definition and Classification

- Microscopic inflammation of the stomach.
- Gastropathies—predominant epithelial and vascular lesions of the gastric mucosa with very low inflammatory infiltrate.

22.2 Upper GI Endoscopy

- Indicated in symptomatic patients (dyspepsia).
- Five biopsies are recommended (two antrum, two body, and one gastric angle), even macroscopic lesions are absent [1].
- *H. pylori* testing (usually rapid urease test).

A.-M. Barbu
University of Medicine and Pharmacy Craiova, Craiova, Romania

S. Iordache (✉)
Department of Gastroenterology, University of Medicine and Pharmacy Craiova, Craiova, Romania

© The Author(s), under exclusive license to Springer Nature Switzerland AG 2023
A. Săftoiu (ed.), *Pocket Guide to Advanced Endoscopy in Gastroenterology*, https://doi.org/10.1007/978-3-031-42076-4_22

22.3   Gastritis Classification

- Acute gastritis.
  - Erosive or hemorrhagic.
  - Nonerosive.
  - Others.
- Chronic gastritis.
  - Infectious.
  - Noninfectious.

22.4   Acute Gastritis

22.4.1 Erosive and Hemorrhage Gastritis

- Causes.
  - NSAIDs intake.
  - Iron-based drugs.
  - Cortico- and chemotherapy.
  - Antibiotics (tetracycline, doxycycline).
  - Strong alcohol intake.
  - Caustic substances.
  - Extensive surgical interventions.
  - Radiotherapy.
  - Respiratory, renal, or hepatic insufficiency.
  - Duodenum-gastric reflux [2–4].
  The most common cause is NSAID intake. Factors associated with a high risk of toxicity for NSAIDs: age, smoking, alcohol, and chronic H. pylori infection. Two main mechanisms:
  - Local mechanism: superficial lesions (detergent effect); weak acids are not ionized and freely penetrate the gastric barrier; direct toxic effect; exhaustion ATP.
  - The systemic mechanism: the reduction of mucosal protective vasodilatory prostaglandin production.
- Diagnosis of erosive/hemorrhage gastritis.
  - Clinical: epigastric pain, nausea, vomiting, or upper GI bleeding.

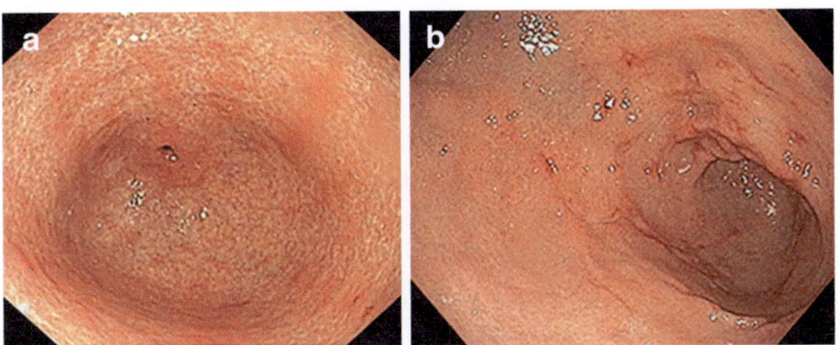

Fig. 22.1 Erosive-hemorrhage gastritis—alcohol-induced (**a**) or NSAIDs (**b**), with multiple erosions in antrum-pyloric area

> - Anamnesis: can identify the etiological agent, frequently NSAIDs, alcohol, and surgical stress.
> - **Endoscopic**: edematous mucosa, petechiae, hemorrhages, and erosions (Fig. 22.1a, b).
- Treatment.
  - Treatment of underlying disease, PPIs, and plasma argon coagulation if necessary [2–4].

22.4.2 Nonerosive Gastritis

H. pylori-induced acute gastritis is rare. Usually, symptoms are absent leading to unobserved infections. Thus, the disease has a progression to chronic gastritis, gastric atrophy, intestinal meta-plasia, and dysplasia (premalignant lesions).

- Diagnosis of *H. pylori-associated* gastritis [5, 6].
  - Clinical: when present there is nausea, vomiting, epigastric pain.
  - **Endoscopic**: antral congestion.
  - Histology: inflammatory infiltrate with PMNs in the sub-mucosa and finding the bacteria.
- Treatment.
  - Eradication of HP [6, 7].

22.4.3 Phlegmonous and Emphysematous Gastritis (Fig. 22.2)

- Diagnosis.
  - Manifested as the acute abdomen or upper GI bleeding.
  - Appears in immunosuppressed patients.
  - Bacterial etiology: *E. coli*, Proteus, *Staphylococcus* and *Streptococcus* species, and *Clostridium perfringens*.
  - Thickening of the gastric wall.
- Treatment.
  - Wide specter antibiotics [2–4].

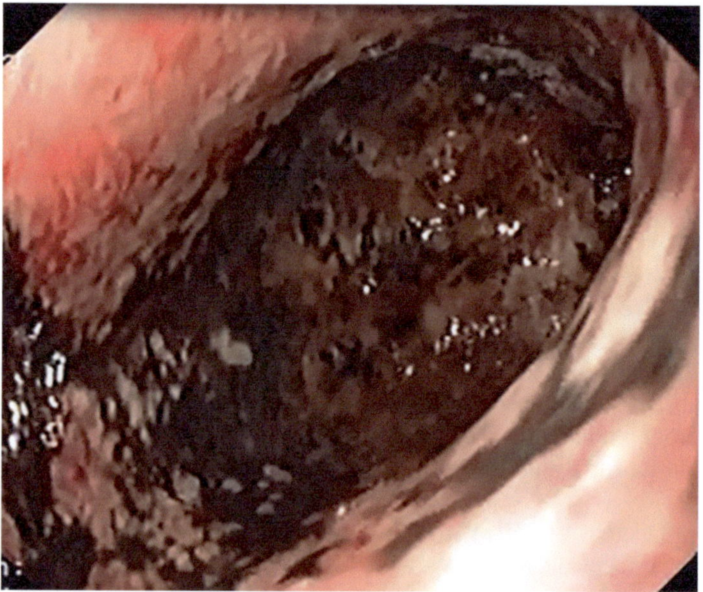

Fig. 22.2 Phlegmonous gastritis: areas of edema, blackish in color corresponding to areas of extensive mucosal necrosis in the stomach

22.4.4 Eosinophilic Gastritis

- Diagnosis.
  - Gastric component of eosinophilic gastroenteritis.
  - Serum immunoglobulin E (Ig E) is elevated, and peripheral eosinophilia is present.
  - Epigastric pain, nausea, and vomiting after the allergen ingestion.
  - Endoscopic findings are nonspecific: friability, erythema, and enlarged gastric folds.
  - Histologically must have >20 eosinophil/high power field.
- Treatment.
  - Oral corticosteroids [2–4]

22.5 Chronic Gastritis

The most frequent causes of chronic gastritis are *H. pylori* chronic infection, NSAIDs, biliary reflux, autoimmunity, and allergens.

22.5.1 Chronic Infectious Gastritis

- *H. pylori* is the most common and most important cause of chronic gastritis [5].
  - A gram-negative bacterium with tropism for gastric mucosa.
  - Fecal-oral, oral-oral, or hydric transmission.
  - HP enzymatic equipment damages the local gastric defense mechanisms and causes inflammation leading to gastritis and then premalignant conditions: gastric atrophy, intestinal metaplasia, and/or dysplasia.
  - Persistent antigenic stimulation can lead to MALT lymphoma.

- Two types of *H. pylori-associated* gastritis:

  Chronic antral gastritis (Fig. 22.3a, b), usually is asymptomatic. Histologically, a diffuse, chronic inflammatory infiltrate.

  Multifocal atrophic gastritis: atrophy and intestinal metaplasia in both antrum and body stomach; endoscopically atrophy appears like a pale mucosa with prominent submucosal vessels (Fig. 22.4a, b).

- Chromoendoscopy is useful to spot lesions and target biopsies [8].
- Histology from five biopsies is the gold standard for diagnosis.
- Of its potential to progress into cancer, the OLGA /OLGIM (operative link on gastritis/intestinal metaplasia) has made a staging system to assess the risk of gastric cancer and follow-up (Table 22.1):

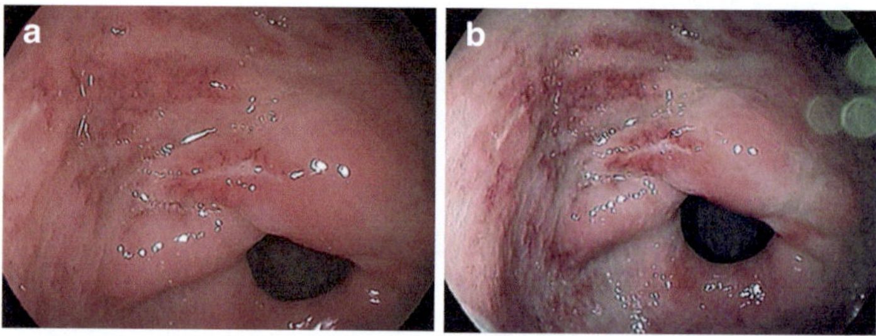

Fig. 22.3 Multiple erosions and antral hyperemia in a patient with chronic *Helicobacter pylori-positive* gastritis, in white light mode (**a**) and I-scan (**b**)

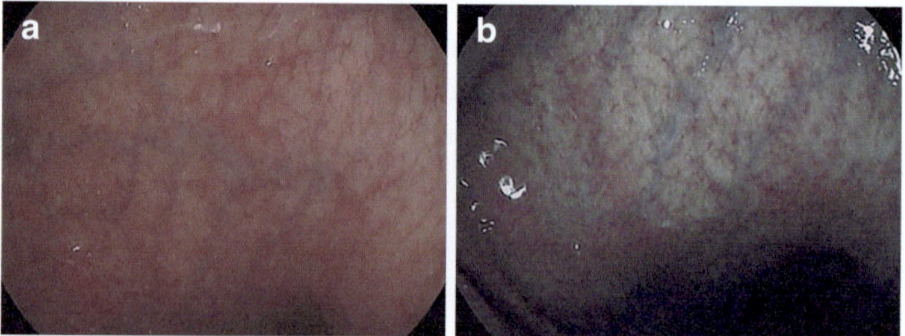

Fig. 22.4 Accentuated vascular pattern of the fornix, visualized in white light (**a**), respectively I-scan 2 (**b**)

Table 22.1 OLGA score for atrophic gastritis [1]

Gastric body					
	Atrophy score	No atrophy	Mild atrophy	Moderate atrophy	Severe atrophy
Antrum	No atrophy	Stage 0	Stage I	Stage II	Stage II
	Mild atrophy	Stage I	Stage I	Stage II	Stage III
	Moderate atrophy	Stage II	Stage II	Stage III	Stage IV
	Severe atrophy	Stage III	Stage III	Stage IV	Stage IV

- The OLGA/OLGIM stages III/IV are proven to be at high risk for gastric cancer.
- Follow-up according to MAPS II 2019 [8, 9]:
  Severe atrophic changes or IM in both antrum and corpus need endoscopic surveillance every 3 years and every 1–2 years in patients associated family history of gastric cancer.
  Limited IM to a single location needs to be surveyed at 3 years only if it is associated with a family history of gastric cancer, incomplete type of IM, persistent H.P. gastritis, or autoimmune gastritis.
  No surveillance is necessary for mild to moderate atrophy restricted to the antrum.
  If dysplasia is found needs to be surveyed at 6 months for high-grade and at 1 year for low-grade dysplasia.
- Other rare infectious causes are TB mycobacteria, gastric syphilis, viral, fungal, and parasitic gastritis in immunosuppressed patients like CMV, Herpes virus, Candida, Aspergillus, etc [4].
  - Tuberculous gastritis: gastric outlet obstruction and ulcerations biopsies show necrotizing granulomas, with acid-fast bacilli (Fig. 22.5).

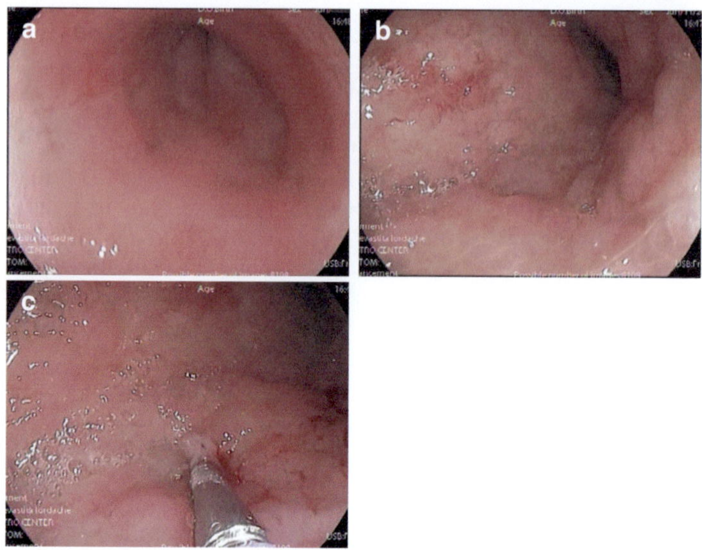

Fig. 22.5 Gastric tuberculosis: tubular aspect of the stomach (**a**), with ulcerations and nodular mucosa (**b**), biopsies from mucosa (**c**) in a patient with extensive TB (intestinal, peritoneum, and stomach)

22.5.2 Noninfectious Chronic Gastritis

- Most frequent is NSAIDs-related gastritis followed by biliary reflux gastritis and autoimmune gastritis but also portal-hypertension gastropathy is seen frequently in cirrhotic patients.
- **NSAIDs chronic gastritis** is considered an adapting way in chronic NSAIDs use:
  - Petechiae and hemorrhages are less often as compared to acute form and usually is asymptomatic.
- Duodenum-gastric bile reflux.
  - Common after partial gastrectomy or pyloroplasty for peptic ulcer or cholecystectomy.
  - **Endoscopy**: edema, redness, erosions, and yellow staining of the gastric mucosa.
  - Treatment: ursodeoxycholic acid.

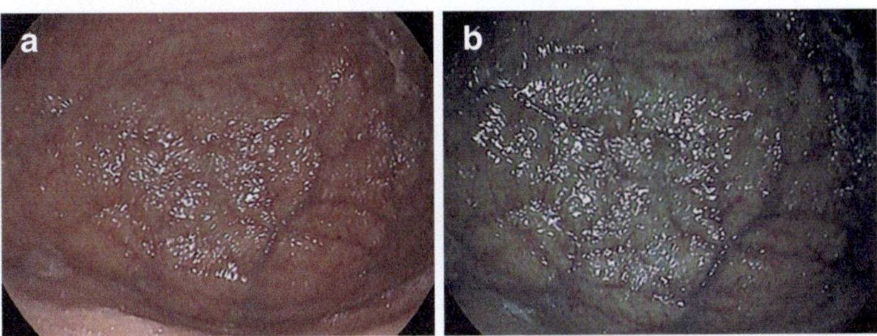

Fig. 22.6 Chronic atrophic gastritis: submucosal vascular pattern clearly visible at the level of the fornix in retroversion in white light mode (**a**) and I-scan 2 (**b**)

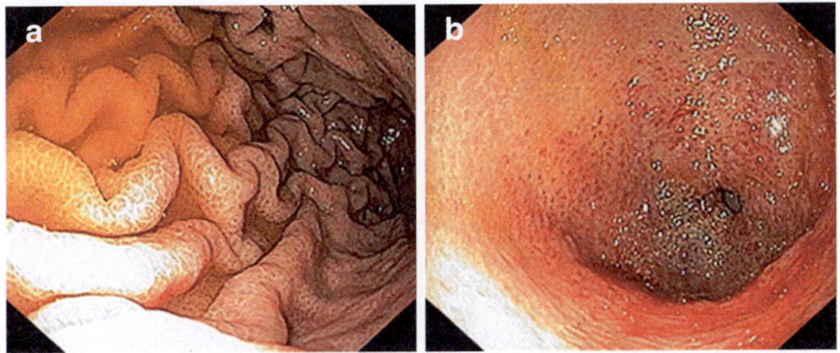

Fig. 22.7 Mild portal-hypertensive gastropathy with gastric mucosa with the appearance of "snake-skin" (**a**) and severe with congested gastric mucosa with multiple petechiae, which bleed slightly (**b**)

- **Autoimmune gastritis** is chronic atrophic gastritis limited to the body and fundus (Fig. 22.6a, b).
  - Associated with circulating anti-parietal cell and anti-intrinsic factor antibodies and B12 vitamin malabsorption.
  - Risk for developing gastric carcinoid tumor because of reactive hypergastrinemia.
  - Endoscopic follow-up every 3–5 years.

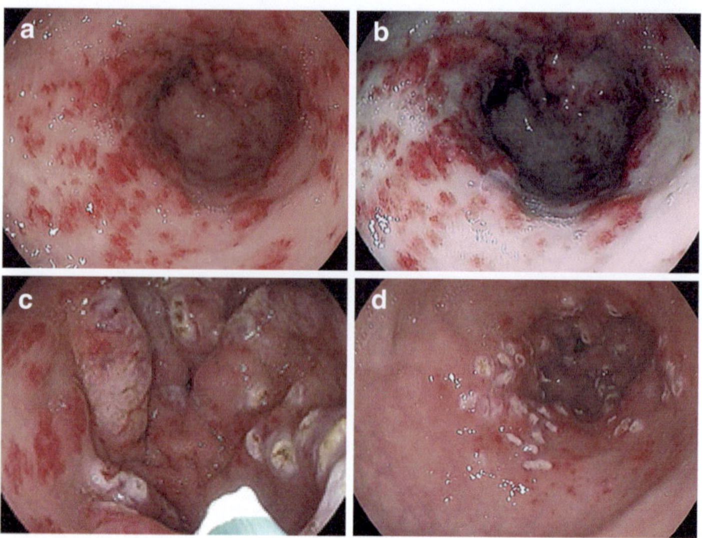

Fig. 22.8 GAVE—examination in WLE (**a**) and I-scan (**b**), plasma argon coagulation (**c**), post-coagulation aspect (**d**)

- Portal-hypertensive gastropathy (PHG).
  - Appears usually in cirrhotic patients (Fig. 22.7a, b).
  - Biopsies show vascular ectasia and congestion in the mucosal layer without a significant inflammatory infiltrate.
  - Treatment: decrease portal pressure.
- Other rare gastritis:
  - Granulomatous gastritis associated with Crohn's disease, sarcoidosis.
  - Lymphocytic and eosinophilic gastritis.
  - Postradiotherapy gastritis.
- GAVE syndrome (gastric antral vascular ectasia) or "watermelon stomach" could be observed (Fig. 22.8a, b) in cirrhotic patients and other conditions.
  - Treatment: plasma argon coagulation (APC) (APC) (Fig. 22.8c, d) or band ligation [2–4].

References

1. Rugge M, Meggio A, Pennelli G, et al. Gastritis staging in clinical practice: the OLGA staging system. Gut. 2007;56:631–6.
2. Yamada T. Textbook of gastroenterology, vol. 40. 5th ed. Hoboken, NJ: Blackwell; 2009. p. 936–73.
3. Varicka S, Wilhemi M. Essentials in gastroenterology and hepatology. 2nd ed. Breisgau: Falk Foundation; 2017. p. 70–87.
4. Feldman M, Friedman L, Brandt L. Sleisenger and Fordtran's, gastrointestinal and liver disease, vol. 1. 9th ed. Philadelphia: Saunders Elsevier; 2010. p. 845–59.
5. Sugano K, Tack J, Kuipers EJ, et al. Kyoto global consensus report on helicobacter pylori gastritis. Gut. 2015;64:1353–67.
6. Mescoli C, Lopez AG, Rojas LT, et al. Gastritis staging as a clinical priority. Eur J Gastroenterol Hepatol. 2018;30:125–9.
7. Malfertheiner P, Megraud F, O'Morain CA, et al. Management of Helicobacter pylori infection—the Maastricht V/Florence consensus report. Gut. 2017;66:6–30.
8. Pimentel-Nunes P, Libânio D, Marcos-Pinto R, et al. Management of epithelial precancerous conditions and lesions in the stomach (MAPS II): European Society of Gastrointestinal Endoscopy (ESGE), European helicobacter and microbiota study group (EHMSG), European Society of Pathology (ESP), and Sociedade Portuguesa de Endoscopia Digestiva (SPED) guideline update 2019. Endoscopy. 2019;51(4):365–88.
9. Dinis-Ribeiro M, Areia M, de Vries AC, et al. Management of precancerous conditions and lesions in the stomach (MAPS): guideline from the European Society of Gastrointestinal Endoscopy (ESGE), European helicobacter study group (EHSG), European Society of Pathology (ESP), and the Sociedade Portuguesa de Endoscopia Digestiva (SPED). Endoscopy. 2012;44:74–94.

Gastric and Duodenal Ulcers

23

Ana-Maria Barbu and Sevastița Iordache

23.1 Definition

- Is a limited loss of gastric or duodenal mucosa (>5 mm in diameter) extending through the muscularis mucosa.

23.2 Epidemiology

- Gastric and duodenal ulcers (GU, DU) usually appear in
    - 3rd–fourth decade for DU and sixth decade for GU
    - Men > women.
    - DU > GU.
    - Decreasing prevalence and incidence in developed countries in last decades due to eradication treatment for *H. pylori* and antisecretory treatment.
    - Increasing incidence for NSAIDs related GU.

A.-M. Barbu
University of Medicine and Pharmacy Craiova, Craiova, Romania

S. Iordache (✉)
Department of Gastroenterology, University of Medicine and Pharmacy Craiova, Craiova, Romania

A. Săftoiu (ed.), *Pocket Guide to Advanced Endoscopy in Gastroenterology*, https://doi.org/10.1007/978-3-031-42076-4_23

23.3   Etiology and Pathogenesis

- Two major causes:
  - *H. pylori* infection (Fig. 23.1a, b).
  - NSAIDs (Fig. 23.2a, b).
- Non-H.P. and non-NSAID causes (rare).
  - Stress ulcers.
  - Infectious.
  - Drugs/toxins (steroids, bisphosphonates, clopidogrel, mycophenolate mofetil, cocaine).
  - Chemotherapy and radiotherapy.
  - Hypersecretory states: Zollinger–Ellison syndrome), systemic mastocytosis, etc.
  - Intestinal obstruction.
  - Idiopathic.
- Risk factors: smoking, alimentation, alcoholism; genetics.
- The imbalance between the aggression factors and the defense of mucosa.
- *Helicobacter pylori*:
  - About 90% of DU and 60% of GU.
  - In the stomach – acute and chronic gastritis, ulcer; normo- or hypochlorhydria.
  - In the duodenum—duodenitis (Fig. 23.3a) and duodenal ulcer (Fig. 23.3b), hyperchlorhydria related.

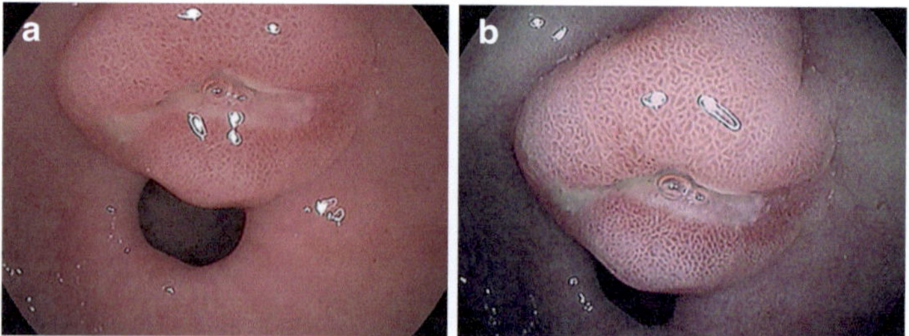

Fig. 23.1 Benign prepyloric ulcer, with central fibrin exudate and marked edema, visualized in white light (**a**) and I-scan mode (**b**). Antrum gastritis associated with rapid urease test *H. pylori* positive

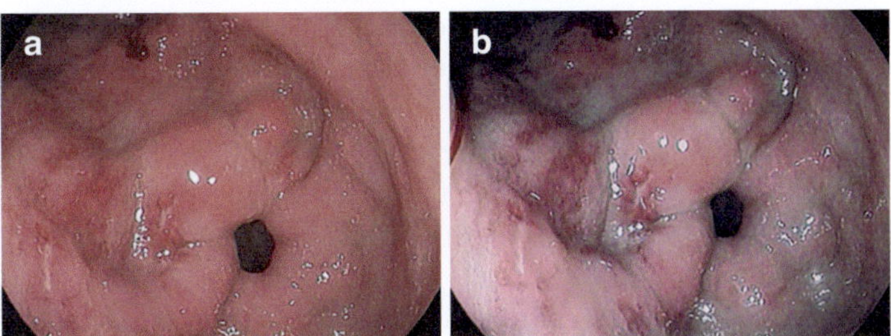

Fig. 23.2 Benign prepyloric ulcerations, with central fibrin exudate and surrounding hyperemia, visualized in white light (**a**) and I-scan mode (**b**). Antrum NSAID gastropathy with rapid urease test *H. pylori* negative

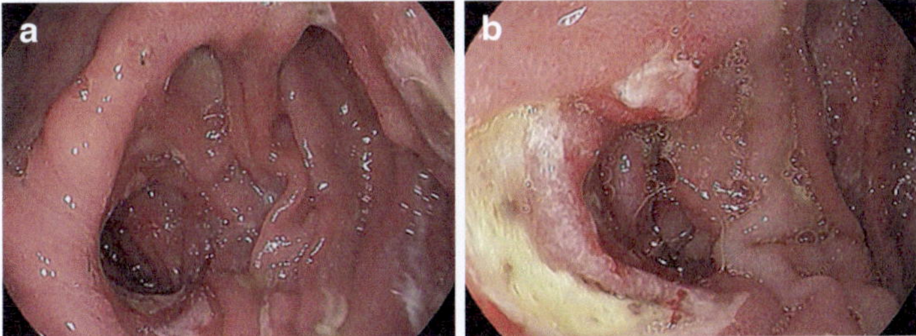

Fig. 23.3 Erosive-hemorrhagic duodenitis with multiple erosions in the duodenal bulb and duodenum 2 (**a**) and duodenal ulcer with central fibrin exudate, edema, and surrounding hyperemia (**b**)

23.4 Diagnosis

- Clinical presentation:
  - Burning epigastric pain usually postprandial present in both ulcers.
  - GU: the epigastric pain has a character of burning or epigastric fullness, and appears early postprandial.
  - DU: burning epigastric "hunger" pain, late postprandial or in the night.
  - Accompanying symptoms: nausea, vomiting, mild weight loss, bloating.

- Biochemical tests—usually normal.
  - Complete blood count, liver chemistries, serum creatinine, serum Ca, and *H. pylori* testing.
- Upper GI endoscopy.
  - The first intention in all symptomatic patients except the youngers without alarm signs (empiric antisecretory treatment at first).
  - In patients with alarm signs (hemorrhage or anemia, early satiety, significant weight loss, recurrent vomiting, HC antecedents of digestive cancer).
  - Mucosal denudation single or multiple.
  - Benign ulcers have smooth, regular, rounded edges with a flat, smooth ulcer base often filled with exudate (Fig. 23.4a, b).
  - Malignant ulcers have surrounding folds that are nodular, clubbed, fused, or stop short of the ulcer margin (Fig. 23.5a, b).

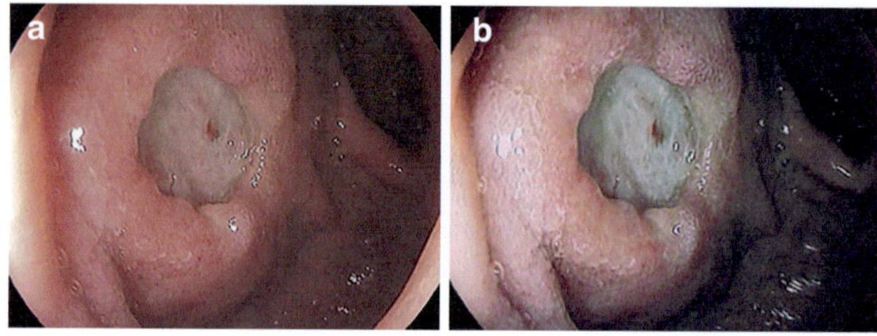

Fig. 23.4 Large duodenal ulcer in a patient with HDS and rapid *H. pylori* positive urease test, visualized in white light (**a**) and I-scan (**b**)

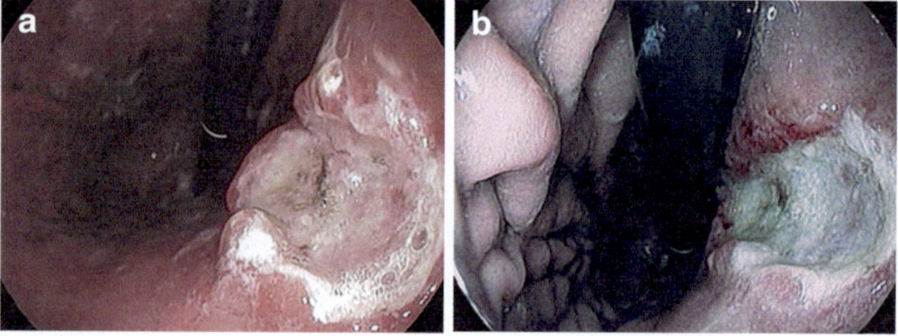

Fig. 23.5 Gastric ulcer of gastric angle with prominent, nodular, and irregular margins, visualized in retroflection, in white light mode (**a**) and I-scan (**b**)

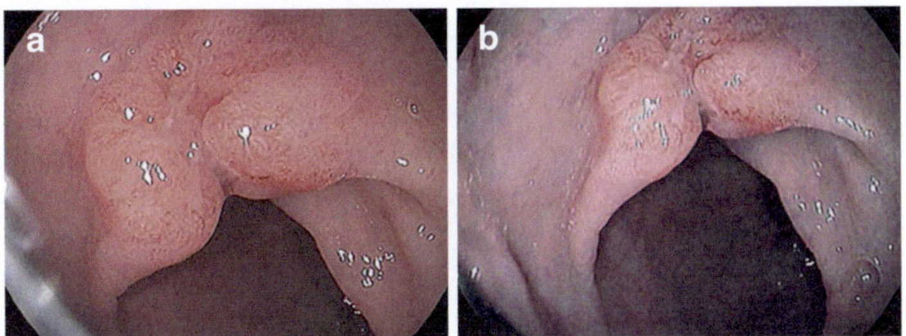

Fig. 23.6 Malignant prepyloric gastric ulcer (early ulcerated adenocarcinoma) with prominent, nodular, and irregular edges, visualized in white light (**a**) and I-scan (**b**)

- Biopsies and endoscopic surveillance in GU (Fig. 23.6a, b).
- DU found in distal duodenum should take into consideration Crohn's disease, ischemic origin, or Zollinger–Ellison syndrome.
- Allows endoscopic treatment for bleeding ulcers and biopsies.
- *H. pylori* testing.
  - In all patients with peptic symptoms or UGIB.
    Invasive: (a) rapid test for urease activity from biopsies or (b) histopathological evidence of bacterial growth.
    Noninvasive: (a) serological tests, rapid capillary, and salivary tests in patients undergoing PPIs and no previous HP treatment (b) dosing fecal antigen and urea breath test—diagnostic and surveillance [1].
- Barium radiological exam.
  - When endoscopy is contraindicated or refused.
  - Defect (crater) with benign or malignant characters.
- Functional exploring of acid secretion—in case of multiple ulcers, distal duodenum ulcers, recurrent and refractory ulcers, or associated with diarrhea, post-vagotomy.
- Others: gastrinemia dosing in Zollinger–Ellison suspicion, CT scan in acute abdominal tenderness.

23.5 Differential Diagnosis

- Gastric cancer: ± alarm symptoms; usually >40 years.
- Non-ulcerous dyspepsia; irritable bowel syndrome.
- Gallbladder and bile ducts diseases.
- Chronic pancreatitis.
- Zollinger–Ellison syndrome.
  - Single or multiple gastric or duodenal ulcers; usually distal duodenum ulcers; recurrent and refractory ulcers with diarrhea.
  - Hyperchlorhydria and hypergastrinemia.
  - Malignant behavior and metastasis.

23.6 Treatment

- Diet: smoking cessation, avoiding fried foods, citrus fruits, carbonated drinks.
- Avoiding NSAIDs.
- Medical.
  - Proton-pump inhibitors (PPI)—therapy of choice: 4–8 weeks standard dose (superior potency, duration, and lack of adverse events compared to other classes of drugs) [2].
  - PPI IV in patients with bleeding ulcers (see Chap. 27).
  - NSAIDs should be stopped in patients with high bleeding or cardiac risk.
  - Sucralfate 4 g per day in gastrectomy patients with anastomotic ulcers [3].
  - *H. pylori* eradication treatment
    First-line therapy
      Areas with low clarithromycin resistance (<15%): standard triple therapy for 10–14 days is recommended as first-line empirical treatment: 2× PPI dose + amoxicillin 1 g × 2 + clarithromycin 500 mg × 2 or metronidazole 500 mg × 2.
      Areas with >15% clarithromycin resistance: bismuth quadruple therapy as first line: PPI× 2+ bismuth subcitrate 240 mg × 4 + metronidazole 500 mg × 3 + tetracycline 500 mg × 3.

Second-line therapy

Bismuth quadruple therapy or fluoroquinolone triple therapy: PPIx2 + amoxicillin 1 g × 2 + levofloxacin 2 × 500 mg.

After second-line failure *H. pylori* culture is required [4].

- Endoscopic treatment.
  - Only Forrest I up to IIb (see Chap. 27),
- Surgery and interventional radiology.
  - Perforation and penetration and failure of repetead endoscopic treatment and/or selective arterial embolization in bleeding ulcers → surgical intervention [5].
  - In perforated and penetrating ulcers surgery is the first option.

23.7 Complications

- Acute or chronic upper GI bleeding.
  - Iron-deficiency anemia or hematemesis and/or melena (see Chap. 27 for management).
- Perforation.
  - NSAIDs associated.
  - The most severe complication.
  - Abdominal defense ± nausea± vomiting ± hemorrhage.
  - Pneumoperitoneum on X-ray.
  - Endoscopy is contraindicated.
- Penetration (Fig. 23.7a, b).
  - Change in ulcer symptoms and rhythmicity.
  - Can be manifested with jaundice, cholangitis, or hemorrhage.
- Stenosis.
  - Late postprandial vomiting, weight loss, early satiety, bloating, and abdominal distension.
  - Endoscopic diagnosis (Fig. 23.8).
  - Usually, juxtapyloric, or duodenal ulcer.
  - Antisecretory treatment in benign ulcers and surgical treatment in malignant lesions after CT scan assessment.

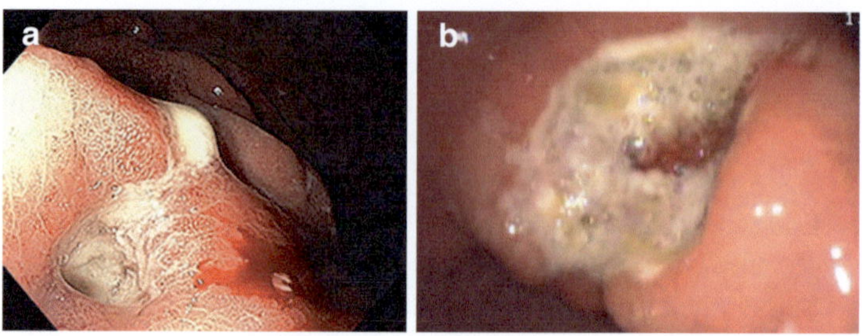

Fig. 23.7 Deep gastric ulcer, penetrating the pancreas

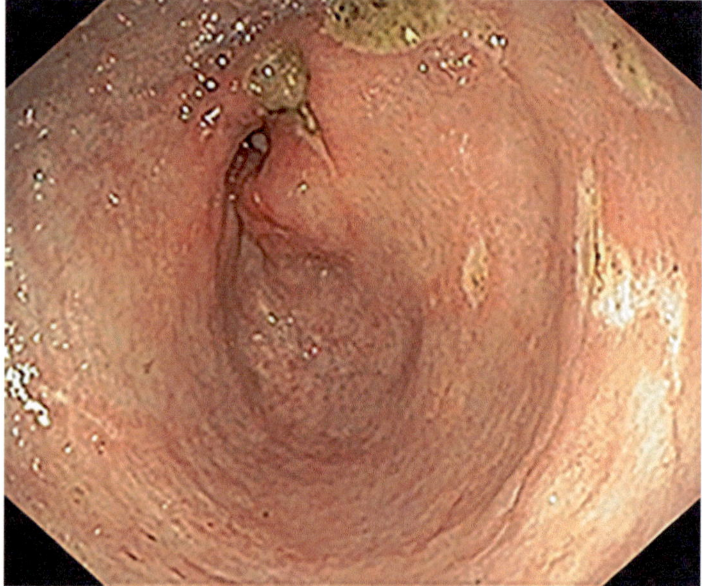

Fig. 23.8 Benign pyloric stenosis in a patient with a long history of the ulcer; the presence of numerous ulcerations in the antrum and pylorus is also noticeable

23.8 Follow-Up

- All gastric ulcers must be surveyed endoscopically at 6–12 weeks after diagnosis, with biopsies if not cured (Fig. 23.9).
- Duodenal ulcers do not require endoscopic follow-up or biopsies.
- *H. pylori* eradication must be proved by fecal antigen >4 weeks after the last antibiotic dose and >2 weeks after the last PPI intake [6].

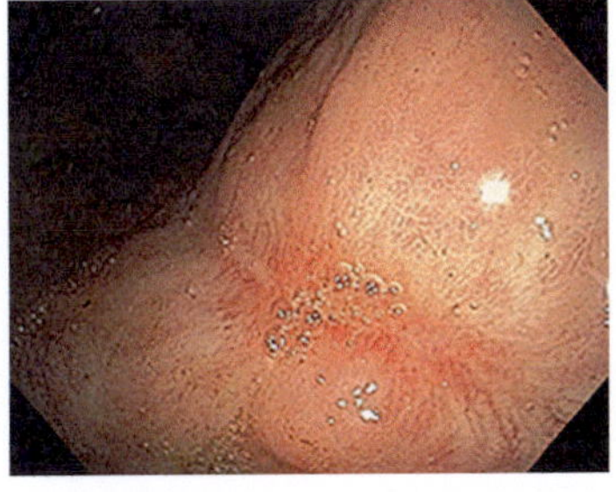

Fig. 23.9 Healed gastric ulcer – endoscopic appearance after 1 month of treatment with PPIs

References

1. Vörhendi N, Soós A, Anne Engh M, Tinusz B, Szakács Z, Pécsi D, et al. Accuracy of the helicobacter pylori diagnostic tests in patients with peptic ulcer bleeding: a systematic review and network meta-analysis. Therap Adv Gastroenterol. 2020;13:1756284820965324.
2. Kavitt RT, Lipowska AM, Anyane-Yeboa A, Gralnek IM. Diagnosis and treatment of peptic ulcer disease. Am J Med. 2019;132:447–56.
3. Feldman M, Friedman L, Brandt L. Sleisenger and Fordtran's, gastrointestinal and liver disease, vol. 1. 9th ed. Philadelphia: Saunders Elsevier; 2010. p. 861–86.
4. Guevara B, Cogdill AG. Helicobacter pylori: a review of current diagnostic and management strategies. Dig Dis Sci. 2020;65:1917–31.
5. Tarasconi A, Ciccolini F, Biffl WL, Tomasoni M, Ansaloni L, Picetti E, et al. Perforated and bleeding peptic ulcer: WSES guidelines. World J Emerg Surg. 2020;15:3.
6. Varicka S, Wilhemi M. Essentials in gastroenterology and hepatology. 2nd ed. Breisgau: Falk Foundation; 2017. p. 70–87.

Esophageal Tumors

Dan Nicolae Florescu and Adrian Săftoiu

24.1 Definition and Classification

- Malignant tumors:
  - Squamous-cell carcinoma (SCC), the most frequent.
  - Adenocarcinoma (AC).
  - Small-cell carcinoma.
  - Adenoid cystic carcinoma.
  - Melanoma.
  - Pseudosarcoma.
  - Primary esophageal lymphoma.
  - Leiomyosarcoma.
- Benign tumors:
  - Epithelial tumors.
      Squamous-cell papilloma.
      Adenoma.
      Inflammatory fibroid polyp.

D. N. Florescu
Department of Gastroenterology, Emergency County Clinical Hospital, University of Medicine and Pharmacy Craiova, Craiova, Romania

A. Săftoiu (✉)
Department of Gastroenterology and Hepatology, Elias Emergency University Hospital, Carol Davila University of Medicine and Pharmacy, Bucharest, Romania

A. Săftoiu (ed.), *Pocket Guide to Advanced Endoscopy in Gastroenterology*, https://doi.org/10.1007/978-3-031-42076-4_24

- Subepithelial tumors.
    Gastrointestinal stromal tumor (leiomyoma).
    Lipoma.
    Hemangioma.
    Granular cell tumor (granular cell myoblastoma; Abrikossoff's tumor).
    Other mesenchymal tumors (fibrolipoma, fibromyxoma, hamartoma).

24.2 Esophageal Cancer

- There are two main subtypes: squamous-cell carcinoma and adenocarcinoma [1–5].

24.2.1 Epidemiology

- Esophageal cancer usually occurs:
  - After 60 years.
  - Men > women; gender ratio (males/females) = 3/1 for SCC and 6/1 for AC, with important geographical variations.

24.2.2 Etiology and Pathogenesis

- Risk factors:
  - Exogenous factors.
      Excessive alcohol consumption.
      Smoking.
      Vitamin (riboflavin, β-carotene) and trace elements (zinc) deficiencies.
      Consumption of foods containing nitrates or moldy foods.
      Thermal aggression of the esophageal mucosa by hot liquids.
      Ingestion of tar or opium derivatives.
      Lower socioeconomic status.

- Endogenous factors and precancerous conditions.
  Gastroesophageal reflux disease (GERD) → Barrett's esophagus (BE) → dysplasia.
  Non-reflux esophagitis:
     Post-caustic esophageal stricture,
     Megaesophagus complicated with stasis esophagitis,
     Plummer–Vinson syndrome.
  Tylosis palmaris et plantaris.
  Human papilloma virus (HPV) infection.
- Squamous-cell carcinoma (SCC):
  - 90% of esophageal cancers worldwide
  - Alcohol consumption and smoking are the most important etiological factors.
  - Located mainly in the upper and middle third.
- Adenocarcinoma (AC):
  - Increasing incidence.
  - More common in obese patients.
  - Usually occurs in the distal esophagus due to GERD and intestinal metaplasia of the epithelium (Barrett's esophagus), through the progression of metaplasia to dysplasia and then adenocarcinoma (Fig. 24.1a, b).
- The pathogenic sequence involves genetic abnormalities with uncontrolled cellular replication under the effect of risk factors, followed by squamous dysplasia or in the area of intestinal metaplasia, so that later SCC and AC appear.

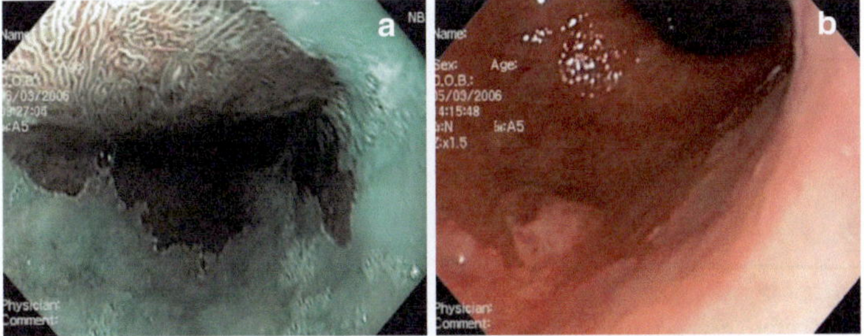

Fig. 24.1 Barrett's esophagus, with characteristic cerebriform pattern of intestinal metaplasia visualized in NBI mode (**a**), with a slightly prominent sessile tumoral mass (Paris IIa) at the level of the mucosa (**b**)

24.2.3 Diagnostic

- Clinical presentation:
  - Progressive dysphagia (initially for solid foods gradually progresses to include liquids) + odynophagia.
  - Neoplastic impregnation syndrome: malaise, anorexia, involuntary weight loss.
  - In advanced stage: sialorrhea, regurgitation, dysphonia, chest pain.
- Physical examination:
  - Cachexia.
  - Dehydrated skin.
  - Signs of metastatic dissemination: left supraclavicular adenopathy Virchow–Troisier, metastatic hepatomegaly.
- Paraclinical examinations:
  - Investigations to confirm the diagnosis.

    EGD—essential diagnostic investigation; highlights the primary tumor and allows multiple biopsies to be taken (Fig. 24.2a, b).

    Upper gastrointestinal series (UGI)—useful for exploring the esophagus in tight malignant stenoses that do not allow the passage of the endoscope, specifies the location of the primary tumor and can highlight the existence of fistulas.

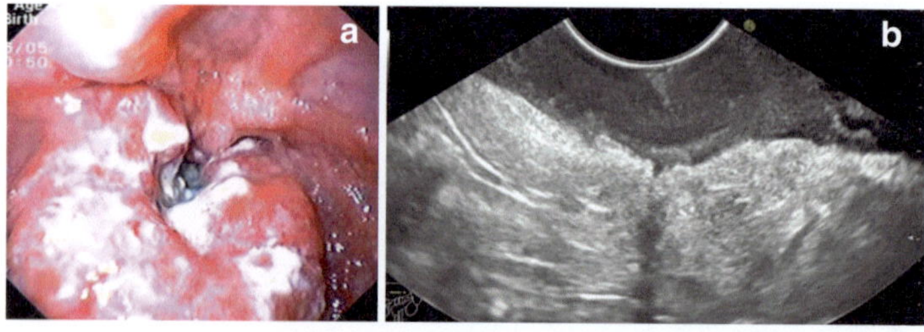

Fig. 24.2 Advanced esophageal squamous-cell carcinoma: EGD appearance of ulcerative-vegetative, stenotic tumor (**a**) and EUS appearance with transmural invasion of the esophageal wall that extends beyond the muscularis propria—T3 (**b**)

- Investigations to assess the extent of the disease.

     CT scan (cervical, thoracic, and abdominal regions) with intravenous and possibly oral contrast—the investigation of choice for highlighting small lung and liver metastases (assessment of M stage).

     EUS—the most useful method to evaluate the loco-regional extension (assessment of T and N stages); allows visualization of the invasion of adjacent organs, mediastinal lymphadenopathy, celiac lymphadenopathy, and permits the confirmation of their malignant invasion by performing endoscopic ultrasound-guided fine-needle aspiration cytology (EUS-FNA) (Fig. 24.3a–d).

     PET/CT—provides superior information to classical tomography, especially for the detection of metastatic disemination; should be considered in patients who may undergo esophagectomy.

24.2.4 Staging (UICC/AJCC, Eighth Edition) [6]

- Primary tumor (T).
    - T_x—Primary tumor cannot be assessed.
    - T_0—No evidence of primary tumor.
    - Tis—Carcinoma in situ/high-grade dysplasia.
    - T_1—Tumor invades lamina propria or submucosa.

         T_{1a}—Tumor invades mucosa or lamina propria or muscularis mucosae.

         T_{1b}—Tumor invades submucosa.
    - T_2—Tumor invades muscularis propria.
    - T_3—Tumor invades adventitia.
    - T_4—Tumor invades adjacent structures.

         T_{4a}—Tumor invades pleura, pericardium, diaphragm or adjacent peritoneum.

         T_{4b}—Tumor invades other adjacent structures such as aorta, vertebral body, or trachea.

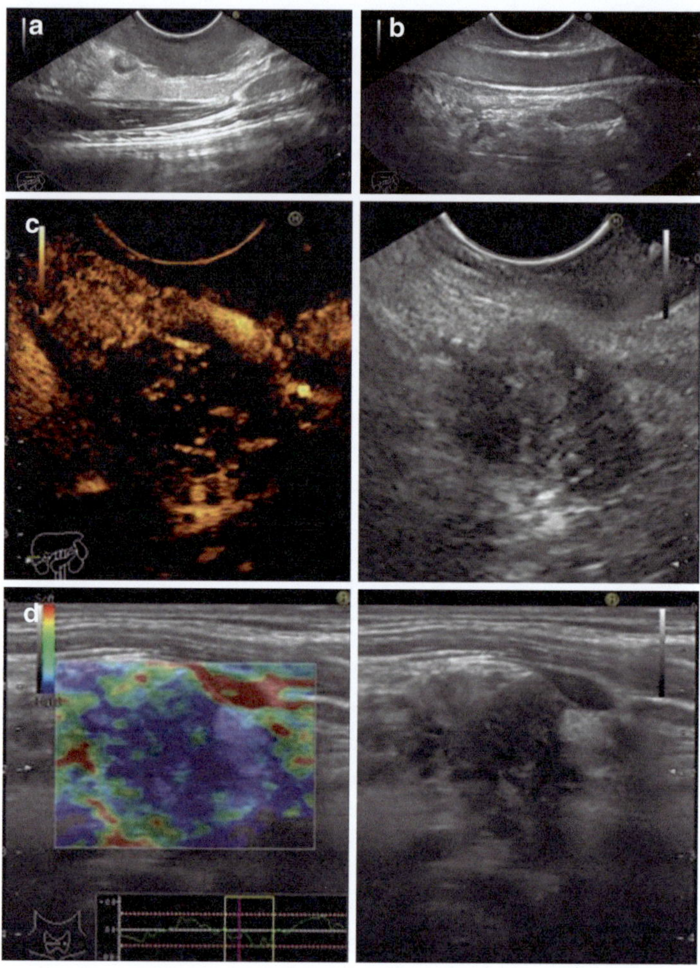

Fig. 24.3 Esophageal squamous-cell carcinoma: EUS appearance with transmural invasion of the esophageal wall that extends beyond the muscularis—T3 (**a**), with small adenopathy near the carotid artery (**b**) and another adenopathy with anarchic vascular pattern, observed on contrast-enhanced endoscopic ultrasonography (**c**), with hard tissue stiffness on strain elastography (**d**)

- Regional lymph nodes (N).
  - Nx—Regional lymph nodes cannot be assessed.
  - N_0—No regional lymph node metastasis.
  - N_1—Metastasis in 1–2 regional lymph nodes.
  - N_2—Metastasis in 3–6 regional lymph nodes.
  - N_3—Metastasis in 7 or more regional lymph nodes.
- Distant metastasis (M).
  - Mx—Distant metastasis cannot be assessed.
  - M_0—No distant metastasis.
  - M_1—Distant metastasis.
- Stage grouping differs depending on:
  - Clinical prognostic.
  - Pathological prognostic.
  - Post-preoperative therapy prognostic.
      Squamous-cell carcinoma.
      Adenocarcinoma.

24.2.5 Treatment [7]

- Limited disease (Stage 0–IB):
  - The treatment of choice is surgery and is practised with curative purposes.
  - Technique: esophagectomy (safety margins of 5 cm below the tumor) + mediastinal and cervical lymphadenectomy + esophagoplasty.
  - In the early stages (Tis, T_{1a} N_0 M_0) endoscopic mucosal resection (EMR) or endoscopic submucosal dissection (ESD) may be performed.
  - For patients unwilling to undergo surgery, combined chemoradiotherapy is superior to radiotherapy alone.
  - Standard chemotherapy: cisplatin +5-fluorouracil.

- Locally advanced disease (Stage IIA–IIIC):
    - Requires neoadjuvant therapy in order to convert to a curable surgical stage.
    - SCC.

        Neoadjuvant chemoradiotherapy followed by surgery **or.**
        Definitive chemoradiotherapy, but with close post-therapeutic follow-up (every 3 months).
        Definitive chemoradiotherapy is recommended for cervically localized tumors.
        Standard chemotherapy: carboplatin + paclitaxel.
    - AC.

        Perioperative chemotherapy followed by surgery **or.**
        Neoadjuvant chemoradiotherapy followed by surgery.
        Standard chemotherapy: platinum-based antineoplastic drug + fluoropyrimidine.
- Metastatic disease (Stage IV):
    - External radiotherapy ± brachytherapy.
    - Chemotherapy is indicated for palliative treatment in selected patients, particularly for patients with AC who have a good performance status.
    - Standard chemotherapy: platinum-based antineoplastic drug + fluoropyrimidine.
    - HER2-positive metastatic AC should be treated with a trastuzumab-containing therapy.
    - Palliative methods:

        Endoscopic esophageal dilation with endoprosthesis (Fig. 24.4a, b) or other endocavitary techniques (argon plasma coagulation, photodynamic therapy).
        Percutaneous or surgical gastrostomy.

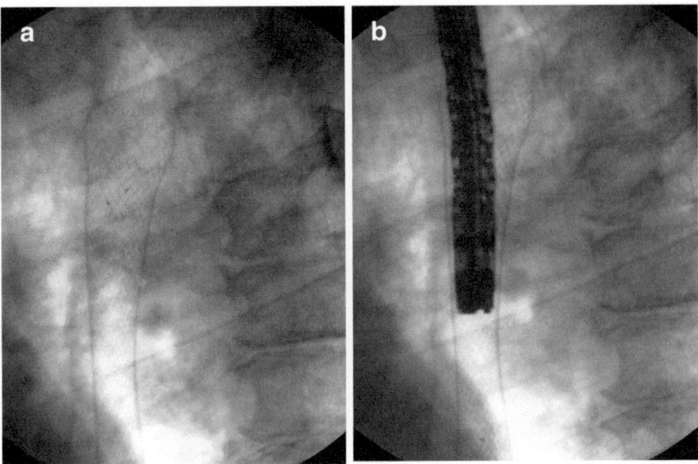

Fig. 24.4 Self-expandable metallic stent placed at the level of a malignant esophageal stenosis, under fluoroscopic (**a**) and endoscopic (**b**) guidance

24.3 Other Primary Esophageal Malignant Tumors

- Small-cell carcinoma.
  - Very aggressive, has early dissemination, and responds poorly to treatment.
- Adenoid cystic carcinoma.
  - Located in the middle third of the esophagus.
  - Early dissemination and unfavorable prognostic.
- Melanoma.
  - Very rare malignant tumor of the esophagus.
- Pseudosarcoma.
  - Composed of two types of cells: an intraluminal polypoid mass containing sarcomatous tissue, and the base is represented by a squamous-cell carcinoma.
  - Treatment of choice: esophagectomy.
  - Unfavorable prognostic.

- Primary esophageal lymphoma and carcinoid tumor.
  - Extremely rare.
  - The diagnosis is confirmed by biopsy with histopathological examination.
- Leiomyosarcoma.
  - Very rare.
  - The diagnosis is confirmed by biopsy with histopathological examination.
  - Surgery is the treatment of choice.

24.4 Esophageal Benign Tumors

24.4.1 Epithelial Tumors

- Squamous-cell papilloma.
  - Pathogenesis: HPV infection or gastroesophageal reflux.
  - Endoscopic features: small white or pink polypoid mass, sessile or pedunculated, with homogeneous appearance (Fig. 24.5a, b).
  - Differential diagnosis: squamous polypoid cancer.
- Esophageal adenomas.
  - Very rare.
  - Potential of malignant degeneration.
  - Endoscopic resection is indicated.

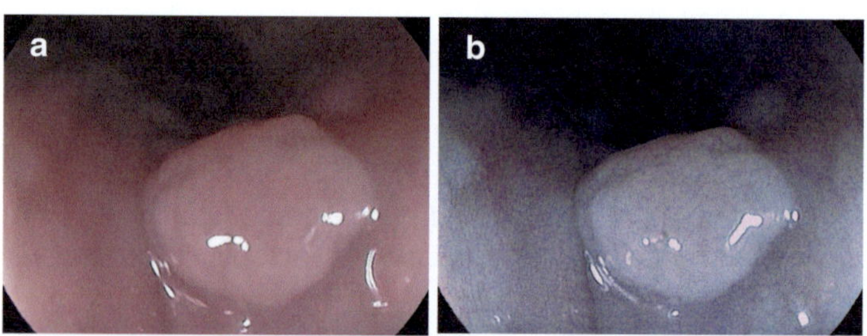

Fig. 24.5 Esophageal papilloma visualized in white light mode (**a**) and I-scan mode (**b**)

- Inflammatory fibroid polyp.
  - Pathogenesis: gastroesophageal reflux.
  - Similar to pseudopolyps in ulcerative colitis.

24.4.2 Subepithelial Tumors

- Gastrointestinal stromal tumor (leiomyoma).
  - Origin usually from muscularis propria (layer 4).
  - Covered by normal squamous epithelium(Fig. 24.6a, b).
  - Rarely, shows ulcerations and bleeding.
- Lipoma.
  - Very rare benign tumor of the esophagus (Fig. 24.7a, b).
  - More common in men.
  - Location in the upper esophagus - > risk of mechanical asphyxia.

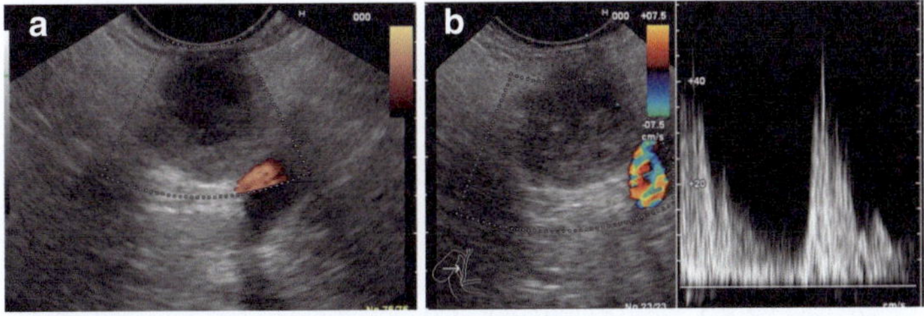

Fig. 24.6 EUS appearance of esophageal leiomyoma originating in layer 4 (muscularis) in power doppler mode (**a**) and color doppler mode + pulsed-wave doppler mode (**b**)

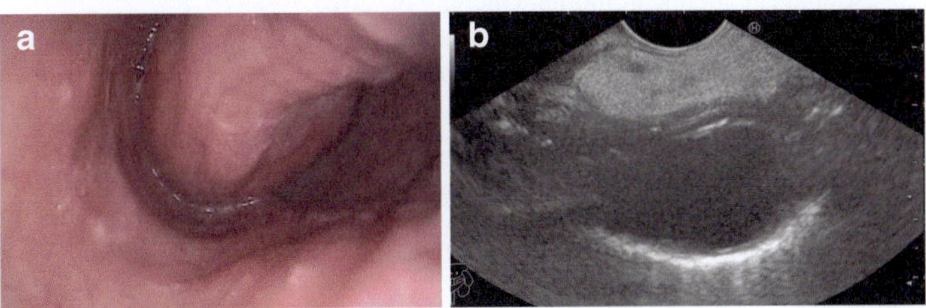

Fig. 24.7 EGD-appearance of esophageal lipoma with normal covering mucosa (**a**) and EUS-appearance originating in layer 2 (submucosa), with characteristic hyperechoic aspect, near the aortic arch (**b**)

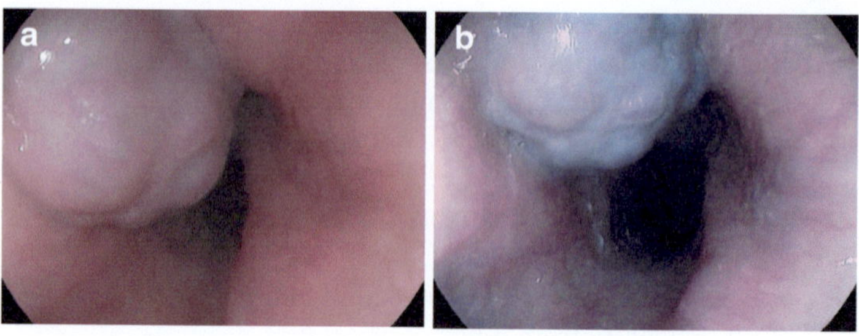

Fig. 24.8 EGD appearance of esophageal hemangioma with normal covering mucosa, in white light mode (**a**) and I-scan mode(**b**)

- Hemangioma.
  - Rare.
  - Frequently causes bleeding (Fig. 24.8a, b).
  - Differential diagnosis: AIDS-associated Kaposi sarcoma.
  - Surgical treatment; endoscopic techniques in selected cases.

References

1. Ciurea T, Săftoiu A, Tumorile esofagului. Bolile aparatului digestiv, sub redacţia Paulina Ciurea, Tudorel Ciurea. Editura Didactică şi Pedagogică; 1999. p. 43–52.
2. Mayer RJ. Gastrointestinal tract cancer. In: Longo DL, Fauci AS, editors. HARRISON'S gastroenterology and hepatology. 2nd ed. New York: McGraw-Hill Education LLC; 2013. p. 518–34.
3. Edgren G, Adami HO, Weiderpass E, Nyren O. A global assessment of the oesophageal adenocarcinoma epidemic. Gut. 2013;62:1406–14.
4. Xie SH, Lagergren J. A global assessment of the male predominance in esophageal adenocarcinoma. Oncotarget. 2016;7:38876–83.
5. Castro C, Bosetti C, Malvezzi M, et al. Patterns and trends in esophageal cancer mortality and incidence in Europe (1980–2011) and predictions to 2015. Ann Oncol. 2014;25:283–90.
6. Amin MB, et al., editors. AJCC cancer staging manual. 8th ed. New York: Springer; 2018.
7. Lordick F, Mariette C, Haustermans K, et al. Oesophageal cancer: ESMO clinical practice guidelines for diagnosis, treatment and follow-up. Ann Oncol. 2016;27(suppl 5):v50–7.

Gastric Tumors

25

Maria Monalisa Filip

25.1 Definition and Classification

- Malignant.
  - Adenocarcinoma.
  - Non-Hodgkin/MALT lymphoma.
  - GIST.
  - Carcinoid tumor.
  - Metastases.
  - Rare tumours (sarcomas, neuroendocrine carcinoma).
- Benign.
  - Mucosal tumors.

    Hyperplastic polyps.

    Inflammatory fibroid polyp.

    Xanthoma/xanthelasma.

    Ectopic pancreas.

    Hamartomatous polyp (Peutz–Jeghers syndrome, juvenile polyps, Cowden disease, Cronkhite–Canada syndrome, Gardner syndrome).

M. M. Filip (✉)
Research Center of Gastroenterology and Hepatology, University of
Medicine and Pharmacy Craiova, Craiova, Romania

© The Author(s), under exclusive license to Springer Nature
Switzerland AG 2023
A. Săftoiu (ed.), *Pocket Guide to Advanced Endoscopy in
Gastroenterology*, https://doi.org/10.1007/978-3-031-42076-4_25

Fundic gland polyp.
Adenomatous polyp.
- Nonmucosal tumors.
   Mesenchymal.
      Gastrointestinal stromal tumors (GIST).
      Lipoma.
      Fibroma.
      Glomus tumor.
   Vascular.
      Hemangioma.
      Lymphangioma [1].

25.2 Adenocarcinoma

25.2.1 Epidemiology

- The fifth most common neoplasm and the third most deadly cancer (GLOBOCAN 2018).
- Men > women.
- Known risk factors:
  - *H. pylori* infection.
  - Tobacco smoking.
  - Dietary factors.
  - Obesity.
  - Gastric surgery.
  - Pernicious anemia.
  - Toxins (various chemicals).

25.2.2 Etiology and Pathogenesis

- Two pathological entities:
  - Intestinal type—characterized by the formation of tubular structures similar to the intestinal glands.
    Closely linked to environmental and dietary risk factors.

- Diffuse form—is less differentiated and has no glandular structures.

  It is found with the same frequency worldwide.

  Occurs at younger ages.

  Associated with a worse prognosis.
- *H. pylori* infection is the main cause of gastric inflammation, being considered an etiological agent of gastric cancer.

25.2.3 Diagnostic

- Symptoms.
  - Dyspeptic, ulcer-like.
  - Weight loss, loss of appetite, dysphagia.
  - Vomiting, gastrointestinal bleeding.
- Physical exam.
  - In the early stages it is normal.
  - Moderate epigastric sensitivity.
  - Palpable abdominal mass.
- Laboratory studies.
  - Hypochromic, microcytic anemia due to occult bleeding with low sideremia/macrocytic anemia due to folate deficiency.
  - CEA, CA 72–4, and CA 19–9 usually elevated.
- Imaging tests.
  - Endoscopy is the initial test.

    Allows visualization of tumor location, surface extension and biopsy for diagnosis, histological classification, and molecular biomarkers, for example, HER2 status.
  - EUS accurate assessment of locoregional extension (T,N).

    Hypoechoic formation that modifies the normal architecture of the gastric wall.
  - CT: for the evaluation of the locoregional extension and the presence of distant metastases [2].

25.2.4 Role of Endoscopy

- Early gastric cancer is defined by its limitation to the mucosa.
- The Murakami Classification of the Japanese Gastric Cancer Society includes the following forms of early gastric cancer:
  - Protruding (type I) appears as a nodular lesion with an irregular surface.
  - Flat (type II).

    Elevated (IIa)—slight mucosal elevation up to 5 mm in height from the surrounding mucosa;

    Flat (IIb)—color changes, usually paler.

    Depressed (IIc)—subleveled surface to the surrounding mucosa.
  - Excavated (III)—ulceration more difficult to differentiate from the benign one (Fig. 25.1a, b).
- Advanced gastric cancer—Borrmann classification:
  - Type I polypoid—tumor that develops inside the gastric lumen, well delimited, not ulcerated, with an irregular, nodular surface, with the surrounding mucosa atrophied.
  - Type II ulceroproliferative—the tumor well delimited, ulcerated, covered with a necrotic material, the adjacent mucosa is pale (Fig. 25.2a, b).
  - Type III ulceroinfiltrative—appears as an inaccurately delimited ulceration with adjacent infiltrated mucosa, rigid when taking biopsies (Fig. 25.3a, b).

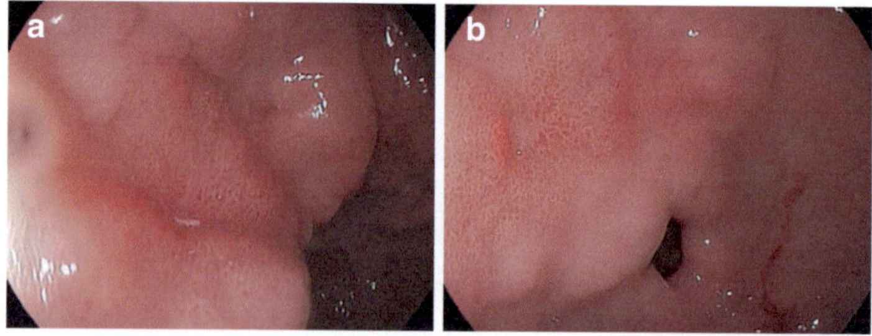

Fig. 25.1 Early gastric adenocarcinoma endoscopic appearance of slightly raised mucosa, with a small central depression (Murakami IIa + IIc) (**a, b**)

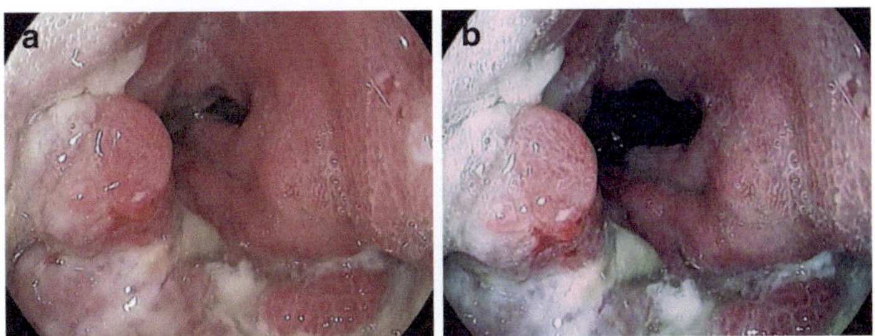

Fig. 25.2 Advanced gastric cancer: endoscopic aspect of an ulceroproliferative tumor, circumferential, visualized in white light mode (**a**) and I-scan mode (**b**)

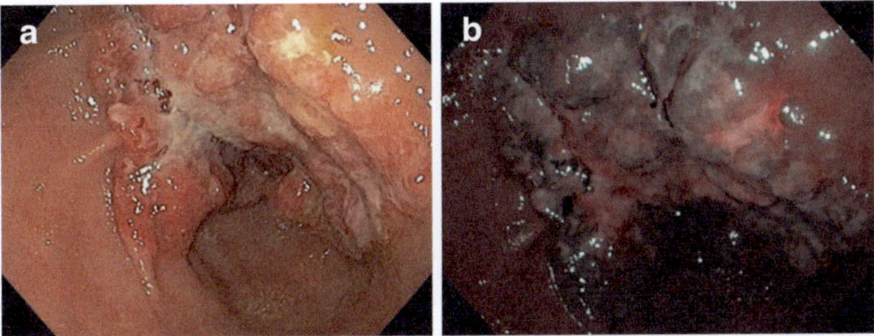

Fig. 25.3 Advanced gastric cancer: endoscopic aspect of an ulceroinfiltrative tumor visualized in white light mode (**a**) and narrow band imaging—NBI (**b**)

- Type IV—diffuse infiltrative form (plastic line)—disappearance of the folds or wide and rigid folds that do not relax on insufflation, the sign of the tent absent, the lack of peristalsis, possibly superficial ulcerations; requires multiple biopsies (Fig. 25.4a, b).
- EUS allows assessment of T and N stage.
  - Low accuracy for differentiating T1a vs. T1b, respectively, T3 vs. T4a (Fig. 25.5a).
  - Regional lymph nodes can be counted and confirmed by EUS-guided puncture (Fig. 25.5b).

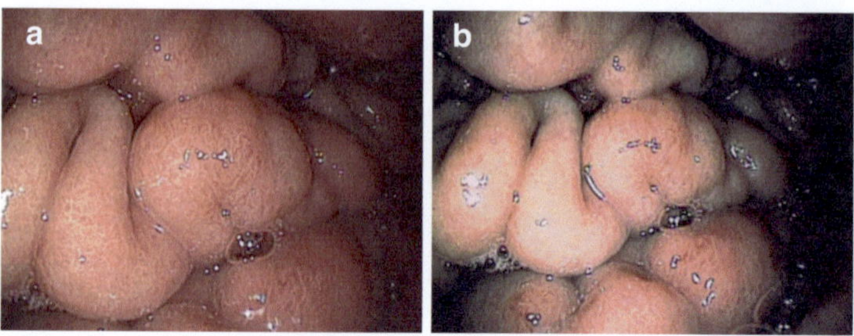

Fig. 25.4 Hypertrophic gastric folds: endoscopic appearance of thickened and stiff folds with diminished peristalsis visualized in white light mode (**a**) and I-scan (**b**)

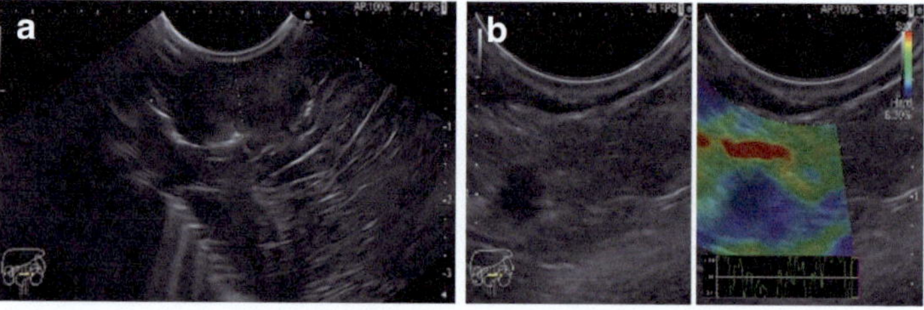

Fig. 25.5 Gastric adenocarcinoma staged by endoscopic ultrasound: hypoechoic mass invading normal layers, including muscularis and serosa (T4a) (**a**), with regional hypoechoic, round nodes with rough elastography appearance (**b**)

- The left liver lobe can be visualized, to identify metastases (M1).
- The presence of ascites may indicate peritoneal carcinomatosis.

25.2.5 Staging (Eighth AJCC)

- Tumor (T).
    - TX—Primary tumor cannot be assessed.
    - T0—No evidence of primary tumor.
    - Tis—Carcinoma in situ: intraepithelial tumor without invasion of the lamina propria.

- – T1a—Tumor invades lamina propria or muscularis mucosae.
- – T1b—Tumor invades submucosa.
- – T2—Tumor invades muscularis propria.
- – T3—Tumor penetrates subserosa without invasion of visceral peritoneum or adjacent structures.
- – T4a–Tumor invades serosa.
- – T4b–Tumor invades adjacent structures.
- Regional lymph nodes (N).
  - – NX – Regional lymph node(s) cannot be assessed.
  - – N0 – No regional lymph node metastasis.
  - – N1 – Metastasis in 1–2 regional lymph nodes.
  - – N2 – Metastasis in 3–6 regional lymph nodes.
  - – N3 – Metastasis in seven or more regional lymph nodes.
  - – N3a – Metastasis in 7–15 regional lymph nodes.
  - – N3b – Metastasis in 16 or more regional lymph nodes.
- Distant metastasis (M).
  - – M0—No distant metastasis.
  - – M1–Distant metastasis.
- Clinical stage TNM (cTNM):
  - – 0–Tis N0 M0
  - – I—T1, T2 N0 M0.
  - – IIA—T1, T2 N1, N2, N3 M0.
  - – IIB–T3, T4a N0 M0.
  - – III–T3, T4a N1, N2, N3 M0.
  - – IVA–T4b Any N M0.
  - – IVB–Any T Any N M1A [3].

25.2.6 Treatment

- Endoscopic resection for very early gastric cancers (T1a) if they are clearly confined to the mucosa, well-differentiated, ≤ 2 cm and non-ulcerated (EMR/ESD).
- For stage IB–III gastric cancer, radical gastrectomy is indicated.

- Perioperative chemotherapy with a platinum/fluoropyrimidine combination is recommended for patients with ≥ stage IB resectable gastric cancer.
- Patients with inoperable locally advanced and/or metastatic (stage IV) disease should be considered for systemic treatment.
- Endoscopic palliative treatment includes placement of expandable stents in stenotic tumors (Fig. 25.6) or argon plasma coagulation (APC) [4].

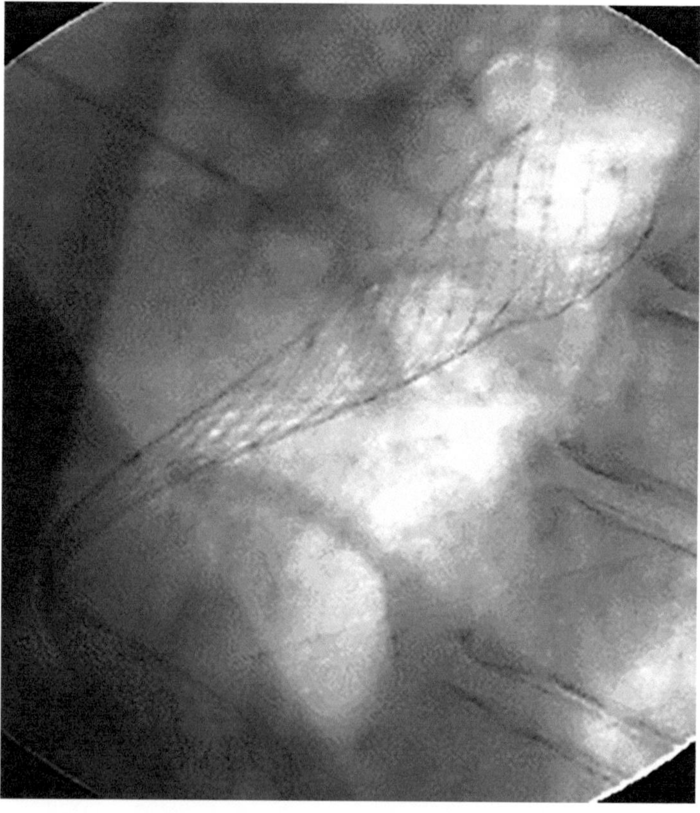

Fig. 25.6 Anastomotic recurrence of a gastric adenocarcinoma operated with curative intent (total gastrectomy): placement of an expandable metallic stent at the level of the malignant stenosis

25.3 Other Gastric Tumors

- Primary gastric lymphoma.
  - 5% of primary gastric neoplasms and 30% to 40% of all extranodal lymphomas
  - The most common are marginal zone B-cell lymphoma of the mucosa-associated lymphoid tissue (MALT) and diffuse large B-cell lymphoma.
  - Gastric MALT lymphomas are strongly associated with *H. pylori* infection.
  - Endoscopic appearance can vary from irregularly shaped superficial erosions, shallow ulcers to enlarged rugal folds, intragastric nodularities, or thickened gastric walls.
  - EUS determine the infiltration of the gastric wall, the involvement of the regional lymph nodes and it is also used in the remission follow-up (Fig. 25.7a, b).
- Gastrointestinal stromal tumors (GISTs).
  - The most common malignant subepithelial lesions.
  - Endoscopic finding—nonspecific smooth bulge covered with normal mucosa.
  - Ulceration may be seen on the large tumor.
  - EUS +/− EUS-FNA is the key test for differential diagnosis and follow-up (Fig. 25.8a, b) [5].

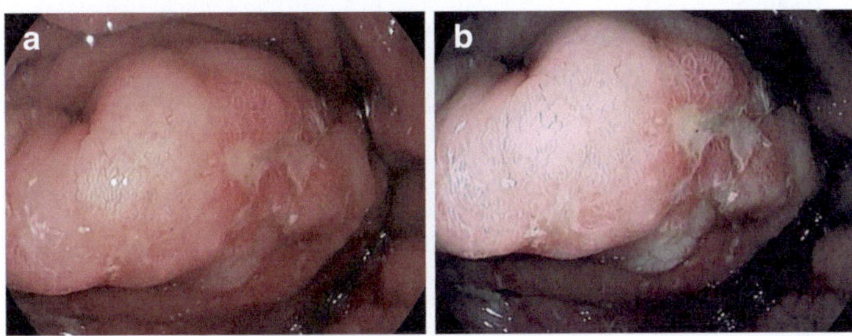

Fig. 25.7 Endoscopic aspect of a gastric lymphoma visualized in white light (**a**) and I-scan mode (**b**) with superficial ulcerations, thickened and rigid folds

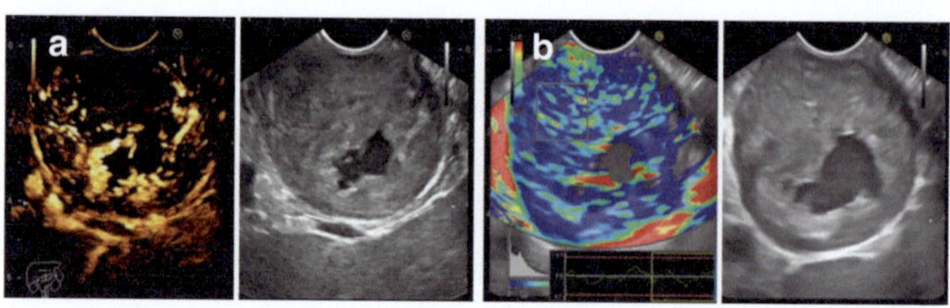

Fig. 25.8 Gastric stromal tumor (GIST), with well-expressed vascularization after the injection of the contrast substance (Sonovue) (**a**), respectively with a hard elastography appearance (**b**)

References

1. Lochhead P, El-Omar E. Gastric tumors: an overview. Atlas Genet Cytogenet Oncol Haematol. 2009;13:761–7.
2. Sitarz R, Skierucha M, Mielko J, et al. Gastric cancer: epidemiology, prevention, classification, and treatment. Cancer Manag Res. 2018;10:239–48.
3. American Joint Committee on Cancer. Digestive System, Amin MB, Edge S, Greene F, Byrd DR, Brookland RK, et al. AJCC cancer staging manual. 8th ed. New York, NY: Springer; 2018.
4. Smyth EC, Verheij M, Allum D, et al. Arnold on behalf of the ESMO guidelines Committee. Gastric cancer: ESMO clinical practice guidelines for diagnosis, treatment and follow-up. Ann Oncol. 2016;27(Supplement 5):v38–49.
5. Akahoshi K, Oya M, Koga T, Shiratsuchi Y. Current clinical management of gastrointestinal stromal tumor. World J Gastroenterol. 2018;24:2806–17.

Duodenal Tumors

26

Dan Nicolae Florescu

26.1 Definition, Classification, Epidemiology

- Benign tumors.
  - Epithelial tumors.
    - Adenoma (tubular, villous, tubulovillous).
    - Brunner's gland adenoma.
  - Mesenchymal tumors.
    - Leiomyoma.
    - Lipoma.
    - Angioma.
  - Within hereditary diseases.
    - Familial adenomatosis polyposis (Fig. 26.1).
    - Gardner's syndrome.
    - Peutz–Jeghers syndrome [1, 2].
- Malignant tumors.
  - Primary malignancies of the duodenum are extremely rare.
  - 0.5% of malignant tumors of the gastrointestinal tract
  - Maximum incidence in the sixth decade of life.
    - Adenocarcinoma, the most frequent.

D. N. Florescu (✉)
Department of Gastroenterology, Emergency County Clinical Hospital,
University of Medicine and Pharmacy Craiova, Craiova, Romania

© The Author(s), under exclusive license to Springer Nature
Switzerland AG 2023
A. Săftoiu (ed.), *Pocket Guide to Advanced Endoscopy in
Gastroenterology*, https://doi.org/10.1007/978-3-031-42076-4_26

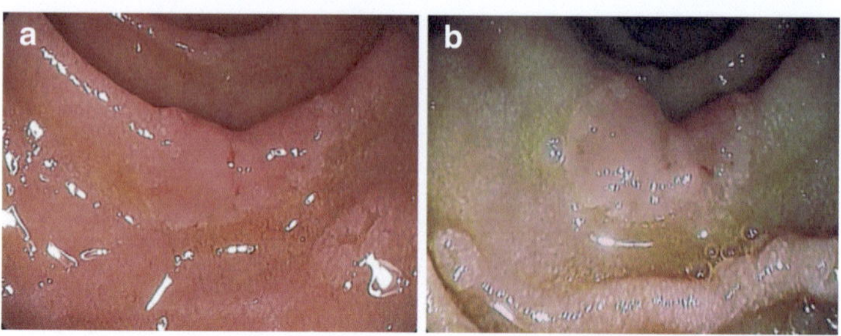

Fig. 26.1 Sessile duodenal polyps visualized in white light mode (**a**) and I-scan mode (**b**) in a patient with familial adenomatosis polyposis

Carcinoid tumors.

Lymphomas.

Leiomyosarcomas.

26.2   Etiology and Pathogenesis

- Brunner's gland adenomas.
  - Represent a hyperplasia of submucosal duodenal glands, possibly in response to gastric acid hypersecretion.
  - Are more common in the proximal duodenum.
  - They were not associated with potential of malignant degeneration.
- Duodenal adenocarcinomas.
  - May develop from duodenal polyps found in familial adenomatosis polyposis or Gardner syndrome, or may be associated with celiac disease.

26.3   Diagnostic

- Clinical presentation.
  - Most patients remain asymptomatic.
  - Nonspecific signs and symptoms.
    Abdominal pain.
    Dyspepsia: nausea, vomiting, bloating.

- Periampullary tumors can lead to complications such as jaundice, angiocolitis or pancreatitis.
- Signs and symptoms of complications (gastrointestinal bleeding, intestinal obstruction).
- Imaging tests.
  - EGD.
    Represents the most useful examination for diagnosis (Fig. 26.2a, b).
    Biopsy allows to establish the definitive diagnosis, especially in malignant tumors [3, 4].
  - EUS.
    Useful in staging duodenal and periampullary malignancies, allowing the assessment of T and N stages.
    Allows the assessment of submucosal tumors, which present normal covering mucosa (Fig. 26.3a, b).

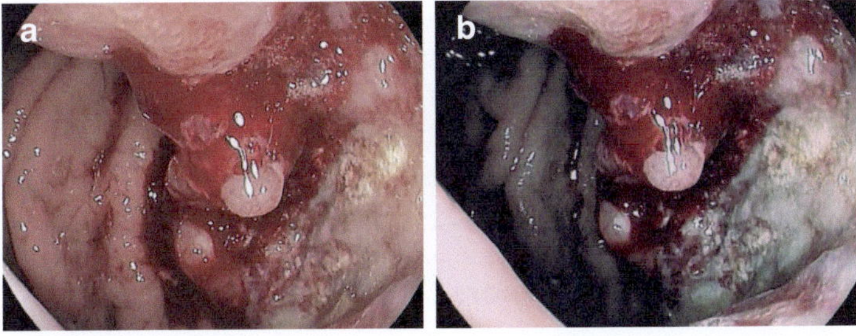

Fig. 26.2 Duodenal ulcerative-vegetative tumor visualized in white light mode (**a**) and I-scan mode (**b**)

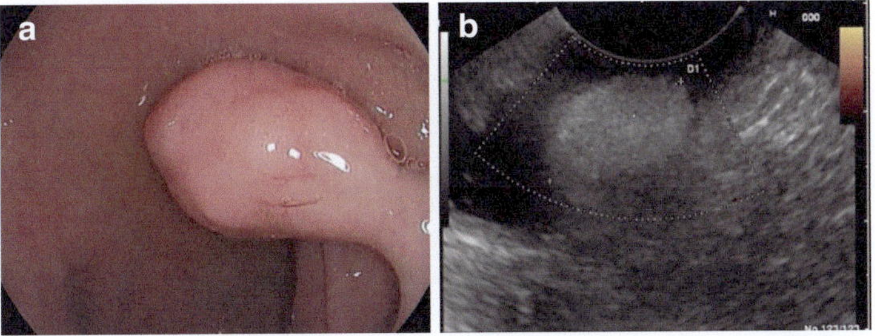

Fig. 26.3 Subepithelial tumoral mass, with normal covering mucosa (**a**), with hyperechoic EUS appearance, highly suggestive of duodenal lipoma (**b**)

## 26.4	Treatment

26.4.1 Benign Tumors

- Endoscopic or surgical resection of benign duodenal tumors remains controversial in the absence of complications.
    - Methods
        - Cold snare polypectomy for tumors <10 mm in diameter.
        - Endoscopic mucosal resection (EMR)—the treatment of choice for polyps <20 mm in diameter.
        - Endoscopic submucosal dissection (ESD) for polyps with size between 20 and 40 mm in diameter.
            - Associated with an increased risk of complications (gastrointestinal bleeding, perforation).
        - Laparoscopic-endoscopic cooperative surgery (LECS) for tumors >20 mm in diameter.
            - Avoids the risk of perforation after ESD.
- Duodenopancreatectomy for any size tumors with suspicion of malignant degeneration.
- Leiomyomas require surgical resection with wide safety margins due to the potential of malignant degeneration [5].

26.4.2 Malignant Tumors

- The treatment of choice:
    - Duodenopancreatectomy + regional lymphadenectomy [5, 6].

References

1. Goh PMY, Lenzi JE. Benign tumors of the duodenum and stomach. In: Holzheimer RG, Mannick JA, editors. Surgical treatment: evidence-based and problem-oriented. Munich: Zuckschwerdt; 2001.
2. Alwmark A, Andersson A, Lasson A. Primary carcinoma of the duodenum. Ann Surg. 1980;191:13–8.

3. Mayer RJ. Gastrointestinal tract cancer. In: Longo DL, Fauci AS, editors. HARRISON'S gastroenterology and hepatology. 2nd ed. McGraw-Hill Education LLC; 2013. p. 518–34.
4. Fagniez PL, Rotman N. Malignant tumors of the duodenum. In: Holzheimer RG, Mannick JA, editors. Surgical treatment: evidence-based and problem-oriented. Munich: Zuckschwerdt; 2001.
5. Ochiai Y, Kato M, Kiguchi Y, Akimoto T, Nakayama A, Sasaki M, Fujimoto A, Maehata T, Goto O, Yahagi N. Current status and challenges of endoscopic treatments for duodenal tumors. Digestion. 2019;99:2126.
6. Yamasaki Y, Uedo N, Takeuchi Y, Ishihara R, Okada H, Iishi H. Current status of endoscopic resection for superficial nonampullary duodenal epithelial tumors. Digestion. 2018;97:45–51.

Upper Gastrointestinal Bleeding

Bogdan Silviu Ungureanu

27.1 Definition

Upper gastrointestinal bleeding (UGIB) is described as blood loss from a gastrointestinal source above the ligament of Treitz. It can manifest as hematemesis, melena, or hematochezia.

27.2 Epidemiology

- UGIB is.
  - More common as people age.
  - Incidence: 40–150 per 100,000 population/year.
  - Men > women.
- Causes:
  - Peptic ulcer (duodenal or gastric).
  - Gastritis/erosive duodenitis.
  - Esophagitis.
  - Mallory–Weiss Syndrome.
  - Esophageal and gastric varices.
  - Esophageal and gastric cancer.

B. S. Ungureanu (✉)
Department of Gastroenterology, University of Medicine and Pharmacy of Craiova, Craiova, Romania

© The Author(s), under exclusive license to Springer Nature Switzerland AG 2023
A. Săftoiu (ed.), *Pocket Guide to Advanced Endoscopy in Gastroenterology*, https://doi.org/10.1007/978-3-031-42076-4_27

- Vascular malformation:
    Portal hypertensive gastropathy.
    Angiodysplasia.
    Gastric antral vascular ectasia (GAVE).
    Dieulafoy's lesion.
- Rare causes:
    Hiatal hernia.
    Crohn's disease.
    Aorto-enteric fistulae.
    Viral infections.

27.3 Diagnosis

- Clinical signs:
    - Hematemesis.
    - Melena.
    - Hematochezia.
    - Dizziness/lipotimia.
- Physical examination:
    - Sweating and pale skin.
    - Tachycardia.
    - Hypotension.
- Laboratory evaluation:
    - Complete blood count (CBC): HGB low; HTC and WBC normal/low.
    - Urea/creatinine: increased.
    - INR, APTT, PT affected by anticoagulant therapy, coagulopathies, liver failure.

27.4 Clinical Evaluation

27.4.1 Objectives

- Stabilize the patient—prevent the complications by protecting the airways and maintaining hemodynamic stability.

- Evaluate the severity of the bleeding.
- Identify the etiology of the bleeding.
- Stop the bleeding.

27.4.2 Patient Stabilization

- Place the patient on the left lateral decubitus position in case of hematemesis.
- Hemodynamic evaluation with clinical signs of bleeding (tachycardia, sweating).
  - Measure: pulse, BP, oxygen saturation.
- Peripheral intravenous access with a minimum of two intravenous lines or, when it is not possible, central venous catheter and crystalloid fluids administration.
- Biological:
  - HGB and HCT levels can be normal at presentation (hemodilution), while a significant decrease may suggest an important bleeding or a superimposition of acute bleeding on chronic bleeding.
  - White blood cell count may be high. Sepsis, which can condition the bleeding, should be considered when very high levels occur.
  - Thrombocytopenia may be the cause of chronic liver disease with hypersplenism, but other conditions associated with thrombocytopenia may also predispose patients to bleeding.
  - Increasing the level of urea may be a sign of renal hypoperfusion or decrease in protein absorbtion in the digestive tract.
- Circulating blood volume resuscitation is based on initial clinical evaluation:
  - If the patient is hypotensive, intravascular volume is low so crystalloid (preferably) or colloid fluids need to be administrated.
  - The objective is to maintain SBP > 100 mmHg.

- – Attention to patients with heart failure because of the risk for pulmonary edema!
- Blood transfusion is indicated in moderate or severe bleeding.
  - – HBG threshold of 7–9 g/dL.
  - – Higher threshold (>9 g/dL) is recommended in case of comorbidities, especially cardiovascular diseases.
- Monitoring vital signs every 15 min and less often once the patient is stable.
- Pacient is not allowed to eat or drink for at least 8 h before endoscopy.
- PPI therapy 80 mg bolus dose followed by a continuous infusion at 8 mg/h for 72 h.
- Terlipressin 2 mg bolus dose followed by 1 mg every 4–6 h is administrated if variceal bleeding is suspected (clinical signs or medical history of portal hypertension).
- Special attention to patients on anticoagulant therapy.
  - – In general, active bleeding presents a higher risk of rebleeding than any other affection whose risk is due to stopping anticoagulant therapy.

27.4.3 The Assessment of Bleeding Severity

Patients can present low or high risk of mortality.

The risk of mortality increases exponentially in the presence of:

- Chronic liver disease.
- Age > 60 years.
- Other comorbidities (cardiovascular, kidney, respiratory diseases).
- Signs of hemorrhagic shock.
- Rebleeding or bleeding in hospitalized patients for another condition.

4.3.1 Glasgow–Blatchford Score (GBS)

	Score
Systolic blood pressure (mmHg)	
100–109	1
90–99	2
<90	3
BUN (mmol/L)	
6.5–7.9	2
8.0–9.9	3
10.0–24.9	4
≥25.0	6
HGB men (g/dL)	
12–12.9	1
10–11.9	3
<10	6
HGB women (g/dL)	
10–11.9	1
<10	6
History and comorbidities	
Pulse >100 beats/min	1
Melena	1
Syncope	2
Hepatic disease	2
Cardiac failure	2

The score is calculated at presentation to evaluate the risk before practising the endoscopy

0–1 = low risk; the patient does not need hospitalization or emergency endoscopy

4.3.2 Rockall Score

Score				
Variable	0	1	2	3
Age (years)	<60	60–79	≥80	
Shock				
SBP (mmHg)	≥100	≥100	<100	
Pulse (beats/min)	<100	≥100	–	

Score				
Comorbidities	No major comorbidities		Cardiac failure, ischemic heart disease, major comorbidities	Kidney failure, liver failure, metastatic cancer
Diagnosis	Mallory–Weiss syndrome, no lesions identified, no evidence of bleeding	All other diagnosis	Malignancy of upper GI tract	
Evidence of bleeding	No stigmata or recent hemorrhage		Blood in upper GI tract, adherent clot, visible vessel, bleeding	

The score varies form 0 to 11; score < 3 low risk of mortality; score ≥ 8 high risk of mortality

27.4.4 Identifying the Etiology

Diagnostic endoscopy

- Prokinetic agents.
  - Erytromycin (250 mg i.v.) is recommended 30–120 min before endoscopy.
  - Metoclopramide (10 mg iv) may be used instead, especially for patients with active or severe UGIB.
  - Increases the endoscopic visualization of the mucosa, reduces the need for a second-look endoscopy, decreases the number of units transfused.
- Hemodynamic resuscitation.
  - After appropriate hemodynamic resuscitation, most patients should undergo endoscopy within 24 h.
  - Early endoscopy, within 12 h after presentation, should be taken into consideration for patients with persistent hemo-

dynamic instability (tachycardia, hypotension) despite aggresive resuscitation, for patients who present bloody emesis or for those who cannot discontinue the anticoagulant therapy.

- Early endoscopy.
  - Should be performed as soon as possible for patients who present signs of active bleeding or when variceal bleeding is suspected.
- Informed Consent
  - It is recommended before the procedure.

27.4.5 The Management of Bleeding

4.5.1 Therapeutic Endoscopy

- When the lesion is identified, therapeutic strategy should be chosen.
- Erytromycin (or metoclopramide) administration and endoscopic reevaluation are recommended if the source is not identified and there is a large amount of blood in the stomach.
- Investigation of the small bowel and colon is recommended in case no potentially bleeding lesion is found.

4.5.2 Bleeding Peptic Ulcer

- Treatment indication according to Forrest classification:
  - Forrest type Ia, Ib or IIa—endoscopic hemostasis (high risk for rebleeding).
  - Forrest type IIb—clot removal and underlying lesion treatment.
  - Forrest type IIc, III—endoscopic treatment is not recommended (low risk for rebleeding); patients can be discharged to administer PPI therapy at home.
- Treatment methods (Figs. 27.1, 27.2, 27.3 and 27.4):
  - Injection of adrenaline 1:10,000 in four quadrants at the periphery and in the centre of the lesion along with another method of hemostasis: mechanical (clips/bands), thermal (contact or noncontact) or sclerotherapy.

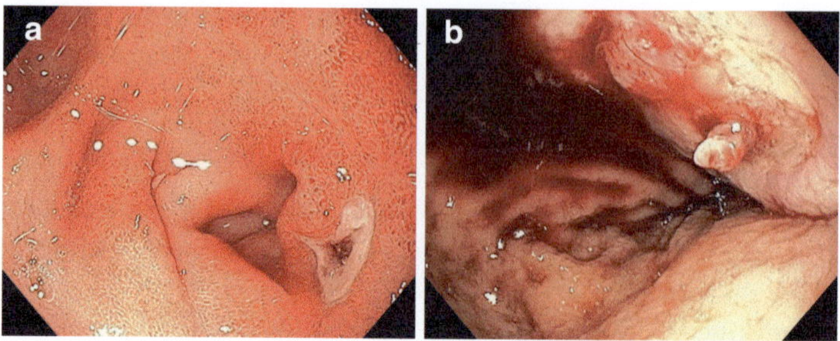

Fig. 27.1 (**a, b**) Forrest IIa duodenal ulcer

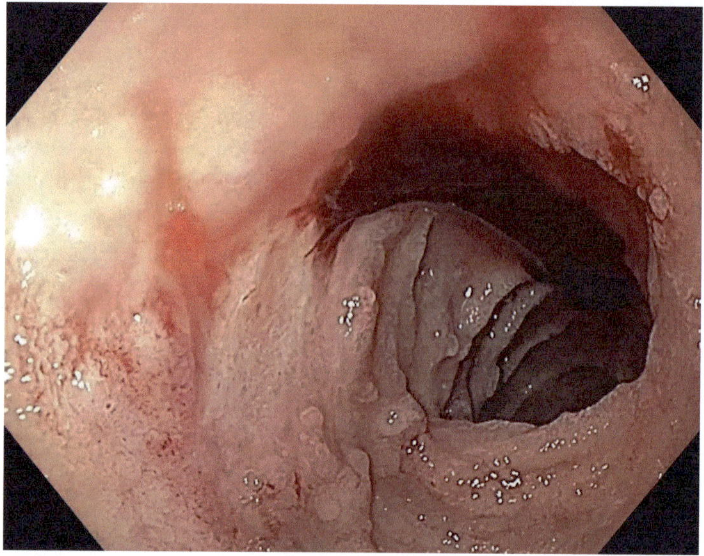

Fig. 27.2 Forrest IIb duodenal ulcer

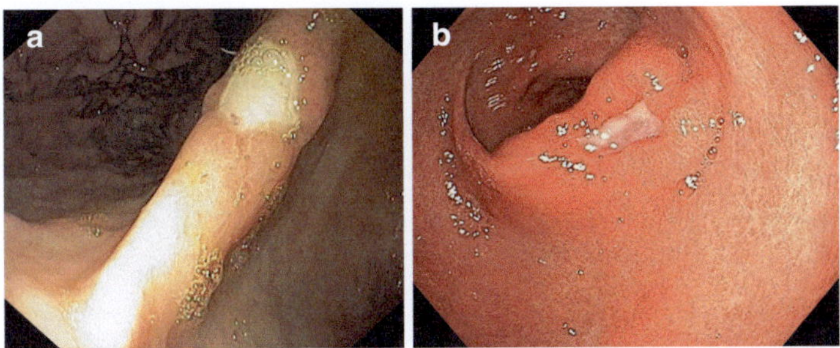

Fig. 27.3 (**a**, **b**) Forrest III gastric ulcer

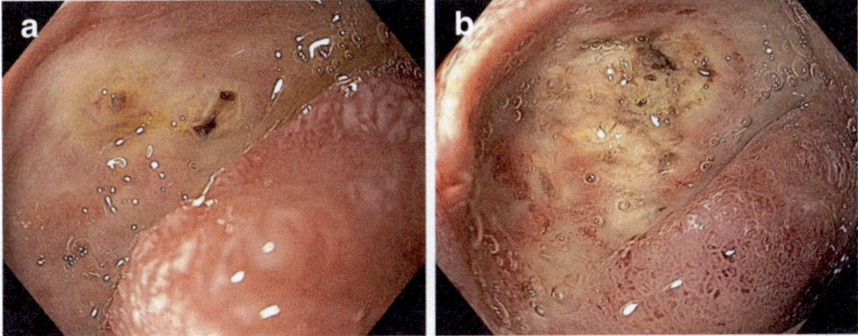

Fig. 27.4 (**a**) Visible vessel of the duodenal ulcer (Forrest IIa); (**b**) post-coagulation aspect of the ulcer

- PPI therapy 80 mg bolus dose followed by 8 mg/h for 72 h after endoscopic hemostasis.
- In case of rebleeding, endoscopic reevaluation with endoscopic hemostasis are recommended.
- In the case of failure of the second attempt at hemostasis, transcatheter angiographic embolization (TAE) or surgery should be considered.

4.5.3 Esophageal and Gastric Varices (Figs. 27.5, 27.6 and 27.7)

- The treatment of esophageal varices includes applying elastic bands on the varices:

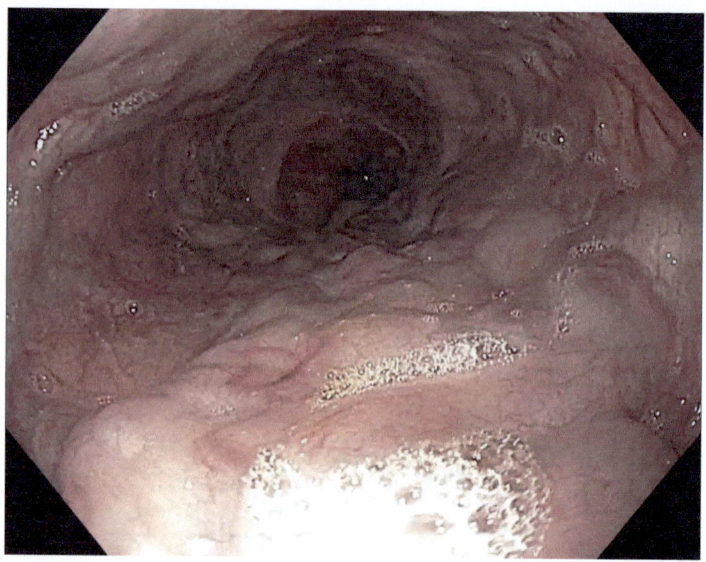

Fig. 27.5 Esophageal varices

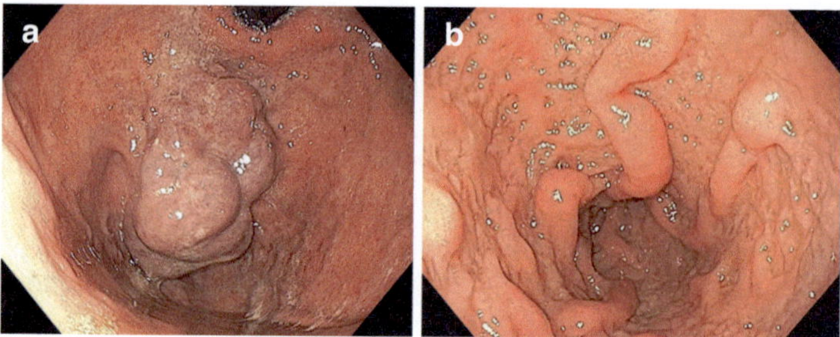

Fig. 27.6 (**a**) Gastric varices; (**b**) duodenal varices

- Application of the bands starts at the bleeding point and then concentrically as the endoscope is withdrawn.
- Endoscopic variceal ligation sesions are repeated at approximately 3 weeks until varices are obliterated.

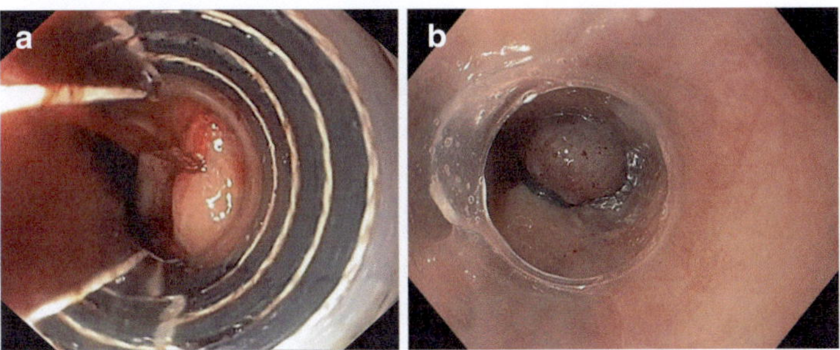

Fig. 27.7 (**a**) Active bleeding from esophageal varices; (**b**) esophageal varices after endoscopic variceal ligation

- In the case of gastric varices, endoscopic or endoscopic ultrasound-guided injection of cyanoacrylate is recommended.
- When edoscopic therapy fails, Blakemore–Sengstaken tube placement and emergency TIPS evaluation are recommended.

4.5.4 Mallory–Weiss Syndrome (Fig. 27.8)
- In most cases the bleeding stops spontaneously:
  - Stopped bleeding > PPI therapy.
  - Active bleeding > endoscopic hemostasis using hemoclips, Blakemore–Sengstaken tube is rarely necessary.

4.5.5 Erosive Gastritis/Duodenitis (Fig. 27.9)
- In most cases the bleeding is stopped during endoscopy:
  - Oozing bleeding may occur > hemostatic powder or different methods of coagulation, including APC, can be used to stop the bleeding.
  - The main treatment is PPI therapy.

4.5.6 Gastric Antral Vascular Ectasia (GAVE)
- Is a condition in which visible columns of red, dilated vessels course along the longitudinal folds of the antrum like the stripes of a watermelon (Fig. 27.10):
  - APC is recommended, but bipolar coagulation and endoscopic band ligation can also be used.

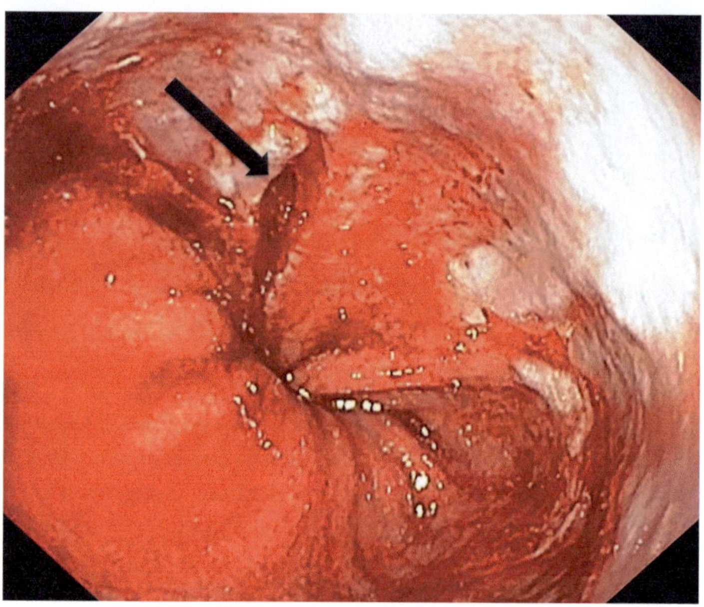

Fig. 27.8 Longitudinal ulceration at the gastroesophageal junction. Mallory Weiss Syndrome

4.5.7   Portal Hypertensive Hastropathy
- It rarely causes clinically significant acute bleeding.
  - Hemostatic powder or thermal coagulation, including APC, are recommended.

4.5.8   Hemobilia
- Most cases of hemobilia are iatrogenic as a consequence of procedures such as liver biopsy or ERCP.
  - (Radiological) embolization or surgery is recommended.

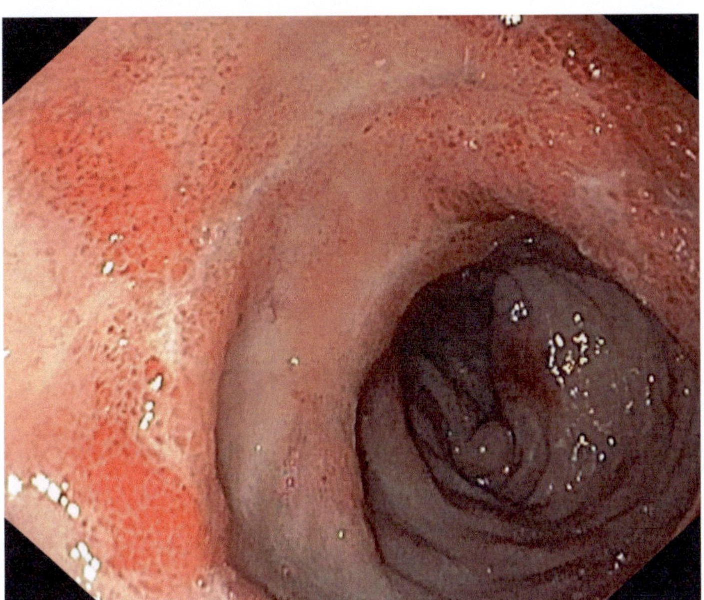

Fig. 27.9 Erosions of duodenal mucoasa, the formation of ulcers on the duodenal wall

4.5.9 Dieulafoy's Lesion (Fig. 27.11)

- It refers to a prominent large caliber vessel which erodes the stomach wall, in the absence of an ulcer.
  - It is most common in the superior portion of the stomach, on the greater curvature, near the esogastric junction, or in the duodenum.
  - Endoscopic hemostasis is recommended as an independent method (hemoclip placement, band ligation) or in combination with endoscopic injection of adrenaline.
  - Embolization or surgery can be attempted in the case of endoscopic hemostasis failure.

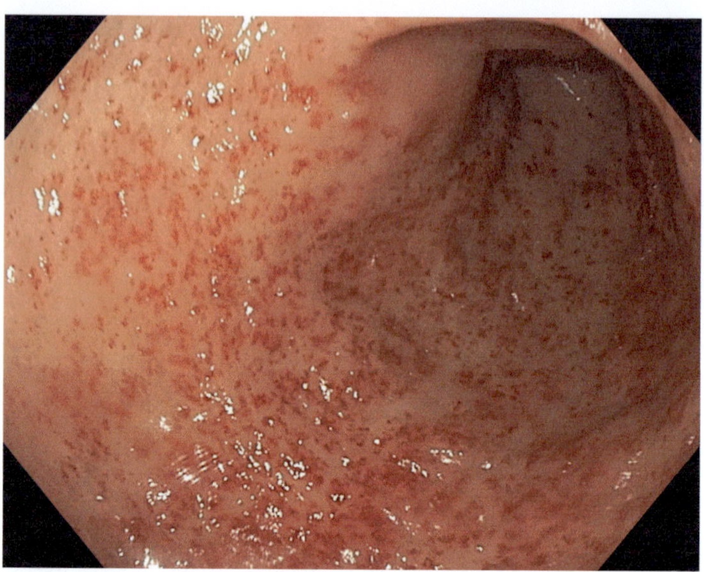

Fig. 27.10 Multiple petechiae developed in the antrum. Aspect of gastric antral vascular ectasia

4.5.10 Angiodysplasia (Fig. 27.12)
- It usually causes chronic bleeding.
  - Active bleeding imposes endoscopic hemostasis.

4.5.11 Esophageal, Gastric, and Intestinal Cancers (Figs. 27.13 and 27.14)
- Can cause UGIB:
  - Endoscopic hemostasis may be used (injection, mechanical, thermal, hemospray) with limited results.
  - The advantages are that it can prevent emergency surgery, it reduces the number of blood transfusions and it may offer a temporary way to oncological therapy and/or selective embolization.

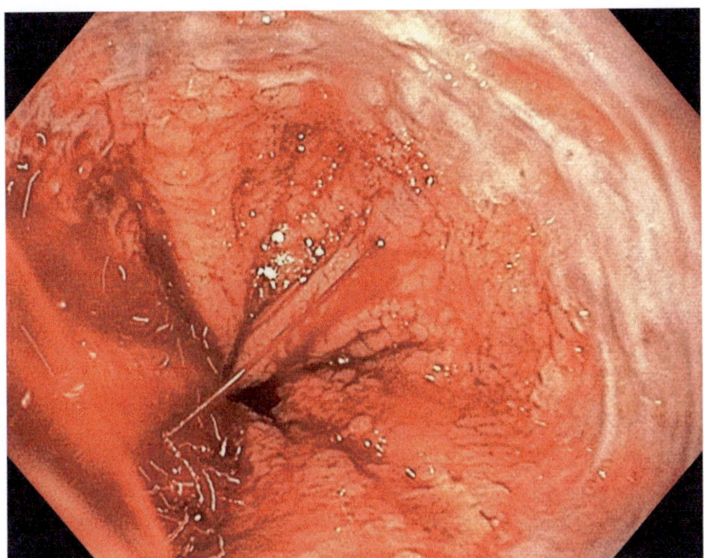

Fig. 27.11 Active spurting bleeding from a superficial vessel erosion. Dieulafoy's lesion

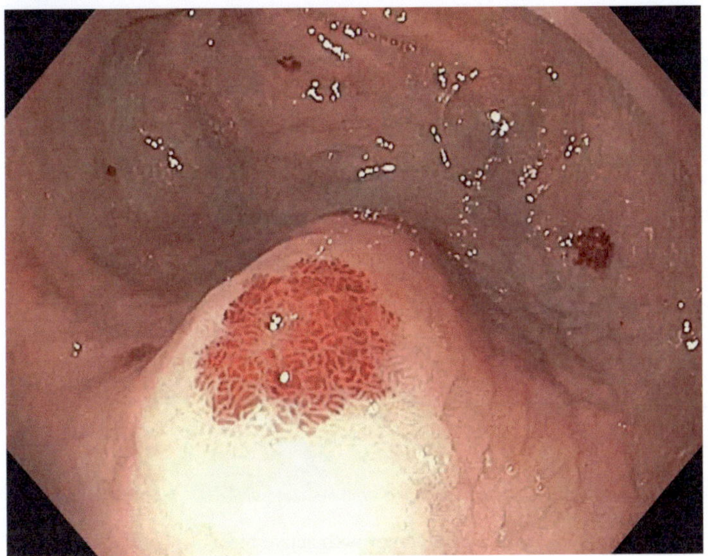

Fig. 27.12 Gastric angiodysplasia

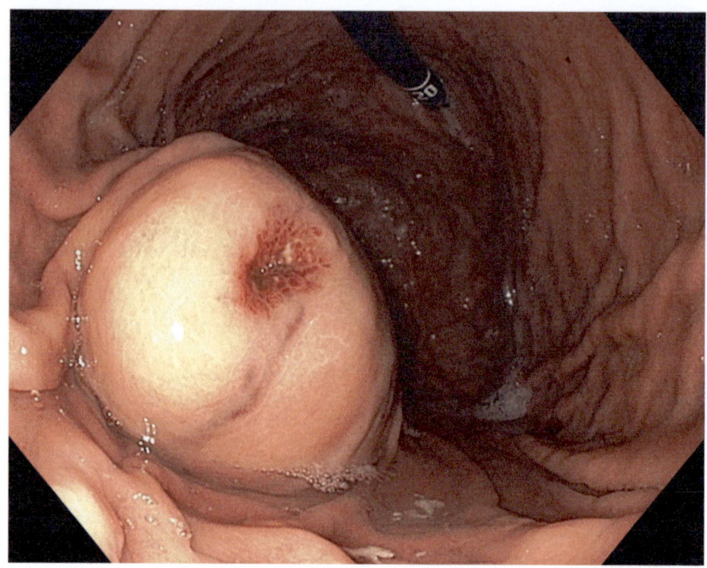

Fig. 27.13 Gastric stromal tumor with recent bleeding

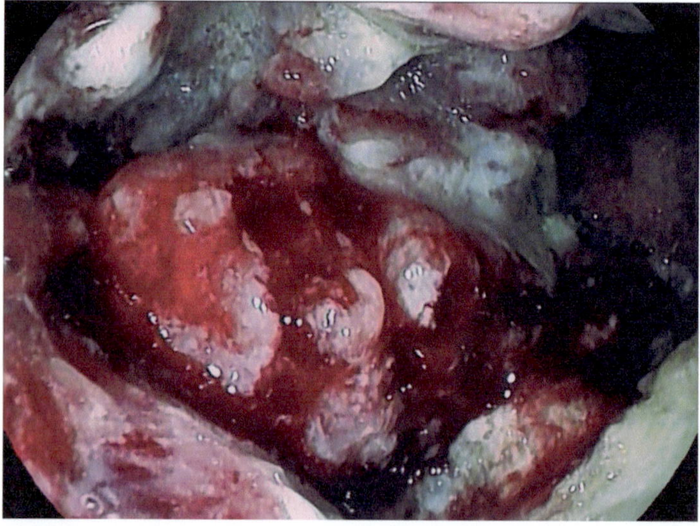

Fig. 27.14 Ulcerating gastric tumor with active bleeding

Lower Gastrointestinal Tract

Inflammatory Bowel Diseases

28

Dan Ionuț Gheonea and Petrică Popa

28.1 Definition

Inflammatory bowel disease (IBD) is a chronic, immune-mediated condition of the digestive tract characterized by inflammation with alternating periods of activity and remission.

- Depending on the location and depth of the intestinal wall damage, BII is divided into two entities:
    - Crohn's disease (BC): can affect any segment of the digestive tract.
        Segmental distribution.
        Transmural damage.
    - Ulcerative colitis (UC):
        Generally affects the rectum.
        Has continuous proximal extension.
        Inflammation limited to the mucosa and submucosa.
    - Unclassified colitis: term reserved for cases that do not allow the differentiation between CU and BC.

D. I. Gheonea (✉) · P. Popa
Gastroenterology Department, University of Medicine and Pharmacy Craiova, Craiova, Romania

A. Săftoiu (ed.), *Pocket Guide to Advanced Endoscopy in Gastroenterology*, https://doi.org/10.1007/978-3-031-42076-4_28

28.2   Epidemiology

- The incidence of IBD differs globally depending on the geographical regions.
  - The number of patients is much higher in highly industrialized countries.
  - In Europe the highest incidence is in Hungary (340 cases/100,000 inhabitants).
  - IBD can occur at any age but there are two peaks of incidence 15–30 years and 60–70 years, respectively.
  - The distribution by sex is approximately equal.

28.3   Etiopathogenesis

- Genetic factors.
  - Approximately 163 loci with a role in the occurrence of IBD are identified.
  - There are involved genes responsible for:
      Innate immunity and autophagy.
      Modulation of metabolic stress.
      Regulation of adaptive immunity.
      Development and resolution of inflammation.
- The microbiome.
  - Diminishing and changing diversity.
  - Growth of enteropathogenic bacteria.
      Escherichia coli.
  - Decrease of bacteria with anti-inflammatory role.
      Ruminnococcaceae.
      Fecalibacterium prausnitzii.
  - Inflamația viral or fungal infections that can activate inflammation.
- Environmental factors.
  - Low fiber diet.
  - High consumption of processed foods.
  - Increased intake of carbohydrates and fats.
  - Insufficient breastfeeding.

- Stress.
- Consumption of nonsteroidal anti-inflammatory drugs and contraceptives.
- Smoking (protective role in UC but not for CD).

28.4   Positive Diagnosis

- Clinical picture.
    - Ulcerative colitis.
        The severity of the symptoms is dictated by the extent of the disease and the degree of inflammation.
        Diarrhea with mucus and/blood (acute or insidious onset).
        Abdominal pain in the form of cramps.
        Feeling of incomplete evacuation.
        Symptoms: dizziness, anorexia, physical asthenia, fever, vomiting, weight loss.
    - Crohn's disease.
        Ileal localization: intense pain, colic in the right iliac fossa, nausea, weight loss, lingering diarrhea weight loss.
        Colonic localization: diarrheal stools with mucus and blood, pain in the colic frame, weight loss, fecal vomiting in the case of gastrocolic or duodenocolic fistulas, rectal tenesmus if the rectum is also affected.
        Perianal localization: pain and burns when passing the fecal bowl, low rectal compliance.
        Localization in the upper digestive tract: pain and discomfort in mastication, dysphagia, odynophagia, retrosternal pain, heartburn; gastroduodenal localization has symptoms similar to peptic ulcers.
        Other symptoms: dizziness, anorexia, physical asthenia, fever or low-grade fever, vomiting, weight loss.
    - Extraintestinal manifestations (characteristic of both conditions):

Joint damage: peripheral arthropathy, scroiliitis, ankylosing spondylitis with progression independent of IBD.
Bone damage: osteopenia, osteoporosis (following malabsorption and corticosteroid treatment).
Skin damage: erythema nodosum, pyoderma gangrenosum, Sweet syndrome.
Eye damage: uveitis, irritation, scleritis, episcleritis, vasculitis, retinal hemorrhage.
Hepato-biliopancreatic involvement: primitive sclerosing cholangitis.
Thromboembolic manifestations: portal vein thrombosis, thromboembolism.

- Clinical exam.
  - Ulcerative colitis:
    May be normal.
    Signs of dehydration, malnutrition.
    Sclero-skin pallor.
    Meteorism.
    Sensitivity in the colic.
    Pain on rectal examination + mucus and blood.
    Signs of extraintestinal manifestations:
      Erickson and Volkmann signs (spondylitis).
      Red-purple subcutaneous nodules on the extension faces of the limbs (erythema nodosum).
      Important skin ulcerative lesions (pyoderma gangrenosum).
      Eyes, eye pain, photophobia (eye damage).
      Pain in the right hypochondrium, scratches, jaundice (primitive sclerosing cholangit.
  - Crohn's disease:
    Similar to UC.
    Ulcerations in the oral cavity (affecting the oral cavity).
    Poor swallowing (esophageal damage).
    Palpable masses usually in the right abdominal quadrant (ileo-colonic damage).
    Fissures, fistulas, abscesses (perianal damage).

- Paraclinical examinations.
  - Serological examinations:
      Markers for inflammation severity: ESR, C-reactive protein, fibrinogen, fecal calprotectin, ferritin.
      Anemia.
      Leukocytosis.
      Thrombocytosis.
      Hypoalbuminemia.
      Hydroelectrolytic imbalances.
      Hypocalcemia.
      Hypophosphataemia.
      p-ANCA antibodies (suggestive of UC),
      Anti-saccharomyces cerevisiae antibodies (suggestive of CD).

28.5   The Role of Endoscopy

- **ESD** is essential for assessing the extent, severity, respectively, for confirming the definite diagnosis and the differential diagnosis (Fig. 28.1a, b).
  - Ulcerative colitis.
      Involves the rectum and extends proximal.
      Can affect the entire colon (pancolitis).

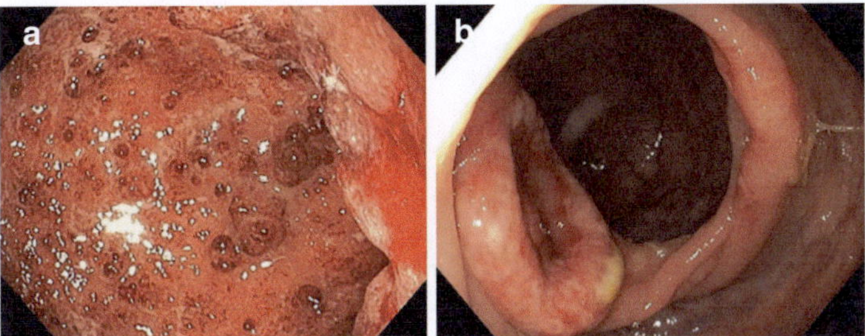

Fig. 28.1 Endoscopic images suggestive of severe ulcerative colitis, with friability, edema, ulceration, and pseudopolyps (**a**), respectively Crohn's disease, with edematous ileocecal valve, with multiple aphthous erosions (**b**)

In pancolitis there may be minimal inflammation on a short portion of the ileum (terminal ileitis – "backwash ileitis").

The lesions are continuous.

When the inflammation is moderate, the colonic mucosa is erythematous, with a fine granular surface.

Severe inflammation is characterized by friable, hemorrhagic, edematous mucosa with erosions and ulcerations (Fig. 28.2a, b).

In long-term evolutions, pseudopolyps appear as a result of regenerative processes.

In fulminant colitis (toxic colitis, toxic megacolon), the mucosa is ulcerated with a thin colonic wall, perforations may occur.

Severe seizure contraindicates colonoscopy; unprepared rectosigmoidoscopy is recommended.

Chromoendoscopic techniques are indicated for the detection of dysplasia and the prevention of colorectal cancer (Fig. 28.3a, b).

– Crohn's disease.

Segmental inflammation of the mucosa.

Small aphthoid ulcerations (1–5 mm) with whitish base and hyperemic halo.

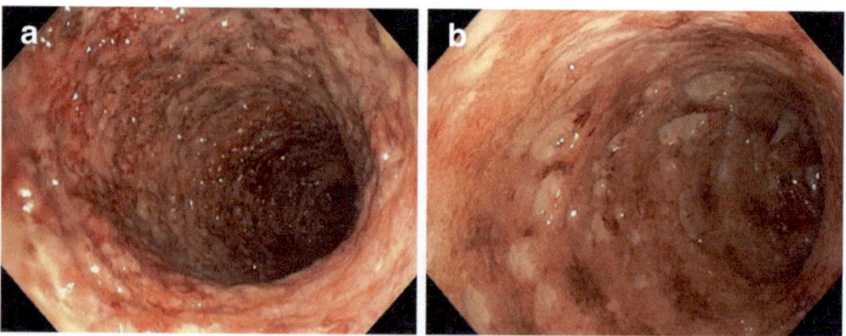

Fig. 28.2 Severe ulcerative colitis, with friable mucosa, edema, erosions and ulcerations, the colon being tubular, completely dehaustrated (**a, b**)

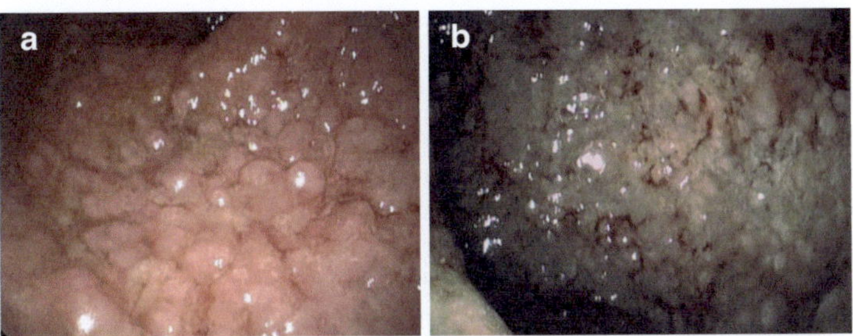

Fig. 28.3 Severe ulcerative colitis, with friable mucosa, edema, erosions and ulcerations, with multiple pseudopolyps visualized in white light (**a**) and I-scan (**b**)

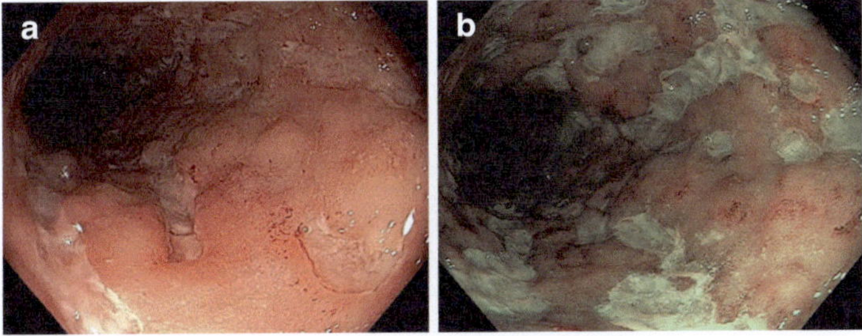

Fig. 28.4 Severe Crohn's disease, with friable mucosa, edema, and deep ulcerations, visualized with white light (**a**) and NBI mode (**b**)

Deep, interconnected ulcers, most often longitudinal, which give the characteristic Appearance of the "paving stone" mucosa (Fig. 28.4a, b).

Erythema, spontaneous bleeding, and severe edema are also common.

In the case of long evolution, stenoses of different degrees and fistular orifices can be detected.

Chromoendoscopic techniques are indicated for the detection of dysplasia and the prevention of colorectal cancer (Fig. 28.5a, b).

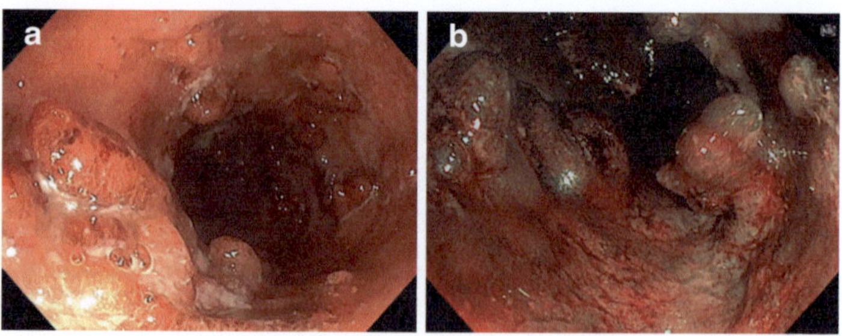

Fig. 28.5 Severe Crohn's disease, with friable mucosa, edema, and pseudo-polipoid lesions, visualized with white light (**a**) and NBI mode (**b**)

Table 28.1 Truelove–Witts classification of ulcerative colitis

Parameter	Mild	Moderate	Severe
Blood stools/day	<4	$\geq$4, <6	$\geq$6
Pulse	<90 beat/min	$\leq$90 beat/min	>90 beat/min
Temperature	<37.5 °C	$\leq$37.8 °C	>37.8 °C
Hb	>11.5 g/dL	$\geq$10.5 g/dL	<10.5 g/dL
ESR	<20 mm/h	$\leq$30 mm/h	>30 mm/h
C-reactive protein	Normal	<30 mg/L	>30 mg/L

- Pathological examination (Tables 28.1, 28.2, 28.3, 28.4, and 28.5).
  - Ulcerative colitis:
    Biopsies are taken in stages, at an interval of 5 or 10 cm depending on the duration of the disease period, the degree of dysplasia described in previous evaluations.
    Inflammation limited to the mucosa and submucosa.
    Deep damage in fulminant forms.
    Crypts are bifid and numerically reduced.
    Inflammatory infiltrate rich in neutrophils, lymphocytes, plasma cells and macrophages.
    Invasion of neutrophils at the level of crypts causes cryptites and cryptic abscesses.

Table 28.2 Mayo score in ulcerative colitis (combines clinical parameters with the endoscopic appearance of the mucosa and doctor's assessment; 0–2 means remission, 3–6 mild severity, 7–9 moderate severity, > 10 significant disease activity)

Mayo score	0	1	2	3
Stool frequency	Normal	1–2/day > N	3–4/day > N	4/day > N
Rectal bleeding	No blood	Traces of blood	Obvious blood	Emission of blood without a stool
Appearance of the mucosa	Normal	Erythema, granularity, decreased vascular pattern, friability	1 + erosions and disappearance of the vascular pattern	2 + spontaneous ulcerations and bleeding
Physician's evaluation	Normal	Mild	Moderate	Severe

Table 28.3 Crohn's disease activity index (CDAI) score

CDAI	Clinical classification
<150	Remission Asymptomatic patient
150–220	Mild to moderate form Good food tolerance No signs of dehydration 3–4 chairs/day ± pathological products Weight loss <10% of initial weight
220–450	Moderate-severe form > 4 chairs/day ± pathological products Abdominal pain Nausea/vomiting Weight loss >10% of initial weight Anemia, fever, chills, palpable ions
>450	Severe fulminating Patients who meet the above criteria but more severe and persistent, associate altered general condition, cachexia, do not respond to the maximum conventional therapy

Table 28.4 Montreal classification of Crohn's disease

Age	A1 < 16 years	A2 17–40 years	A3 > 40 years	
Location	L1: Ileal	L2: Colonic	L3: Ileocolonic	L4: Isolated upper disease
Behavior	B1 (non-stenotic, non-penetrating)	B2 (stenotic)	B3 (penetrating)	P (perianala disease)

Table 28.5 Appreciated clinical response after modification of CDAI score

	Response	CDAI
1	Clinical response	CDAI decrease by>70 points
2	Clinical remission	CDAI <150 puncte

- Crohn's disease:

   Biopsies are taken in stages, at an interval of 5 or 10 cm depending on the duration of the disease period, the degree of dysplasia described in previous evaluations.

   Inflammation is transmural.

   Aphthoid ulcers and cryptic abscesses are the initial lesions.

   Epithelioid granuloma resulting from agglutination of epithelioid cells, macrophages, monocytes, lymphocytes and eosinophils, without central necrosis, is the characteristic lesion of CD.

   The granuloma is detected in less than 30% of the biopsies taken endoscopically.

   Transmural fibrosis that causes stenosis, occurs late in the course of the disease.

   neighboring adipose tissue is affected by inflammation, Lymph nodes occur frequently and specific granuloma lesions can be encountered.

28.6   Imaging Examinations

- Simple abdominal radiography: useful in diagnosing complications (occlusion, perforation, megacolon).
- CT / MRI: evaluation of extramural complications, assessment of severity depending on wall thickness and vascularization, characterization of stenoses (Fig. 28.6a, f) and fistulas.
- Ultrasonography: diagnosis and surveillance.

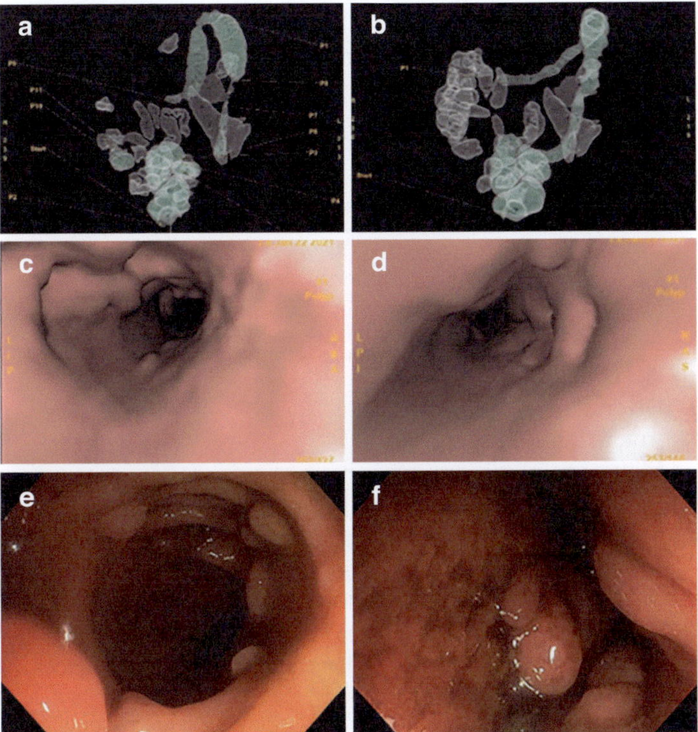

Fig. 28.6 Severe colonic Crohn's disease, with stenosis in the descending colon visualized by CT virtual colonography, with 3D reconstructions (**a**, **b**), fly-through images (**c**, **d**) and colonoscopic correspondent (**e**, **f**). Colon fistula demonstrated by the passage of inhaled gas into the anterior and posterior pararenal space (**a**, **b**)

- Evaluates the wall thickness (<5 mm).
- Evaluates the integrity of the five layers of the intestinal wall and vascularization.
- Stenoses and post-stenotic dilatations can be visualized.
- Identifies lymphadenopathy and abscesses.
- The results are operator-dependent.
- Video capsule
  - Useful in the diagnosis of small bowel CD.
  - Avoid administration if any stenosis is suspected.

28.7 Differential Diagnosis

- Appendicitis.
- Intestinal tuberculosis.
- Infectious colitis.
- Intestinal lymphoma.
- Colorectal cancer.
- Lactose intolerance.
- Celiac disease.
- Irritable bowel syndrome.
- Ischemic colitis.
- Diverticulitis.
- Irradiation colitis.
- Microscopic colitis.
- NSAID-induced enteropathy [1].

28.8 Principles of Treatment

- **Therapeutic goals** in IBD have changed with advances in understanding pathogenesis.
- **The goal** is to induce and maintain clinical and endoscopic remission without corticosteroid therapy, preventing complications and repeated hospitalizations.
- **General treatment measures.**
  - In the onset of the disease: hypercaloric, hyperprotein diet, rich in vitamins and minerals.

- Foods that accelerate intestinal transit or are irritating the intestines (sweets, spices, intolerant foods) are eliminated from the diet.
- Parenteral nutrition is reserved for complications (perforation, toxic megacolon).
- Correction of anemia by administration of erythrocyte mass and Fe-injectable preparations.
- Prophylaxis of thromboembolism in the phases of disease activity.
- Prophylaxis of osteoporosis through exercise, administration of calcium and vitamin D3 supplements.

- **Drugs** used in the treatment of IBD.
  - Aminosalicylates.
      Anti-inflammatory effect in doses of 2–4 g/day.
      Are usually very well tolerated by patients.
      Dose-dependent side effects are nausea, headache, vomiting, folate malabsorption.
      Dose-independent effects (hemolytic anemia, cholestasis, rash, neutropenia, male infertility).
      It is indicated in inducing and maintaining remission in mild forms of the disease.
  - Corticosteroids.
      Potent anti-inflammatory and immunosuppressive effect.
      It is indicated in inducing remission in severe forms of the disease (40–60 mg methyl-Prednisolone per day/400 mg HHC per day).
      Long-term use is not recommended.
  - Immunomodulators,
      Used to maintain remission (azatiprine, 6-mercaptopurine, cyclosporine).
      Maximum effect after about 3–6 months.
      It is necessary to monitor the blood count, liver and pancreatic tests.
      Cyclosporine is the second line of treatment in case of failure of corticosteroid remission induction therapy after 72 h, alternative to infliximab.

- Biological agents.

     The most efficient in inducing and maintaining remissions.

     Depending on the mode of action are divided into:
          Anti-TNFα antibodies (infliximab, adalimumab).
          Anti-integrin antibodies (vedolizumab).
          Anti-IL12/23 antibodies (ustekinumab).
          JAK-kinase inhibitors (tofacitinib).

     Is recommended for the induction and maintenance of remission in moderate and severe forms of the disease that have not responded to corticosteroid therapy associated with immunosuppressants.

     Discontinuation of treatment and non-association with immunosuppressants may be hampered by the development of antibodies against biological agents that will compromise the response to resumption of administration.

     Biological treatment is associated with an increased risk of contracting opportunistic infections.

          Extended screening is recommended to detect infections before starting treatment.

- Surgical treatment is indicated in:
  - Acute fulminant colitis without response to drug therapy.
  - Perforations/toxic megacolon/severe bleeding.
  - Severe forms of the disease that do not respond to medication or have severe extraintestinal manifestations.
  - Detection of high-grade dysplasia or colorectal cancer [1, 2].
- **Ulcerative colitis**—differentiated treatment according to extension and severity.
  - Proctita.

     Medium and mild forms are treated with mesalazine suppositories, in the standard dose of 1 suppository per day (1 g). Forms that do not respond can receive 2–3 suppositories per day.

Therapy may be discontinued after induction of remission.

If relapses are frequent, chronic therapy with 1 g of intrarectal mesalazine per day is instituted.

Severe forms benefit from the induction of remission with systemic corticotherapy,

- Proctosigmoiditis (damage <50 cm):

    Medium and light forms are treated with mesalazine foam enemas.

    The combination of oral mesalazine has superior effects.

    Severe forms benefit from the induction of remission with systemic corticotherapy,

- Left colitis.

    Mild or moderate forms may respond to combination treatment with enemas with mesalazine (> 1 g/day) and oral mesalazine (3–4 g/day).

    Mild and moderate forms that do not respond to combination therapy with mesalazine, benefit from systemic corticosteroid therapy (40 mg/day) to achieve remission, with doses gradually decreasing by 5–10 mg/week and remission is maintained with mesalazine (approximately 2–3 g/day).

    In patients with frequent exacerbations, thiopurines are associated.

    Maintenance of remission in patients who were induced with biological therapy will be achieved with the same preparation.

- Pancolita.

    For the forms with medium severity, the first intention is to try the response to the combined therapy with mesalazine administered topically and orally (2–4 g orally +1 g enema).

    If the response does not appear after 3–4 weeks, systemic corticosteroid therapy is instituted (40 mg/day for 7 days with subsequent 5 mg/week dose reduction).

Alternatives to systemic corticosteroid therapy: budesonide (topical release in the colon) and beclomethasone.

Maintenance of remission is based on the administration of aminosalicylates.

- Severe colitis.

  Requires high doses of steroids to induce remission (60 mg/day).

  Lack of response after 3 days of treatment means failure of treatment.

  Rescue therapies with infliximab, cyclosporine, or more recently with vedolizumab or tofacitinib are required.

  If remission is induced with biological therapy, it will be kept for maintenance.

  An immunosuppressant (azathioprine) can be combined to increase efficiency and decrease immunogenicity.

  When a biological preparation loses its effectiveness, it is recommended to increase the doses until changing with another biological preparation, preferably with a different mechanism of action [1, 3, 4].

- **Crohn's disease**—differentiated treatment by extension and severity.

  - Mild ileal, ileo-colonic, colonic (limited to ascending colon) damage:

    The latest recommendations suggest the administration of budesonide 9 mg/day, with induction of clinical remission after 8 weeks.

    Mesalazine has no better effects than placebo and is not recommended.

    Rifaximin 800 mg/day may help induce remission, but not monotherapy.

  - Ileal, ileo-colonic, moderately active colonic damage.

    Attempts are made to induce remission by administration of budesonide or conventional corticosteroid therapy.

For unanswered forms or intolerant patients, it is recommended to initiate biological therapy.

- Ileal, ileo-colonic, severe colonic damage.

Systemic corticosteroid therapy is of choice for inducing remission.

In case of repeated outbreaks >2/year, it is recommended to initiate biological therapy that will be maintained and to maintain remission + the association of an immunosuppressant, recommended for better response and decreased immunogenicity.

Remission obtained with corticosteroid therapy will be maintained by administration of immunosuppressants (azathioprine, methotrexate); if the remission is prolonged, it is recommended to give up the immunosuppressant.

For patients who have lost the therapeutic response to years-TNFα agents it is recommended to use biological agents with another mechanism of action (ustekinumab/vedolizumab).

- Fistulizing CD.

Simple fistulas can respond to antibiotic treatment (metronidazole, ciprofloxacin) without the need for fistulotomes/seton placement.

For complex and recurrent fistulas, biological treatment is recommended from the beginning, associated or not with immunosuppressant [1, 5–7].

28.9 Complications

- Toxic megacolon (transverse colon diameter >6 cm):
  - In severe outbreaks of extensive IBD.
  - Can be precipitated by:

    Hydroelectrolytic imbalances (hypokalemia).

    Opiate use.

    Colonoscopy or colon preparation for colonoscopy.

- Obstructive complications.
  - Common in CD with localization in the small intestine but can occur in any segment of the digestive tract.
  - May occur in severe UC with long evolution.
- Severe lower gastrointestinal bleeding.
  - May require hemostasis colectomy.
- Colitis with Clostridium difficile.
  - Is frequently associated and increases mortality.
- Fistulas and abscesses.
  - About 1 in 3 patients with IBD will develop an abscess in the course of the disease.
  - Fistulas, characteristic of CD, can develop anywhere in the affected digestive tract.
    The perianal ones can even appear as a manifestation of onset.
- Cytomegalovirus colitis.
  - Refractory to corticosteroid treatment and difficult to diagnose (biopsy and highlighting of viral inclusions).
- Colorectal cancer.
  - The risk of development is proportional to the duration of the disease.
  - Hereditary-collateral antecedents, disease extension, presence of strictures, and pseudopolyps play an important role.
  - Most commonly located in the right colon.
  - There is an increased risk for the development of synchronous cancers.
  - After 8–10 years of disease, a screening colonoscopy is recommended every 1–2 years.
- Bone and kidney complications.
  - The consequence of malabsorption of calcium, Ca salts, and vitamin D.
- Thromboembolic complications.
  - Occur especially in hospitalized patients with severe disease outbreaks.
  - Anticoagulant treatment with low-molecular-weight heparins is indicated.

28.10 Prognosis

- IBD have an undulating evolution, with periods of activity that alternate with periods of remission.
- Clinical remission (absence of symptoms) is not synonymous with disease control.
- During evolution, 30% of patients need surgery to control the condition.
  - Consecutively, short bowel syndrome or even the need for a colostomy may occur.
  - Surgeries are not curative, IBD recurrence may occur.
  - Factors associated with an unfavorable prognosis:
    Age less than 30 years at the time of diagnosis.
    Extended disease.
    The presence of deep ulcers.
    Fistulizing or stenotic forms of the disease.
    Surgical resections in the history of the disease.
    Severe perianal and/or rectal damage.
- Mortality of patients with IBD is not significantly increased compared to the general population.
- However, the quality of life is significantly lower [1, 5, 6].

References

1. Trifan A, Gheorghe C, Dumitrascu D, Diculescu M, Gheorghe L, Sporea I, Tantau M, Ciurea T. Gastroenterologie și Hepatologie Clinică, București; 2018.
2. AGA medical position statement. Guidelines on osteoporosis in gastrointestinal disease. Gastroenterology. 2003;124:791–4.
3. Coward S, Kuenzig ME, Hazlewood G, et al. Comparative effectiveness of mesalamine, sulfasalazine, corticosteroids, and budesonide for the induction of remission in Crohn's disease: a Bayesian network meta-analysis: republished. Inflamm Bowel Dis. 2017;23:E26–37.
4. Colombel JF, Shin A, Gibson PR. AGA clinical practice update on functional gastrointestinal symptoms in patients with inflammatory bowel disease: expert review. Clin Gastroenterol Hepatol. 2019;17:380–390.e1.

5. Steinhart AH, Panaccione R, Targownik L, et al. Clinical practice guideline for the medical management of perianal fistulizing Crohn's disease: the Toronto consensus. Inflamm Bowel Dis. 2019;25:1–13.
6. Panés J, Rimola J. Perianal fistulizing Crohn's disease: pathogenesis, diagnosis and therapy. Nat Rev Gastroenterol Hepatol. 2017;14:652–64.
7. Moja L, Danese S, Fiorino G, Del Giovane C, Bonovas S. Systematic review with network meta-analysis: comparative efficacy and safety of budesonide and mesalazine [mesalamine] for Crohn's disease. Aliment Pharmacol Ther. 2015;41:1055–65.

Irritable Bowel Syndrome

29

Irina F. Cherciu Harbiyeli
and Adrian Săftoiu

29.1   Definition

- Chronic, functional frequently debilitating gastrointestinal disorder.
- Recurrent abdominal pain associated with defecation changes.

29.2   Classification [1]

- On the basis of the patient's stool characteristics, as defined by the Bristol stool form scale (BSFS):
    - IBS with constipation (IBS-C): >25% of bowel movements associated with BSFS 1 or 2, <25% of bowel movements BSFS 6 or 7.
    - IBS with diarrhea (IBS-D): >25% of bowel movements associated with BSFS 6 or 7, < 25% of bowel movements with BSFS 1 or 2.

I. F. Cherciu Harbiyeli (✉)
Research Center of Gastroenterology and Hepatology Craiova,
University of Medicine and Pharmacy of Craiova, Craiova, Romania

A. Săftoiu
Department of Gastroenterology and Hepatology, Elias Emergency
University Hospital, Carol Davila University of Medicine, Bucharest,
Romania

A. Săftoiu (ed.), *Pocket Guide to Advanced Endoscopy in
Gastroenterology*, https://doi.org/10.1007/978-3-031-42076-4_29

- IBS with mixed bowel habits (IBS-M): >25% of bowel movements associated with both BSFS 1 or 2 and BSFS 6 or 7.
- Un-subtyped IBS(IBS-U): insufficient abnormality of stool consistency to meet criteria.
- On clinical grounds:
  - Based on symptoms:
    IBS with predominant bowel dysfunction.
    IBS with predominant pain.
    IBS with predominant bloating.
  - Based on precipitating factors:
    Postinfectious (PI-IBS).
    Food-induced (meal-induced).
    Stress-related.

29.3 Pathophysiology [2]

- Multifactorial.
- Key roles are played by:
  - Disorders of intestinal motility.
  - Disorders of gut-brain interactions.
  - Dysregulation of intestinal microbiota.
  - Mucosal inflammation.
  - Neurotransmitters and endocrine substances.
  - Diet rich on poorly absorbed, easily fermentable oligo-, di-, monosaccharides and polyols (FODMAPs).
  - Stress, coexisting psychological or psychiatric conditions.
  - Genetics.

29.4 Epidemiology [1, 2]

- The prevalence.
  - Depends on sex, age, residential area, or occupation.
  - In the global population is estimated at 11%.

- – In women is about twice as high as in men.
- – Is not higher among obese individuals.
- IBS mainly occurs between the ages of 15–65 years.
- Half of patients report their first symptoms before the age of 35. In some cases, symptoms may date back to childhood.
- The first presentation of patients to a physician is usually in the 30–50 years old age group.
- PI-IBS develops in 8–31% of patients with a previous acute infectious episode of gastrointestinal inflammation.

29.5 Diagnosis

- A positive diagnostic approach is recommended versus the exclusion diagnostic strategy for optimizing the time to initiate a proper therapy and cost-effectiveness.
- Diagnostic cascade for IBS: taking a thoughtful history, clinical examination, exclusion of alarm symptoms, taking into consideration psychological disorders.

29.6 Clinical Manifestations [3–5]

- Common:
  - – Abdominal pain (relieved by defecation).
  - – Abdominal bloating (reported by up to 96% of patients with IBS), tenesmus.
  - – Abnormal stool form (hard and/or loose), stool frequency (less than three times per week/over three times per day), straining at defecation, urgency, sensation of incomplete evacuation, passage of mucus per rectum.
- Associated noncolonic symptoms:
  - – Dyspepsia, nausea, heartburn, lethargy, fatigue, backache and other muscle and joint pains, fibromyalgia, headache, urinary symptoms (nocturia, frequency and urgency of micturition, incomplete bladder emptying), dyspareunia in women, insomnia, low tolerance to medications in general.

29.6.1 Rome IV Diagnostic Criteria

- Recurrent abdominal pain on average at least 1 day/week in the last 3 months, associated with two or more of the following*:
  - Related to defecation.
  - Accompanied by a change in frequency of stool.
  - Accompanied by a change in form (appearance) of stool.

*Criteria should be fulfilled for the last 3 months with symptom onset over 6 months prior to diagnosis.

29.6.2 History

- The patients:
  - Should be allowed to tell their story in their own words.
  - Approximately half the consulting patients believe they have serious disease such as cancer.
  - Ensure that they feel the doctor has understood their concerns and expectations are met, as previous consultations may have been unsatisfactory in this respect.
- The clinician:
  - Inquires about the family history of IBS or colon cancer (particularly below the age of 50).
  - Should make an effort to understand the psychosocial factors which might have led the patient to seek help at this particular time.
  - Ensure optimal eye contact, adopts a body language which conveys empathy, elaborates open-ended questioning designed to elicit the patient's ideas.
  - Forming a nice patient-doctor relationship impacts the evolution of IBS.
  - Such practice can reduce reconsultation rates.

29.6.3 Behavioral Features Helpful in Recognizing IBS

- Symptoms occur for >6 months.
- Stress is aggravating symptoms.
- Frequent consultations for nongastrointestinal symptoms.
- History of previous medically unexplained symptoms.
- Aggravation of symptoms after meals, associated anxiety, and/or depression.
- Parental reinforcement of illness behavior and children borrowing their parent's behavior.

29.6.4 Physical Examination

- A physical examination reassures the patient and helps detect possible organic causes.
- General examination for signs of systemic disease should be followed by abdominal examination.
  - This includes asking the patient to demonstrate the area of pain.
- Examination of the perianal region and digital rectal exam.
- Physical examination usually reveals no significant abnormality.

29.7 Paraclinical Investigations [2, 3, 5]

- First level:
  - Full blood count.
  - Erythrocyte sedimentation rate.
  - C-reactive protein.
  - Coeliac serology (endomysial antibodies—EMA or tissue transglutaminase—TTG).
  - Liver function tests.

- Second level:
  - Ultrasonography.
  - Rigid or flexible sigmoidoscopy.
  - Colonoscopy and biopsy.
  - Barium enema.
  - Thyroid function test.
  - Stool studies (white blood cells, ova, parasites).
  - Fecal occult blood test.
  - Hydrogen breath test.
  - Calprotectin or lactoferrin.
  - Selenium homocholic acid taurine test (SeHCAT).

29.7.1 Colonoscopy

- Carries a high diagnostic value as it both excludes organic diseases and reveals the presence of pathophysiological mechanisms compatible to IBS (due to visceral hypersensitivity, the insufflations of air during the colonoscopic procedures might reproduce the pain).
- It is indicated only in justified cases, when coexisting red flag signs:
  - Age > 50 years.
  - Family history for colon cancer, celiac disease, inflammatory bowel diseases.
  - Recent treatment with antibiotic.
  - Trips in endemic regions with infectious or parasitic diseases.
  - Short duration of symptoms.
  - Occurrence of symptoms at night.
  - Unintentional weight loss.
  - Fever.
  - Bleeding from the lower gastrointestinal tract.
  - Abdominal tumor or mass.
  - Ascites.
  - Anemia.

- It allows collecting biopsy specimen, hence the histopathological examination of the gut mucosa. Increased mucosal permeability with increased number of mast cells, enterochromaffin cells and inflammatory cells, are characteristics supporting IBS features and the exclusion of collagenous colitis or celiac disease.

Esophagogastroduodenoscopy and distal duodenal biopsy in patients with diarrhea is useful:

- To rule out celiac disease, tropical sprue, giardiasis.
- In patients with abdominal pain and discomfort located predominantly in the upper abdomen.

29.7.2 Other Gastroenterological Imaging Examinations

- Abdominal ultrasonography, abdominal computer tomography scan, abdominal magnetic resonance imaging or plain X-ray of the abdomen, barium enema.
  - Are useful for differentiating IBS from organic diseases in some cases.

29.7.3 Examinations of Gastrointestinal Function

- Anorectal or colonic manometry, gastrointestinal transit or hydrogen breath test:
  - Are not universally available.
  - Are suitable for differentiating IBS from anorectal dysfunction or SIBO.
  - Anorectal physiology testing should be directed toward the patients with IBS and symptoms recalling a pelvic floor disorder and/or constipation refractory to conventional medical therapy and dietary changes.

29.7.4 Signs Suggesting Another Disease Than IBS

- Age > 40 years.
- History <6 months.
- Weight loss and anorexia.
- Waking at night with pain/diarrhea.
- Mouth ulcers.
- Abnormal investigation findings.

29.8   Differential Diagnosis [5]

- Celiac disease.
- Bile acid malabsorption.
- Lactose malabsorption.
- Inflammatory bowel disease.
- Colorectal carcinoma.
- Microscopic (lymphocytic and collagenous) colitis.
- Acute or chronic diarrhea caused by protozoa or bacteria, giardiasis, tropical sprue.
- Diverticulitis.
- Endometriosis.
- Pelvic inflammatory disease.
- Ovarian cancer.
- Colitis associated with NSAIDs.
- Small bowel bacterial overgrowth.

29.9   Management

- Diet and lifestyle might trigger or aggravate symptoms.
- Highlight the importance of self-reliance in efficiently managing IBS.
- Offer information on lifestyle and nutrition, physical activity, and medication addressing symptoms.

29.10 Treatment [2, 5, 6]

- The aim of therapy is the improvement of IBS symptoms.
- **Diet therapy**:
    - Have regular meals and take time to eat.
    - Avoid missing meals or leaving long gaps between eating.
    - Eliminating high-fat foods and avoiding spicy foods.
    - Embracing low fermentable oligo-di-monosaccharide and polyol (FODMAP) diet.
    - Drink at least eight cups of fluid per day (water, herbal teas).
    - Restrict black tea and coffee to three cups per day.
    - Reduce intake of alcohol and fizzy drinks.
    - Limit fresh fruit to three portions per day (a portion = aproximately 80 g).
    - People with diarrhea should avoid sorbitol, found in sugar-free sweets and drinks, in some diabetic and slimming products.
    - People with wind and bloating could benefit from eating oats (oat-based breakfast cereal or porridge) and linseeds (up to one tablespoon per day).
    - Excess high fiber may exacerbate symptoms→review fiber intake and adjust it according to symptoms (should be limited to 12 g a day).
    - It is recommended the use of soluble fibers or bulking polymers (psyllium, ispaghula, and polycarbophil calcium), but not insoluble fiber (ineffective and even worsened IBS symptoms in some patients).
    - Reduce the intake of "resistant starch," which is often found in processed or re-cooked foods.
    - Consider referral to a dietitian for advice on avoidance of single foods and an exclusion diet.
- Behavioral modifications.
    - Eliminating alcohol and smoking, exercise, properly sleeping, taking rest.
    - Are effective at reducing IBS symptoms.

- **Antispasmodics** for colic and bloating.
  - Trimebutine maleate, mebeverine, hyoscine butylbromide, butylscopolamine, alverine citrate.
- **Anti-diarrheal agents** are effective for some patients with IBS-D.
  - Bulking agents and loperamide hydrochloride (2 mg after each loose stool).
- Probiotics.
  - Are recommended for IBS.
  - Patients should administer the product for at least 4 weeks while monitoring the effect.
- Laxatives.
  - Are effective for some patients with IBS-C.
  - Macrogols, polyethylene glycol, lactulose, sorbitol, magnesium oxide.
  - The long-term use of anthraquinone derivatives (e.g., senna) should be done with caution because of its undesirable side effects: electrolyte abnormalities, development of tolerance, colon pigmentation (pseudo-melanosis coli).
  - The dose should be titrated in accordance with stool consistency, aiming to achieve a soft, well-formed stool (corresponding to Bristol Stool Form Scale type 4).
- **Enemas,** as rescue medication, are effective for some patients with IBS-C.
- **Antimicrobial agents.**
  - Rifaximin may be effective in reducing global symptoms of IBS-D, the benefit lasting up to 10 weeks after treatment.
- **Mucosal epithelium modifiers**.
  - Are recommended for treating IBS-C.
  - Chloride channel activators (lubiprostone), help peristalsis, determine coordinated muscle contractions.
  - Guanylate cyclase activators (linaclotide), accelerate the movement of the gastrointestinal tract content and block painful signals.
- **Bile acid sequestrants** should not be used to treat global IBS-D symptoms.

- **5-HT35-HT3 receptor antagonists**.
  - Effective in treating IBS-D.
  - Ramosetron improves stool consistency, health-related quality of life and reduces abdominal pain/bloating.
  - Alosetron is used to relieve global symptoms in women with severe symptoms who have failed conventional therapy. It blocks the transmission of painful/painless sensations from the intestines to the brain.
- **5-HT45-HT4 receptor agonists**.
  - Effective in IBS-C patients whose bowel symptoms are refractory to usual laxatives.
  - Prucalopride may improve stool consistency and quality of life, reduces abdominal pain/bloating.
- Antidepressants.
  - Tricyclic antidepressants (TCA) or selective serotonin reuptake inhibitors (SSRIs) are recommended for some patients with IBS, being aware of the side effects.
  - Consider TCA as second-line treatment for abdominal pain or discomfort if laxatives, antispasmodics, or loperamide have been unhelpful.
  - Consider SSRIs for people with IBS only if TCAs are ineffective.
- **Anxiolytics** are recommended only for patients with high levels of anxiety, experiencing IBS for a short period of time.
- **Psychological interventions**.
  - Cognitive behavioral therapy, hypnotherapy, and/or psychotherapies should be considered for people with IBS who do not respond to pharmacotherapy after 12 months and who develop a continuing symptom profile (refractory IBS).
  - May help patients cope with their symptoms without necessarily abolishing it.
- **Comprehensive alternative medicine**.
  - Except for peppermint oil, it is almost entirely noneffective in treating IBS.
- **Placebo** is effective on approximately 40% patients with IBS.

29.11 Prognosis

- Symptoms of IBS are likely to decline after the age of 50.
- Subtypes of IBS show transition over time.
- Comorbidities: functional dyspepsia, GERD, extraintestinal disorders (fibromyalgia, chronic fatigue syndrome), chronic idiopathic constipation, celiac disease, IBD, anxiety, depression.

References

1. Quigley EM, Fried M, Gwee KA, et al. World Gastroenterology Organisation global guidelines irritable bowel syndrome: a global perspective update September 2015. J Clin Gastroenterol. 2016;50:704–13.
2. Spiller R, Aziz Q, Creed F, et al. Guidelines on the irritable bowel syndrome: mechanisms and practical management [published correction appears in gut 2008; 57: 1743]. Gut. 2007;56:1770–98.
3. Song KH, Jung HK, Kim HJ, et al. Clinical practice guidelines for irritable bowel syndrome in Korea, 2017 revised edition. J Neurogastroenterol Motil. 2018;24:197–215.
4. Fukudo S, Kaneko H, Akiho H, et al. Evidence-based clinical practice guidelines for irritable bowel syndrome. J Gastroenterol. 2015;50:11–30.
5. National Institute for Health and Clinical Excellence. Irritable bowel syndrome in adults. Diagnosis and management of irritable bowel syndrome in primary care. London: NICE; 2008. www.nice.org.uk/CG061.
6. Lacy BE, Pimentel M, Brenner DM, et al. ACG Clinical Guideline: Management of Irritable Bowel Syndrome [published online ahead of print, 2020 Dec 14]. Am J Gastroenterol. 2021;116:17–44. https://doi.org/10.14309/ajg.0000000000001036.

Malabsorbtion Syndrome

30

Irina F. Cherciu Harbiyeli
and Adrian Săftoiu

30.1 Definition [1]

- Complex clinical entity
  - symptoms secondary to maldigestion and/or malabsorption, emerging when the extension of the condition surpasses the ability of intestine compensation
- Malabsorbtion represents the deteriorated nutrient absorption at any anatomic level
- Maldigestion is the deteriorated nutrient digestion within the intestinal lumen or at the brush border

I. F. Cherciu Harbiyeli (✉)
Research Center of Gastroenterology and Hepatology Craiova,
University of Medicine and Pharmacy Craiova, Craiova, Romania

A. Săftoiu
Department of Gastroenterology and Hepatology, Carol Davila
University of Medicine, Bucharest, Romania

A. Săftoiu (ed.), *Pocket Guide to Advanced Endoscopy in
Gastroenterology*, https://doi.org/10.1007/978-3-031-42076-4_30

30.2   Classification [2]

- **Global malabsorbion**
  - poor absorption of almost all nutrients due to diffuse damage of the small bowel mucosa or reduction of the absorption surface
- **Partial or isolated malabsorption**
  - results from diseases that interfere with the absorption of specific nutrients

30.3   Epidemiology

- Malabsorption affects millions of people worldwide
  - the prevalence and incidence are ambiguous due to the multiple etiologies of malabsorption syndromes

30.4   Etiology

- Malabsorption syndromes:
  - originate from dysfunction at any level of digestion or absorption
  - arise from the liver, pancreas, stomach, or intestines
  - can result from congenital/acquired defects or after surgery

30.5   Pathophysiology [2, 3]

- Malabsorption and maldigestion are pathophysiologically dissimilar although the processes of digestion/absorption are codependent (Table 30.1)
- There are three stages of nutrient absorption possibly affected
  - the luminal phase involves mechanical and enzymatic degradation of food
  - the parietal phase demands an intact and functional mucosal brush border

Table 30.1 Examples of pathologies associated with malabsorption and maldigestion

	Examples
Malabsorption	Celiac disease, tropical sprue, Whipple's disease, chronic mesenteric ischemia, short bowel syndrome, small intestinal bacterial overgrowth, lymphatic obstruction, Crohn's disease, biliopancreatic pathologies, gastric surgery, giardiasis, HIV enteropathy
Maldigestion	Decreased bile salts (cirrhosis, bile duct obstruction, ileal resection), pancreatic dysfunction (chronic pancreatitis, cystic fibrosis, duct obstruction)

- the intracellular (postabsorptive) phase is enabled by an undamaged blood supply and lymphatic system
- The etiopathogenetic mechanisms:
  - degradation of digestive processes
  - deterioration of uptake and transport, triggered by alteration or reduction of absorption surface
  - mixed

30.5.1 Celiac Disease

- Small intestine malabsorption
  - provoked by gluten ingestion in genetically susceptible patients, often of European descent
  - can initially present as a watery diarrhea that may be confused with IBS
  - classically associates chronic diarrhea, fatigue, weight loss and hypochromic, microcytic, hyposideremic anemia

30.5.2 Small Intestinal Bacterial Overgrowth (SIBO)

- Characteristics
  - patients with anatomical or functional abnormalities of the oro-cecal transit have been reported to be at increased risk for SIBO

- predisposing factors
    diabetes
    scleroderma
    intestinal pseudo-obstruction
    prior surgery (gastric surgery involving a blind loop, terminal ileal resection)
    diverticulosis
- is associated with achlorhydria (in old age patients or therapy with proton-pump inhibitors)
- the difficulty in establishing a positive diagnosis of SIBO is the lack of a standardized investigation tool (currently breath test, small intestine aspirate, and fluid culture)
- bacterial overgrowth, mainly due to coliforms and enterococci, could occur in seemingly healthy individuals with no sign of malabsorption

30.5.3 Short Bowel Syndrome

- Characteristics
    - a condition commonly found in patients who have undergone an extensive surgical resection of the small bowel
    - decreased absorption of macronutrients and/or water and electrolytes, impaired synthesis of gastrointestinal hormones, and accelerated intestinal transit are responsible for malabsorption
    - clinical manifestations are various and depend on the localization and extension of resection
    - the most common causes are Crohn's disease, mesenteric ischemia, radiation enteritis, and postoperative complications

30.6 Diagnosis [4, 5]

- Malabsorption is associated with multifactorial disorders, making diagnosis difficult

- symptoms are nonspecific and are frequently mistaken for other conditions, resulting in a missed diagnosis
- Signs and symptoms
  - chronic diarrhea is the most common symptom, steatorrhea, weight loss, flatulence, postprandial abdominal pain
  - stool description: bulky, pale, with a glossy/greasy appearance, floating in water, malodorous; additionally, patients may report oil droplets in the toilet
  - non-gastrointestinal manifestations can include elevated levels of liver function markers, anemia, skin conditions, infertility, bone disease
- History
  - should review
      duration of symptoms and the time of onset
      characteristics of pain (presence/absence, location/irradiation/location changes, intensity, and its variations)
      stool appearance and changes in bowel habits
      associated symptoms
  - additional questions
      medical history (e.g., peptic ulcer)
      family history (systemic and gastrointestinal disorders)
      medication
      surgical interventions
      irradiation
      caustic substances ingestion
      allergies
      smoking, alcohol or drugs use
- Physical exam
  - hyper/hypoactive bowel sounds
  - abdominal distention or tenderness
  - pallor
  - rashes
  - ecchymosis
  - poor wound healing
  - hypotrophy
  - cardiac arrhythmia

- skeletal deformities
- abnormal deep tendon reflexes
- auditory disturbances
- decreased visual acuity
- cognitive impairment
- peripheral neuropathy
- Blood tests
  - complete blood count
  - CRP
  - complete metabolic panel (electrolyte disturbances, liver function tests, renal function tests) + lipid studies
  - thyroid function tests
  - coeliac serology (IgA/IgG anti-endomysial, tissue transglutaminase (tTG) IgA/IgG, anti-gliadin IgA/IgG antibodies)
  - vitamin levels (vitamin A, C, D, E, B12) + serum microelements (Mg, Zn, Se, Cu, Mn)
  - assessment of anemia (iron level, total iron-binding capacity, iron saturation, folate)
  - serum D-lactate
  - SeCHAT scan for the absorption capacity of bile acids
  - genetic testing (lactose/fructose intolerance)
- Stool tests
  - stool microscopy and culture
  - *C. difficile* antigen
  - fecal occult blood test
  - fecal calprotectin
  - stool pH
  - fecal fat globules
  - fecal alpha1 antitrypsin (a1-AT)
  - fecal elastase
- Breath tests
  - hydrogen breath test
  - ± lactose tolerance test
  - ± urine galactose
  - 13C-mixed-chain triglyceride breath test

- Imaging
  - endoscopy (duodenal biopsies, terminal ileum biopsies, jejunal aspirate for culture)
  - abdominal ultrasonography
  - abdominal X-ray/CT/MRCP
  - Technitium-99m scintigraphy

30.7   The Role of Endoscopy [6, 7]

- Useful for distinguishing malabsorptive from functional/inflammatory forms of diarrhea
- Inflammatory lesions, polyps, strictures, and other sources of bleeding can be visualized
- Endoscopy with biopsy
  - has some limitations because complete visualization of the small intestines is not usually possible
  - duodenal biopsies should be collected from the patients in whom small bowel malabsorption is suspected on clinical grounds, even if serology is negative, in order to evaluate the existence of other small bowel enteropathies

    obtaining a minimum of four duodenal biopsy specimens is recommended for evaluation of suspected celiac disease

    biopsy specimens obtained from the second or third portion of the duodenum with standard forceps are usually sufficient

    most experts recommend that a positive serologic test result for celiac disease should be confirmed with a biopsy of the intestinal mucosa
  - small bowel biopsies can target tissue that appears abnormal, but histologically lacks specificity, requiring further evaluation
  - it is possible to exclusively establish the diagnosis of malabsorption based on the endoscopic biopsy of a specific lesion

- limited data is published regarding the diagnostic performance of upper endoscopy in patients with diarrhea suspected to be associated to malabsorption
- Video capsule endoscopy (VCE)
  - is useful in detecting mucosal abnormalities of Crohn's and celiac disease
  - is often used as part of the diagnosis of anemia
  - it lacks the ability to obtain biopsy, hence to make a tissue diagnosis
  - because of the risk of retention, VCE is used with caution in conditions in which malignancy or stricturing Crohn's disease are suspected
- Although a diagnosis of celiac disease cannot be definitively made based on the endoscopic appearance of the small bowel (e.g., flattened/erased mucosal folds), magnification endoscopy may enhance the diagnostic yield and may be helpful in highlighting the diseased area for targeted biopsy
- Endoscopic ultrasound (EUS) is able to identify mild parenchymal and ductal abnormalities associated with chronic pancreatitis
- Endoscopic retrograde cholangio-pancreatography (ERCP) is a key diagnostic and management method for patients with hepatobiliary and pancreatic disorders
- The role of aspiration of enteric contents for quantitative bacterial culture is unclear

30.8   Management [8]

- Identification and treatment of underlying disease
- Treatment of diarrhea and other symptomatology
- Identification and correction of nutritional deficits

30.9   Treatment

- Celiac disease
  - discontinuation of gluten intake

- oral or intravenous iron, folate for anemia
  - vitamin C and D supplementation for osteopenia
- Short bowel syndrome:
  - intravenous fluid resuscitation
  - total parental nutrition
  - nutrient supplementation, pancreatic enzyme replacement
  - proton pump inhibitors, loperamide
  - surgical treatment (procedures to slow the passage of nutrients or to lengthen the intestine, intestinal transplantation)
- Exocrine pancreatic insufficiency:
  - pancreatic enzyme replacement therapy and replacement of fat-soluble vitamins
- Small bowel bacterial overgrowth (SIBO):
  - empirical antibiotic therapy (rifaximin, neomycin, metronidazole, tetracyclines, fluoroquinolones, etc.) in the absence of intestinal aspirate cultures
  - nutritional support: B_{12} and fat-soluble vitamins, calcium, and magnesium
  - surgical reparatory treatment, where appropriate
- Crohn's disease
  - nutritional supplementation: fats, iron, calcium, magnesium, vitamins (A, D, E, K, B12), folic acid, sodium, potassium

30.10 Prognosis [8]

- Malabsorption syndromes generally are not life-threatening
- Life-threatening or even fatal complications:
  - severe malnutrition from prolonged pancreatic exocrine insufficiency
  - life-threatening electrolyte disturbances from prolonged, intractable diarrhea
  - bowel perforation
  - hematologic disorders: anemia, coagulopathy
  - cardiovascular disease: cardiac arrhythmias
  - visual impairment

References

1. Clark R, Johnson R. Malabsorption syndromes. Nurs Clin North Am. 2018;53:361–74.
2. Montalto M, Santoro L, D'Onofrio F, et al. Classification of malabsorption syndromes. Dig Dis. 2008;26:104–11.
3. Keller J, Layer P. The pathophysiology of malabsorption. Viszeralmedizin. 2014;30:150–4.
4. Arasaradnam RP, Brown S, Forbes A, Fox MR, Hungin P, Kelman L, Major G, O'Connor M, Sanders DS, Sinha R, Smith SC, Thomas P, Walters JRF. Guidelines for the investigation of chronic diarrhoea in adults: British Society of Gastroenterology, 3rd edition. Gut. 2018;67(8):1380–99.
5. Nikaki K, Gupte GL. Assessment of intestinal malabsorption. Best Pract Res Clin Gastroenterol. 2016;30:225–35.
6. Shen B, Khan K, Ikenberry SO, Anderson MA, Banerjee S, Baron T, Ben-Menachem T, Cash BD, Fanelli RD, Fisher L, Fukami N, Gan SI, Harrison ME, Jagannath S, Lee Krinsky M, Levy M, Maple JT, Lichtenstein D, Stewart L, Strohmeyer L, Dominitz JA, ASGE Standards of Practice Committee. The role of endoscopy in the management of patients with diarrhea. Gastrointest Endosc. 2010;71(6):887–92.
7. Al-Toma A, Volta U, Auricchio R, Castillejo G, Sanders DS, Cellier C, Mulder CJ, Lundin KEA. European Society for the Study of Coeliac Disease (ESsCD) guideline for coeliac disease and other gluten-related disorders. United European Gastroenterol J. 2019;7(5):583–613.
8. Zuvarox T, Belletieri C. Malabsorption syndromes. In: StatPearls. Treasure Island: StatPearls Publishing; 2022. Available from https://www.ncbi.nlm.nih.gov/books/NBK553106/.

Acute Diarrhea

Irina F. Cherciu Harbiyeli

31.1 Definition [1, 2]

From a clinical perspective, diarrhea can be defined as the passage of:

- Three or more loose or liquid stools per 24 h, and/or
- Stools that are more frequent than normal, lasting <14 days, and/or
- Stool with increased water content, weighing >300 g/day

31.2 Classification [1, 2]

- Based on duration, diarrhea is classified as:
    - Acute (≤14 days)
    - Persistent (>14 days), or
    - Chronic (>4 weeks)
- Based on the cause, diarrhea is classified as:
    - Infectious, due to viruses, bacteria, and, less often, parasites. Viral infections are the most common cause of acute

I. F. Cherciu Harbiyeli (✉)
Research Center of Gastroenterology and Hepatology Craiova,
University of Medicine and Pharmacy Craiova, Craiova, Romania

© The Author(s), under exclusive license to Springer Nature Switzerland AG 2023
A. Săftoiu (ed.), *Pocket Guide to Advanced Endoscopy in Gastroenterology*, https://doi.org/10.1007/978-3-031-42076-4_31

Table 31.1 Classification and characteristics of diarrheal syndromes

Diarrheal syndromes	Noninflammatory	Inflammatory
Etiology	– Usually viral – Can be bacterial or parasitic	– Generally invasive or toxin-producing bacteria
History and examination findings	– Nausea, vomiting – Normothermia – Abdominal cramping – Stool: larger volume, nonbloody, watery – milder disease	– Fever – Abdominal pain, tenesmus – Stool: smaller volume, bloody – More severe disease
Laboratory findings	– Absence of fecal leukocytes	– Presence of fecal leukocytes
Common pathogens	Enterotoxigenic *Escherichia coli, Clostridium perfringens, Bacillus cereus, Staphylococcus aureus, Rotavirus, Norovirus, Giardia, Cryptosporidium, Vibrio cholerae*	*Salmonella* (non-Typhi species), *Shigella, Campylobacter,* Shiga toxin-producing *E. coli,* enteroinvasive *E. coli, Clostridium difficile, Entamoeba histolytica, Yersinia*

diarrhea. Bacterial infections are more often associated with travel, comorbidities, and foodborne illness.
- Noninfectious, due to medication adverse effects, acute abdominal processes, gastroenterological disease, and endocrine diseases.
• Clinically, acute infectious diarrhea is classified into:
  - Noninflammatory/watery diarrhea
  - Inflammatory/dysenteric diarrhea (mostly invasive or with toxin-producing bacteria, see Table 31.1)

31.3 Patient History [1, 2]

• Epidemiological clues: international travel, contaminated food and water supplies, sexual activity, daycare attendance, nursing home residents, recently hospitalized patients, animal exposure, outbreaks

- Recent use of antibiotics and other medications
- Exposure to other sick contacts
- Medical history:
  - gastroenterologic underlying conditions or surgery
  - endocrine or autoimmune disease
  - radiation to the pelvis
  - human immunodeficiency virus infection
  - long-term steroid use
  - chemotherapy
  - immunoglobulin A deficiency
  - pregnant women have a 12-fold increased risk of listeriosis
- Sexual practices increase the possibility of direct rectal inoculation and fecal-oral transmission

31.4 Physical Examination [2, 3]

- The primary goal is to assess the patient's degree of dehydration:
  - Generally ill appearance, dry mucous membranes, delayed capillary refill time, increased heart rate, blood pressure, respiratory rate and abnormal orthostatic vital signs, decreased urine output, thirst, dizziness, change in mental status
- The onset, duration, severity, volume and frequency of diarrhea, particular attention to stool character (e.g., watery, bloody, mucus-filled, purulent, bilious)
- Enteric symptoms:
  - Nausea, abdominal pain/cramps, fecal urgency, moderate to severe flatulence
  - Vomiting is more suggestive of viral illness or illness caused by ingestion of a preformed bacterial toxin
  - Fever, tenesmus, and grossly bloody stool are more suggestive of invasive bacterial (inflammatory) diarrhea

- The abdominal examination is important to assess for pain and acute abdominal processes
- A rectal examination may be helpful in assessing for blood, rectal tenderness, and stool consistency

31.5 Diagnostic Testing [2–4]

- Most watery diarrhea is self-limited: testing is usually not indicated
- Routine testing for ova and parasites in acute diarrhea is not necessary in developed countries
- Stool cultures should be reserved for: grossly bloody stool, severe dehydration, signs of inflammatory disease, moderate-severe illness, symptoms lasting >7 days, immunosuppression, men who have sex with men, suspected nosocomial infections, community outbreaks
- Testing for *Clostridium difficile* toxins A and B should be performed in patients who develop unexplained diarrhea after 3 days of hospitalization
- Individuals presenting fever or bloody diarrhea should be tested for enteropathogens counting *Salmonella enterica* subspecies, *Shigella* and *Campylobacter*
- The watery diarrhea subgroup with clinical dehydration will have to exclude cholera by stool examination with dark field microscopy confirmed later by stool culture
- For detection of bacterial infections, if a timely diarrheal stool sample cannot be collected, a rectal swab may be used
- Molecular techniques generally are more sensitive and less dependent than culture on the quality of specimen
- For identification of viral, protozoal agents and *C. difficile* toxin fresh stool is preferred
- Fecal leukocyte evaluation and stool lactoferrin detection are not recommended to be used for determining the etiology of acute infectious diarrhea
- There are insufficient data available to make a recommendation on the value of fecal calprotectin measurement in people with acute infectious diarrhea

31.6   Differential Diagnosis [3, 4]

- Conditions presenting as acute diarrhea ± signs of peritonitis:
  - Appendicitis
  - Adnexitis
  - Diverticulitis
  - Peritonitis secondary to bowel perforation
  - Systemic infections: malaria, measles, typhoid, etc.
  - Inflammatory bowel disease
  - Ischemic enterocolitis
  - Mesenteric artery/venous occlusion

31.7   The Role of Endoscopy in the Diagnosis and Management of Acute Diarrhea [3–6]

- Is limited
- Endoscopic evaluation may be considered if:
  - diagnosis is unclear after routine blood and stool tests
  - empiric therapy is ineffective
  - symptoms persist
  - worsening clinical course remains unresponsive to management
  - certain underlying medical conditions (as clinical colitis, proctitis, AIDS)
- Routine use of upper gastrointestinal endoscopy in self-limited illnesses is not indicated
  - Acute diarrheal illnesses are generally caused by infectious agents involving the lower part of the GI tract
- Colonoscopy should be considered if:
  - the findings at flexible sigmoidoscopy are inconclusive
  - the symptoms persist
  - there is large-volume blood loss
  - inflammatory bowel disease (IBD) or colorectal cancer is suspected

- Colonoscopy with biopsy and culture can be helpful in:
  - patients with diarrhea and suspected tuberculosis or diffuse colitis (as in C. difficile colitis)
  - determining noninfectious causes of acute diarrhea (inflammatory bowel disease, ischemic colitis, enteropathy related to nonsteroidal anti-inflammatory drug use, cancer)
- Duodenal aspirate may be considered for diagnosis of suspected *Giardia*, *Strongyloides*, *Cystoisospora*, or microsporidia infection
- Endoscopy with small bowel biopsy is useful for diagnosis of *Mycobacterium avium* complex and Microsporidiosis
- Flexible sigmoidoscopy:
  - may be a suitable initial investigation for the evaluation of acute diarrhea in patients with suspected diffuse colitis
  - biopsy may assist in differentiating infectious colitis from inflammatory bowel disease, CMV disease or *C. difficile* colitis
- Endoscopy is not recommended for patients with persisting symptoms (14 up to 30 days) and negative stool workup

31.8 Treatment [1–5]

- The first step to treating acute diarrhea is rehydration, preferably oral rehydration
- Diet: the majority of patients with acute diarrhea can maintain a proper level of fluids and electrolytes by ingesting water, sports drinks, juices, oral rehydration solutions, broths, soups, and saltine crackers. Dairy products, alcohol, caffeine, carbonated drinks, high-fiber foods should be avoided
- Antimotility agents (see Chap. 32) should not be administered in severe acute colitis as it might precipitate the toxic megacolon
- The loperamide/simethicone combination might provide more rapid and complete relief of symptoms related to acute nonspecific diarrhea/gas than either drug alone

- Probiotics or prebiotics are not recommended for the management of acute diarrhea in adults, excluding the cases of antibiotic-associated diarrhea
- Bismuth subsalicylates:
  - have moderate effectiveness
  - can be administered to control rates of passage of stool
  - may help travelers function better during episodes of mild-to-moderate illness
  - may be considered for travelers who do not have any contraindications to use and can adhere to the frequent dosing requirements
- Antibiotic:
  - Antibiotic prophylaxis has moderate to good effectiveness and may be considered in high-risk groups for short-term use
  - Most of the community-acquired diarrhea are viral in origin (norovirus, rotavirus, adenovirus); hence, the use of empiric antimicrobial therapy should be discouraged as it would not shorten the diarrhea episode
  - Patients receiving antibiotics for traveler's diarrhea should complementary receive loperamide in order to reduce the duration of diarrhea and increase the chance of cure
  - Antibiotics (usually azithromycin, fluoroquinolones, rifaximin) reduce both the duration and severity of traveler's diarrhea, where the high probability of bacterial pathogens might justify the prospective side effects of antibiotics
  - The bloody diarrhea should be treated with antibiotics either empirically (azithromycin) or after stool examination and culture; antimotility agents, quinolones (due to increasing antibiotic resistance) and sulfatrimethoprim will be avoided
  - Nosocomial diarrhea: antimicrobial drugs should be discontinued; consider oral metronidazole and/or vancomycin for severely affected or immunocompromised patients

- If patients do not improve after the first visit and specific pathogens causing diarrhea are identified, specific antibiotics should be administered according to the sensitivity results or data from the community

31.9 Prevention [1–3]

- Good hygiene, hand washing, safe food preparation, and access to clean water are key factors in preventing diarrheal illness
- Public health interventions to promote handwashing can reduce the incidence of diarrhea by 1/3
- Effective and safe vaccines exist for rotavirus, typhoid fever, and cholera
  - Vaccines for *Campylobacter*, enterotoxigenic *E. coli*, and *Shigella* infections are under investigation
  - Vaccine development remains a high priority for disease prevention, particularly for those in the developing world
- To contain disease outbreaks, designated diseases should be reported to public health authorities
- Individuals should undergo pretravel counseling

References

1. Barr W, Smith A. Acute diarrhea. Am Fam Physician. 2014;89(3):180–9. PMID: 24506120.
2. Farthing M, Salam MA, Lindberg G, Dite P, Khalif I, Salazar-Lindo E, Ramakrishna BS, Goh KL, Thomson A, Khan AG, Krabshuis J, LeMair A, WGO. Acute diarrhea in adults and children: a global perspective. J Clin Gastroenterol. 2013;47(1):12–20. https://doi.org/10.1097/MCG.0b013e31826df662. PMID: 23222211.
3. Riddle MS, DuPont HL, Connor BA. ACG clinical guideline: diagnosis, treatment, and prevention of acute diarrheal infections in adults. Am J Gastroenterol. 2016;111(5):602–22. https://doi.org/10.1038/ajg.2016.126. Epub 2016 Apr 12. PMID: 27068718.

4. Shane AL, Mody RK, Crump JA, Tarr PI, Steiner TS, Kotloff K, Langley JM, Wanke C, Warren CA, Cheng AC, Cantey J, Pickering LK. 2017 Infectious diseases society of America clinical practice guidelines for the diagnosis and management of infectious diarrhea. Clin Infect Dis. 2017;65(12):e45–80. https://doi.org/10.1093/cid/cix669. PMID: 29053792; PMCID: PMC5850553.

5. Manatsathit S, Dupont HL, Farthing M, Kositchaiwat C, Leelakusolvong S, Ramakrishna BS, Sabra A, Speelman P, Surangsrirat S, Working Party of the Program Committee of the Bangkok World Congress of Gastroenterology 2002. Guideline for the management of acute diarrhea in adults. J Gastroenterol Hepatol. 2002;17(Suppl):S54–71. https://doi.org/10.1046/j.1440-1746.17.s1.11.x. PMID: 12000594.

6. Shen B, Khan K, Ikenberry SO, Anderson MA, Banerjee S, Baron T, Ben-Menachem T, Cash BD, Fanelli RD, Fisher L, Fukami N, Gan SI, Harrison ME, Jagannath S, Lee Krinsky M, Levy M, Maple JT, Lichtenstein D, Stewart L, Strohmeyer L, Dominitz JA, ASGE Standards of Practice Committee. The role of endoscopy in the management of patients with diarrhea. Gastrointest Endosc. 2010;71(6):887–92. https://doi.org/10.1016/j.gie.2009.11.025. Epub 2010 Mar 25. PMID: 20346452.

Chronic Diarrhea

32

Irina F. Cherciu Harbiyeli

32.1 Definition [1, 2]

- The persistent production of loose/altered stools
- Stool consistency between types 5 and 7 on the Bristol stool chart
- Increased stool frequency for more than 4 weeks duration

32.2 Prevalence [1, 2]

- Estimated to affect approximately 5% of the population
- One of the most common reasons for referral to a gastroenterology clinic

32.3 Clinical Classification

- Watery diarrhea (osmotic, secretory, or functional)
- Fatty diarrhea (steatorrhea)
- Inflammatory diarrhea

I. F. Cherciu Harbiyeli (✉)
Research Center of Gastroenterology and Hepatology Craiova,
University of Medicine and Pharmacy Craiova, Craiova, Romania

A. Săftoiu (ed.), *Pocket Guide to Advanced Endoscopy in
Gastroenterology*, https://doi.org/10.1007/978-3-031-42076-4_32

32.4   History

- Family history: neoplastic, inflammatory bowel, or celiac disease
- Epidemiological factors (travel before the onset of illness, exposure to potentially contaminated food or water, illness in other family members)
- Recent antibiotic therapy and *Clostridium difficile* infection
- Sexual history: HIV infection, anal intercourse risk factor for proctitis

32.5   Etiology [1–3]

- **Common causes**
  - IBS diarrhea
  - Bile acid diarrhea
  - Diet: FODMAP malabsorption, artificial sweeteners, lactase deficiency, excess alcohol, caffeine, liquorice
  - Colonic neoplasia
  - Inflammatory bowel disease: ulcerative colitis, Crohn's disease, microscopic colitis
  - Celiac disease
  - Medication: antibiotics (especially macrolides, e.g., erythromycin), hypoglycemic agents (e.g., metformin, gliptins), antihypertensives (e.g., furosemide), antiarrhythmics, nonsteroidal anti-inflammatory drugs (NSAIDs), products containing magnesium, anticancer agents
  - Overflow diarrhea
- **Infrequent causes**
  - Small intestine bacterial overgrowth (SIBO), mesenteric ischemia, radiation enteropathy, lymphoma, surgical causes (gastric surgery and jejunoileal bypass interventions, extensive resections of the ileum and right colon, small bowel resections, shorter resections of the terminal ileum, cholecystectomy, procedures for fecal incontinence, or internal

fistulae), chronic pancreatitis, pancreatic carcinoma, hyperthyroidism, diabetes, cystic fibrosis, giardiasis, and other chronic infections
- **Rare causes**
  - Whipple's disease, Addison's disease, amyloidosis, tropical sprue, protein losing enteropathy, diabetic autonomic neuropathy, factitious or Brainerd diarrhea, hypoparathyroidism, hormone-secreting tumors

32.6 Clinical Assessment [1–4]

- Onset of diarrhea (congenital, abrupt, or gradual)
- Pattern of diarrhea (continuous or intermittent)
- Duration of symptoms (abdominal pain, bloating, discomfort)
- Stool characteristics (watery, bloody, or fatty)
- The presence of:
  - Fecal incontinence
  - Abdominal pain (as in inflammatory bowel disease, IBS, mesenteric ischemia)
  - Substantial weight loss (nutrient malabsorption, neoplasm, or ischemia)
- Aggravating factors (diet and stress)
- Mitigating factors, such as alteration of diet and use of drugs
- Factitious diarrhea determined by clandestine laxative ingestion (history of eating disorders or malingering)

32.7 Organic Vs. Functional Diarrhea Symptoms [1–4]

- **Organic disease**: duration of diarrhea <3 months, primarily nocturnal or constant symptoms, important weight loss
- **Functional altered bowel motility**: long history of intermittent diarrhea, absence of organic symptoms, positive symptoms (Rome II criteria), normal physical examination

32.8 Osmotic/Secretory Vs. Malabsorptive Vs. Inflammatory Forms of Diarrhea [1–4]

- Osmotic: diarrhea ceases once the patients fasts/stops ingesting the poorly absorbed edibles
- Secretory: diarrhea usually persists during a 48–72 h fast
- Malabsorption: steatorrhea and the passage of bulky, malodorous, difficult- to -flush, pale stools
  - Milder forms may not generate any obvious stool abnormality
- Inflammatory: liquid/loose stools with blood or mucous discharge

32.9 Physical Examination [2–5]

- Main conclusions to draw: the extent of fluid and nutritional depletion
- Clinical aspects with diagnostic value: skin flushing or rashes, oral ulcers, arthritis, thyroid or abdominal masses, hepatomegaly, ascites, edema, wheezing, heart murmurs
- Special attention to anorectal examination: anal sphincter tone/contractility, the presence of perianal fistula/abscess

32.10 Differential Diagnosis [2, 6, 7]

32.10.1 Watery Diarrhea

- **Osmotic diarrhea**: ingestion of osmotic laxatives (magnesium citrate/phosphate/sulfate), sugar alcohols frequently found in foods (mannitol/sorbitol/xylitol), lactose/fructose malabsorption, celiac disease
- **Secretory**: alcoholism, bacterial enterotoxins (cholera), bile acid malabsorption, Crohn's disease (early ileocolitis), hyperthyroidism, medications (quinine, antibiotics, antineoplastics, biguanides, calcitonin, digitalis, colchicine, prostaglandins,

ticlopidine), non-osmotic laxatives (senna, docusate sodium), microscopic colitis, neuroendocrine tumors (gastrinoma, vipoma, carcinoid tumors, mastocytosis)
- **Functional**: IBS, diabetis, postgastrectomy, bile salt, or hyperthyroidism-induced diarrhea

32.10.2 Fatty Diarrhea

- **Malabsorption syndromes:** gastric bypass, mesenteric ischemia, short bowel syndrome, SIBO, intestinal parasites (e.g., Giardia), celiac disease, tropical sprue, Whipple disease, drugs (e.g., orlistat)
- **Maldigestion:** hepatobiliary disorders, inadequate luminal bile acid, pancreatic insufficiency

32.10.3 Inflammatory Diarrhea

- Inflammatory bowel disease: Crohn's disease, ulcerative colitis, diverticulitis, ulcerative jejunoileitis
- Invasive infections: *Clostridium difficile* colitis, bacterial infections (tuberculosis, yersiniosis), parasites (Entamoeba), ulcerating viral infections (cytomegalovirus, herpes simplex virus)
- Neoplasms: colon cancer, lymphoma, villous adenocarcinoma
- Radiation colitis

32.11 Initial Investigations [2–4] Should Include

- Complete blood count, iron studies, folate, B12 to examine for infection and anemia
- Erythrocyte sedimentation rate and C-reactive protein to look for infections
- Thyroid function tests to screen for hyperthyroidism
- Coeliac serology (antiendomysium antibodies)

- Complete metabolic profile to search for electrolyte abnormalities, renal function
- Total protein and albumin to look for signs of protein malnutrition
- Stool laboratory assessment (culture and microscopy)
  - Stool electrolytes will categorize the diarrhea into osmotic or secretory, based on the calculation of the stool osmotic gap
  - Fecal leukocytes (leukocytes/calprotectin/lactoferrin are markers of inflammation)
  - Fecal chymotrypsin and elastase can be found in the stool in the setting of pancreatic insufficiency
  - Quantitative stool fat (48–72 h timed collection is ideal)
  - Fecal occult blood test
  - *C. difficile* toxin

32.12 Secondary Assessment [2–4]

- HIV infection should be excluded in those who are immuno-compromised and present with chronic diarrhea
- Specific tests for malabsorbtion (see Chap. 8)
- Blood and urine hormone levels for neuroendocrine tumors
- Urine levels of 5—HIAA for carcinoid
- Barium studies: for detecting fistulae, strictures, surgical bypasses
- Ultrasonography of the small bowel:
  - Attractive due to its noninvasive nature and absence of radiation exposure
  - Has a limited diagnostic role
  - Cannot be routinely recommended (unless other modalities are unavailable)
- Referral for endoscopy is necessary if alarm features:
  - Symptom onset after 50 years of age
  - Rectal bleeding/melena
  - Nocturnal pain or diarrhea

- Progressive abdominal pain
- Unexplained weight loss, fever, other systemic symptoms
- Laboratory abnormalities such as iron deficiency anemia, elevated ESR/CRP, elevated fecal calprotectin, positive test for fecal occult blood
- First-degree relative with inflammatory bowel disease or colorectal cancer

32.13 Endoscopic Assessment [2, 6]

- **Upper gastrointestinal endoscopy**
  - Should be considered in patients with chronic diarrhea, in the absence of significant findings on laboratory studies and colonoscopy
    The differential diagnosis in these patients: celiac disease, Giardia infection, Crohn's disease, eosinophilic gastroenteropathy, Whipple's disease, intestinal amyloid, pancreatic insufficiency
  - Upper endoscopy/enteroscopy with biopsies of the duodenum/jejunum should be performed in patients with unexplained steatorrhea
  - Mucosal biopsies of the small intestine should be completed even if normal endoscopic appearance
    It is important to include the clinical suspicion in the pathology request form in order to perform special histochemical and immunohistochemical stains
  - Evaluation of the further distal small bowel may be beneficial in selected patients (persistent symptoms in suspected celiac disease/small-bowel lymphoma)
  - Patients at high risk of Giardia infection and negative findings on stool studies might require duodenal biopsies for touch preparation and/or duodenal aspirates to identify trophozoites
  - Upper endoscopy with quantitative culture of small-bowel biopsies or aspirate is useful for the diagnosis of SIBO

- Endoscopy-assisted pancreatic function tests for the diagnosis of exocrine pancreatic insufficiency in chronic pancreatitis
- **Flexible sigmoidoscopy**
  - In patients <40 years with normal fecal calprotectin test and suspected functional bowel disorder, flexible sigmoidoscopy may be sufficient as the initial endoscopic test
    In this age group, the diagnostic yield differs little from the use of colonoscopy
  - Even when the mucosa appears normal, biopsies should be performed in order to exclude microscopic colitis or other etiologies
  - In HIV patients with diarrhea, flexible sigmoidoscopy or colonoscopy is recommended if laboratory assessment is nondiagnostic
- **Colonoscopy**
  - All patients with chronic diarrhea should undergo colonoscopy with biopsy if:
    The findings at flexible sigmoidoscopy are inconclusive
    The symptoms persist, there is large-volume blood loss
    Unexplained diarrhea or inflammatory bowel disease (IBD), microscopic inflammatory disorders, colorectal cancer is suspected
  - The candidates for routine CRC screening/surveillance who associate chronic diarrhea should undergo a diagnostic colonoscopy to evaluate the diarrhea and satisfy their cancer screening/surveillance requirements
  - Routine ileoscopy further adds to the value of colonoscopy
  - Colonoscopy with mucosal biopsy is valuable in inflammatory and secretory diarrheas
  - There are insufficient data to determine whether biopsy of an endoscopically normal-appearing terminal ileum should be routinely performed, but the yield of this is likely low
  - Regarding patients with acute or chronic diarrhea, the differential diagnosis of atypical endoscopic and histologic findings in the terminal ileum takes into account: Crohn's

disease, NSAID-induced enteropathy, adenocarcinoma, carcinoid, tuberculosis, lymphoma
- Histology:
    Is essential for excluding or confirming etiologies that are not macroscopically obvious (inactive IBD, microscopic colitis, eosinophilic colitis, amyloidosis)
    Multiple biopsy samples should be taken from both the right and left sides of the colon (the distribution of microscopic colitis can be patchy)
- The type of bowel preparation for colonoscopy in the evaluation of diarrhea:
    Should be determined on an individual basis
    Sodium phosphate – based bowel preparations may cause mucosal changes that can be confused with the macroscopic appearance of IBD, most commonly in the distal colon
- NSAIDs-induced enteropathy can cause terminal ileal mucosal changes that mimic IBD
- **Video capsule endoscopy (VCE)**
  - Is not recommended for the routine evaluation of chronic diarrhea because of the limited diagnostic yield, inability to obtain tissue, risk of capsule retention
  - Should be the first-line investigation for diagnosing small-bowel inflammation, rather than CT
- **Enteroscopy**
  - There is limited data on the diagnostic value of enteroscopy solely for the evaluation of diarrhea
  - Is not recommended for the routine evaluation of chronic diarrhea
  - Its main role is targeting predefined small-bowel lesions (through radiographic imaging or VCE)
  - Total colonoscopy with ileoscopy might represent the gold standard for excluding inflammatory disease in the ascending colon and terminal ileum. While in some cases endoscopy will be incomplete, further imaging of the terminal ileum and proximal colon may be necessary

32.14 Treatment [2, 4, 5, 7]

- Empiric treatment is justified when testing does not find a specific diagnosis, when a specific diagnosis has no specific treatment or treatment has failed
- Antimotility agents:
  - Loperamide: a safe, typical first-line empiric therapy (2–4 mg, 4 times a day)
  - Clonidine: option for diarrhea secondary to opioid withdrawal or to loss of noradrenergic innervation in patients with diabetes, has limitations due to the antihypertensive effect (0.1–0.3 mg, 3 times a day)
  - Opiates: morphine (2–20 mg, 4 times a day), codeine phosphate (additive potential)
  - Anticholinergic medications: tricyclic antidepressants for coexisting diarrhea
- Bile acid-binding resins: cholestyramine (4 g up to 4 times a day)
- Octreotide (50–250 mg 3 times a day, subcutaneously)
- Fiber supplements (calcium polycarbophil 5–10 g daily, psyllium 10–20 g daily)
- Other agents: bismuth subsalicylate, adsorbents, bulk forming agents

32.14.1 N.B

- It is important that subjects with an organic disorder are properly investigated in order to find a potentially curable disease.
- Patients with a functional bowel disorder should not unnecessarily undergo extensive investigations.
- Repeat the history and physical examination, reexamine previous evaluations whenever possible, before additional tests are ordered.
- Failure to establish a diagnosis is rather due to overlooking a common cause than omitting a rare etiology of chronic diarrhea.

References

1. Stotzer PO, Abrahamsson H, Bajor A, Kilander A, Sadik R, Sjövall H, Simrén M. Are the definitions for chronic diarrhoea adequate? Evaluation of two different definitions in patients with chronic diarrhoea. United European Gastroenterol J. 2015;3(4):381–6. https://doi.org/10.1177/2050640615580219. PMID: 26279847; PMCID: PMC4528211.
2. Arasaradnam RP, Brown S, Forbes A, et al. Guidelines for the investigation of chronic diarrhoea in adults: British Society of Gastroenterology, 3rd edition. Gut. 2018;67:1380–99.
3. Thomas PD, Forbes A, Green J, Howdle P, Long R, Playford R, Sheridan M, Stevens R, Valori R, Walters J, Addison GM, Hill P, Brydon G. Guidelines for the investigation of chronic diarrhoea, 2nd edition. Gut. 2003;52(Suppl 5):1–15. https://doi.org/10.1136/gut.52.suppl_5.v1. PMID: 12801941; PMCID: PMC1867765.
4. Fine KD, Schiller LR. AGA technical review on the evaluation and management of chronic diarrhea. Gastroenterology. 1999;116:1464–86.
5. Schiller LR, Pardi DS, Sellin JH. Chronic diarrhea: diagnosis and management. Clin Gastroenterol Hepatol. 2017;15(2):182–193.e3. https://doi.org/10.1016/j.cgh.2016.07.028. Epub 2016 Aug 2. PMID: 27496381.
6. Shen B, Khan K, Ikenberry SO, Anderson MA, Banerjee S, Baron T, Ben-Menachem T, Cash BD, Fanelli RD, Fisher L, Fukami N, Gan SI, Harrison ME, Jagannath S, Lee Krinsky M, Levy M, Maple JT, Lichtenstein D, Stewart L, Strohmeyer L, Dominitz JA, ASGE Standards of Practice Committee. The role of endoscopy in the management of patients with diarrhea. Gastrointest Endosc. 2010;71(6):887–92. https://doi.org/10.1016/j.gie.2009.11.025. Epub 2010 Mar 25. PMID: 20346452.
7. Descoteaux-Friday GJ, Shrimanker I. Chronic diarrhea. In: StatPearls. Treasure Island: StatPearls Publishing; 2020.

Small Bowel Tumors

33

Dan Nicolae Florescu

33.1 Definition and Classification

- Malignant tumors
  - primary
    - adenocarcinoma, the most frequent
    - carcinoid tumor
    - lymphoma
    - gastrointestinal stromal tumors: leiomyosarcoma
  - metastatic
- Benign tumors
  - Epithelial tumors
    - adenoma
    - hyperplastic polyps
  - Nonepithelial tumors
    - gastrointestinal stromal tumors: leiomyoma, the most frequent
    - lipoma
    - hemangioma
    - fibroma

D. N. Florescu (✉)
Gastroenterology Department, University of Medicine and Pharmacy Craiova, Craiova, Romania

© The Author(s), under exclusive license to Springer Nature Switzerland AG 2023
A. Săftoiu (ed.), *Pocket Guide to Advanced Endoscopy in Gastroenterology*, https://doi.org/10.1007/978-3-031-42076-4_33

33.2 Epidemiology

- 2% of primary gastrointestinal tumors
- Maximum incidence: sixth decade of life
- Slight predominance in males
- Metastatic tumors are more common than primary malignancies [1, 2]

33.3 Etiology and Pathogenesis

- Conditions associated with the risk of developing small-bowel cancer
  - Celiac disease
  - Regional enteritis
  - Polyposis syndromes
  - Crohn's disease
  - AIDS [2, 3]

33.4 Diagnostic

- Clinical presentation
  - Asymptomatic >50% of cases
  - Nonspecific signs and symptoms
    Cramping periumbilical pain
    Dyspepsia: nausea, vomiting, bloating
  - Neoplastic impregnation syndrome:
    malaise

    anorexia

    involuntary weight loss
  - Signs and symptoms of complications (intestinal obstruction, gastrointestinal bleeding, perforation)
- Physical examination
  - Pallor (in case of anemia)

- Abdominal pain caused by palpation
- Palpable abdominal mass in case of large tumors
- Signs of metastatic dissemination: metastatic hepatomegaly, ascites, jaundice
- Laboratory studies
  - Microcytic hypochromic anemia (in case of occult bleeding)
- Imaging tests
  - Endoscopic examination
      Video capsule endoscopy (VCE)
         Risk of capsule retention and intestinal obstruction
      Double-balloon enteroscopy (DBE)/single-balloon enteroscopy (SBE)
         Biopsy may pe performed during these procedures
         Some therapeutic techniques may be performed (polypectomy, hemostasis)
  - Radiologic examination
      Computed Ttmographic enterography, magnetic esonance enterography and enteroclysis
      They allow the assessment of the intestinal wall
  - Transabdominal ultrasound
      It may visualize some large tumors (>4 cm) [3–5]

33.5 Treatment

- Benign tumors
  - Endoscopic resection (small, superficial tumors) **or**
  - Surgical resection
- Malignant tumors
  - The treatment of choice: surgical resection
      Segmental and mesenteric resections depending on the location of the primary tumor + regional lymphadenectomy [5, 6]

33.5.1 Malignant Small-Bowel Tumors

- Adenocarcinoma
  - Usually affects the distal duodenum and the proximal jejunum
  - Tends to ulcerate
  - Possible complications: bleeding, intestinal obstruction
- Primary small-bowel lymphomas
  - The ileum is most frequently affected, then the jejunum and the duodenum
  - Conditions associated with an increased risk of developing primary small-bowel lymphomas

    Celiac disease → enteropathy-associated T-cell lymphoma (EATL)

    Diffuse nodular lymphoid hyperplasia

    Crohn's disease

    Regional enteritis

    AIDS

    Immunodeficiency associated with organ transplantation, autoimmune diseases
  - The diagnosis needs to be confirmed by biopsy with histopathological examination
  - These are non-Hodgkin's lymphomas
  - Recommended treatment: surgical resection + adjuvant chemoradiotherapy
  - *Immunoproliferative small intestinal disease (IPSID)*

    It diffusely affects the entire small intestine

    Clinical features

      Chronic diarrhea

      Steatorrhea

      Vomiting

      Abdominal cramps

      Clubbing of the digits

    Laboratory studies

      The existence of an abnormal IgA that presents a shortened α heavy chain in the blood and intestinal secretions

Treatment

Prelymphomatous stage: tetracycline or metronidazole for 6–24 months

Advanced stage: anthracycline-based chemotherapy

- Small-bowel carcinoid tumors
  - Develop from argentaffin cells of the crypts of Lieberkühn
  - Typically appear in the distal ileum
  - Represent the most common cause of carcinoid syndrome
  - Surgery should be preceded by the administration of a somatostatin analog to prevent a carcinoid crisis
- Leiomyosarcomas
  - Frequently have dimensions >5 cm
  - Usually occur in the jejunum and the ileum
  - May often complicated by bleeding, obstruction, or perforation
  - Present mutations of the c-kit gene
  - The treatment of non-resectable tumors or with proven distant metastasis

    Imatinib mesylate or

    Sunitinib, in case of imatinib failure
- Small-bowel metastatic tumors
  - Melanoma is the most common neoplasm that metastasizes to the small bowel [6, 7]

33.5.2 Benign Small Bowel Tumors

- Can be found as isolated lesions or in hereditary gastrointestinal polyposis syndromes (Peutz–Jeghers syndrome; familial adenomatous polyposis—Gardner's syndrome; juvenile polyposis)
- Adenomas
  - Located predominantly in the proximal bowel
  - Sessile or pedunculated
  - Histologically, there are tubular adenomas, villous adenomas, or tubulovillous adenomas

    Villous adenomas are associated with a higher malignancy risk than tubular ones

- Hyperplastic polyps
  - No risk for malignant degeneration
- Leiomyomas
  - Are usually intramural tumors
  - May present ulcerations of the mucosa that can cause gastrointestinal bleeding
  - Risk for malignant degeneration
  - Require surgical resection with wide safety margins
- Lipomas
  - Higher frequency in the distal segment of the ileum
  - May cause intestinal obstruction
- Hemangiomas
  - Frequently cause gastrointestinal bleeding
  - Are most common in the jejunum
  - Angiography can be useful for diagnosis, and also may be a solution to stop active bleeding by embolization [8]

References

1. Ludwig E, Kurtz RC. Tumors of the small intestine. In: Feldman M, Brandt LJ, editors. Sleisenger and Fordtran's gastrointestinal and liver disease: pathophysiology, diagnosis, management, vol. 1. 9th ed. Philadelphia: Saunders; 2010. p. 2145–53.
2. Schottenfeld D, Beebe-Dimmer JL, Vigneau FD. The epidemiology and patho-genesis of neoplasia in the small intestine. Ann Epidemiol. 2009;19:58–69.
3. Bilimoria KY, Bentrem DJ, Wayne JD, et al. Small bowel cancer in the United States changes in epidemiology, treatment, and survival over the last 20 years. Ann Surg. 2009;249:63–71.
4. Gill SS, Heuman DM, Mihas AA. Small intestinal neoplasms. J Clin Gastroenterol. 2001;33:267–82.
5. Liao Z, Gao R, Xu C, Li ZS. Indications and detection, completion, and retention rates of small-bowel capsule endoscopy: a systematic review. Gastrointest Endosc. 2010;71:280–6.
6. Schnadig I, Blanke C. Gastrointestinal stromal tumors: imatinib and beyond. Curr Treat Options in Oncol. 2006;7:427–37.

7. Demetri G, van Oosterom A, Garrett C, et al. Efficacy and safety of suni-
    tinib inpatients with advanced gastrointestinal stromal tumour after fail-
    ure of imatinib: a randomised controlled trial. Lancet. 2006;368:1329–38.
    [German].
8. Benson AB, Venook AP, Al-Hawary MM, et al. Small bowel adenocarci-
    noma, version 1.2020, NCCN clinical practice guidelines in oncology. J
    Natl Compr Cancer Netw. 2019;17:1109–33.

Colorectal Polyps

34

Vlad-Florin Iovănescu and Adrian Săftoiu

34.1 Definition

Protruding masses that arise from the wall of the colorectum and project into the lumen

34.2 Classification

- Epithelial polyps
    - adenoma (tubular/villous/tubulovillous)
    - carcinoma
    - serrated
        hyperplastic
        sessile serrated lesions (SSLs)
        traditional serrated adenomas (TSAs)

V.-F. Iovănescu (✉)
University of Medicine and Pharmacy of Craiova, Craiova, Romania
e-mail: vlad.iovanescu@umfcv.ro

A. Săftoiu
Department of Gastroenterology and Hepatology, Elias Emergency
University Hospital, Carol Davila University of Medicine and Pharmacy,
Bucharest, Romania

© The Author(s), under exclusive license to Springer Nature
Switzerland AG 2023
A. Săftoiu (ed.), *Pocket Guide to Advanced Endoscopy in
Gastroenterology*, https://doi.org/10.1007/978-3-031-42076-4_34

- hamartoma
    juvenile
    Peutz–Jeghers
- inflammatory
- Non-epithelial polyps (subepithelial lesions)
    - lipoma/liposarcoma
    - leiomyoma/leiomyosarcoma
    - fibroma/fibrosarcoma
    - hemangioma/hemangiosarcoma
    - stromal tumors (GISTs)
    - neuroendocrine tumors (NETs)
    - schwannoma
    - colitis cystica profunda
    - pneumatosis cystoides coli
    - granular cell tumors
    - metastatic neoplasms

34.3 Epidemiology

- Adenomas
    - 75% of epithelial polyps
    - incidence increases with age and male gender
- Serrated [1]
    - hyperplastic:
        25% of epithelial polyps
        80% of serrated lesions
        incidence increases with age
    - sessile serrated lesions:
        approximately 20% of serrated lesions
        more prevalent in older individuals
        gender prevalence equal for men and women
    - traditional serrated adenomas
        rare

- Juvenile
    - rare lesions mostly occur in children
- Lipoma (Fig. 34.1a, b)
    - the colon is the most frequent location in the gastrointestinal tract
- GISTs
    - rare in colon and rectum
- NETs (Fig. 34.2a, b)
    - rare in colon, frequent in rectum

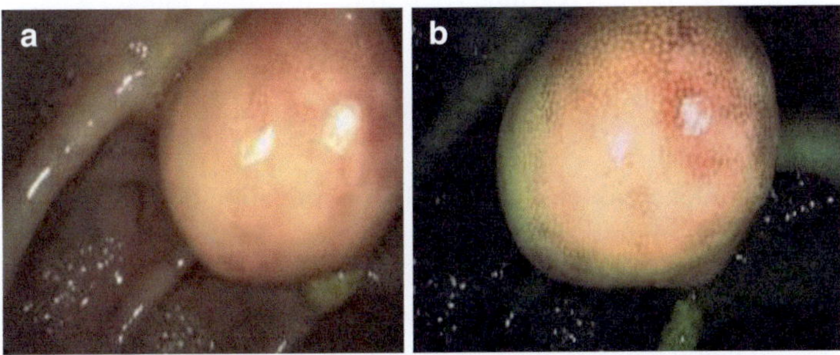

Fig. 34.1 Colonic lipoma, with a yellow hue, visualized in white-light mode (**a**) and i-SCAN, with visible normal colonic crypts at the surface (**b**)

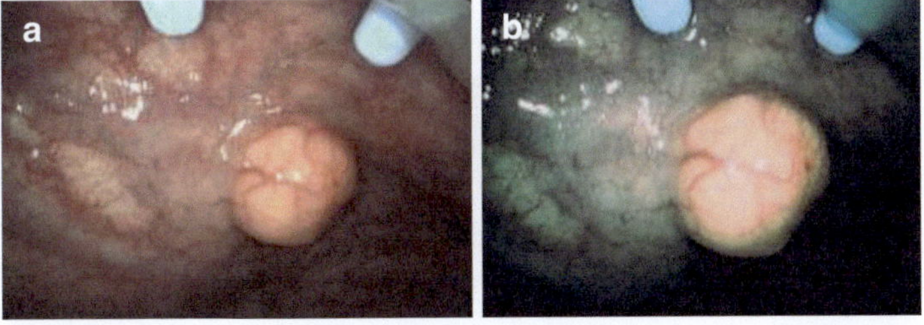

Fig. 34.2 Rectal neuroendocrine tumor, with a yellow hue, visualized in white-light mode (**a**) and i-SCAN (**b**)

## 34.4	Pathogenesis

- Adenomas (adenomatous polyps) (Fig. 34.3a, b)
  - known risk factors [2]:
      family history of adenoma/colorectal cancer (genetic factors)
      obesity (debated)
      type II diabetes mellitus
      alcohol consumption
      smoking
      alimentary regimen (rich in fat, low fiber intake)
  - other known associations:
      ureterosigmoidostomy
      bacterial endocarditis with *S. bovis*
  - location
      adenomas <1 cm located predominantly distal
      >1 cm uniformly distributed throughout the colorectum
  - pathogenesis includes failure of proliferative regulatory mechanisms resulting in abnormal growth and dysplasia
  - genetic alterations include three known pathways
      mutations of the APC and KRAS genes
      "microsatellite instability"
      hypermetilation

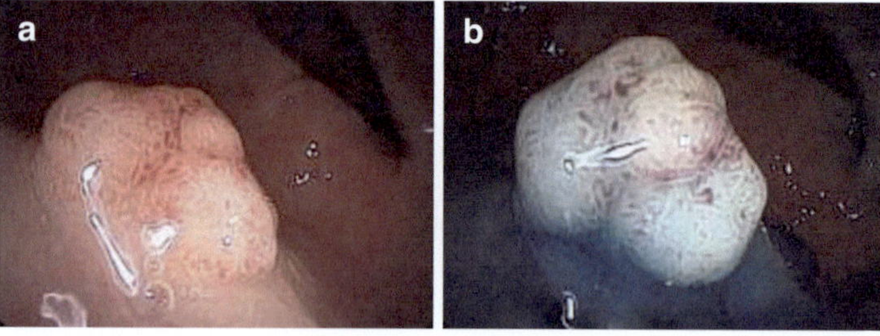

Fig. 34.3 Adenomatous colonic polyp with a cerebriform pit-pattern, visualized in white-light mode before (**a**) and after adrenaline 1:10,000 + methylene blue injection (**b**)

- risk of evolving to adenocarcinoma (risk depends on histology)
- Hyperplastic:
  - similar pathogenesis to adenomas yet no dysplasia
  - reduced or no malignant potential
      pathogenic sequences involve BRAF/KRAS gene mutations
  - located predominantly distally
- Sessile serrated lesions
  - frequently located in the proximal colon (Fig. 34.4a, b)
  - may contain dysplasia
  - malignant potential

- Traditional serrated adenoma
  - located in the distal colon
  - malignant potential
- Inflammatory polyps
  - occur in severe inflammatory diseases of the colon and rectum: ulcerative colitis, Crohn's disease, tuberculous colitis etc.
  - no malignant potential

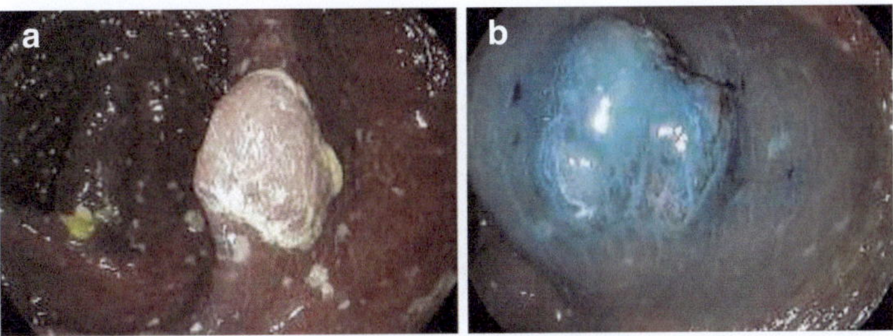

Fig. 34.4 Sessile serrated colonic polyp, with adherent mucus, visualized in contrast to the colonic mucosa with pseudomelanosis coli (laxative abuse), in white-light mode before (**a**) and after adrenaline 1:10,000 + methylene blue injection (**b**)

34.5   Diagnosis

- Clinical signs
  - most often asymptomatic; symptoms are usually present in large polyps (>1 cm)
  - bleeding per rectum (frequent in juvenile polyps)
  - constipation (in the case of large polyps that cause obstruction)
  - diarrhea (large villous adenomas localized in the distal colon)
  - abdominal pain: not characteristic; sometimes in large polyps that cause obstruction
- Physical exam
  - usually unremarkable
  - rectal examination may rarely reveal blood/a palpable mass (polyp)
- Laboratory studies
  - usually unremarkable
  - microcytic hypochromic anemia (rare)
  - fecal occult blood testing (FOBT): low sensibility and sensitivity
  - fecal immunohistochemical testing (FIT): superior to FOBT; low sensitivity for small adenoma detection
- Imaging tests
  - lower gastrointestinal endoscopy (colonoscopy)
  - CT colonography (virtual colonoscopy)
    useful when colonoscopy in not possible/incomplete

34.6   Role of Colonoscopy

- Colonoscopy is the main diagnostic and therapeutic procedure
  - allows the assessment of polyp type and suitability of resection by using the **Paris classification** [3]
    protruding lesions
        Ip—pedunculated polyp (Fig. 34.5a, b)
        Ips—subpedunculated polyp

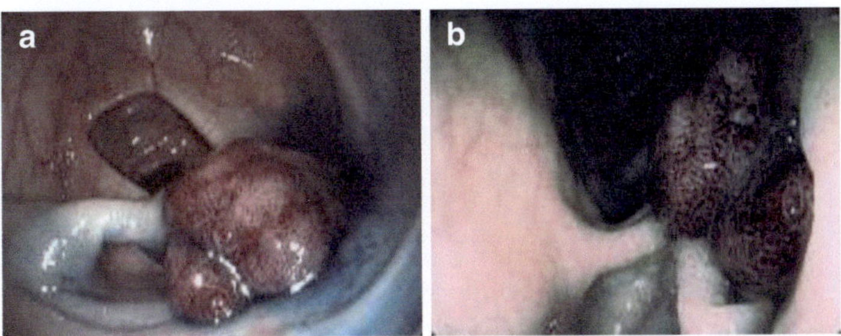

Fig. 34.5 Pedunculated sigmoid polyp, visualized in white-light mode after adrenaline 1:10,000 + methylene blue injection (**a**) and in i-SCAN mode (**b**)

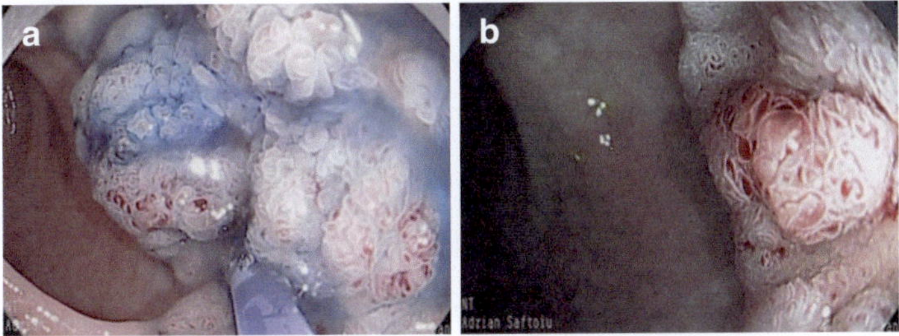

Fig. 34.6 Semicircumferential sessile rectal polyp, visualized in white-light mode after adrenaline 1:10,000 + methylene blue injection (**a**) and in i-SCAN mode (**b**)

Is—sessile polyp (Fig. 34.6a, b)

flat-elevated lesions

0-IIa—flat elevated lesion (Fig. 34.7)

0-IIa/c—flat elevated lesion with central depression

flat-depressed lesions

0-IIb—completely flat lesion

0-IIc—depressed lesion

0-III—excavated/ulcerated lesion, with prominent margins

- allows enhanced optical diagnosis for prediction of polyp histology with the contribution of advanced imaging: HD white-light endoscopy and virtual chromoendoscopy using the **JNET (Japan NBI Expert Team) classification**

- JNET 1 (Fig. 34.8a, b)
- JNET 2A/B (Figs. 34.9a, b and 34.10a, b)
- JNET 3 (Fig. 34.11a, b)
    - granular/nongranular lateral spreading tumors (LST-G/NG) represent a distinct category of adenomatous polyps (Fig. 34.12a, b)
    - optical magnification endoscopes provide additional information regarding mucosal and vascular patterns (Fig. 34.13a, b)

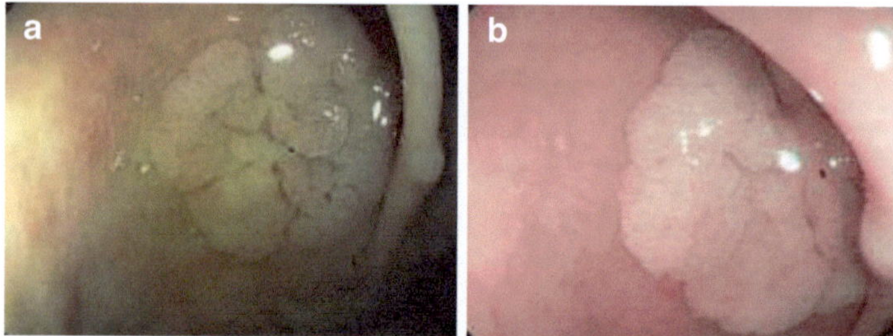

Fig. 34.7 Flat cecal polyp visualized in i-SCAN (**a**) and OE (optical enhancement) i-SCAN mode (**b**)

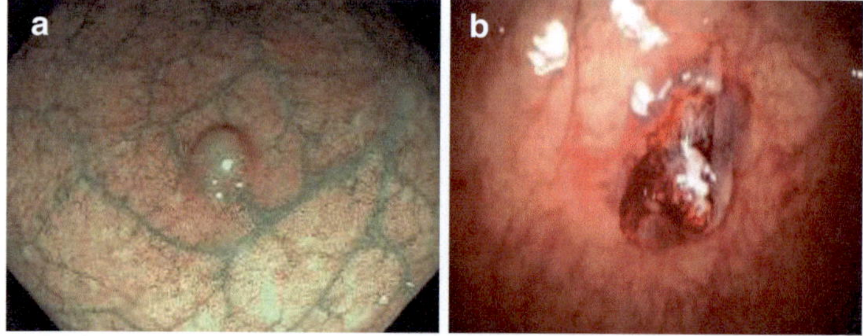

Fig. 34.8 Diminutive translucid JNET1-type sigmoid polyp, visualized in NBI mode (**a**) and after cold-snare polypectomy (**b**), with central-gathered submucosa and minimal bleeding that stopped spontaneously

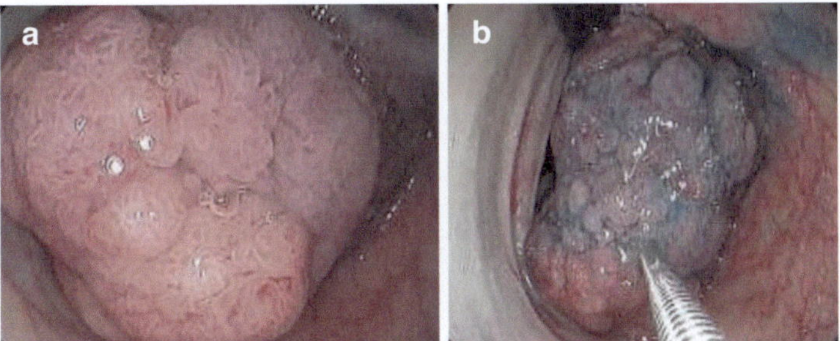

Fig. 34.9 JNET 2A colonic polyp, visualized in white-light mode (**a**) and during adrenaline 1:10,000 + methylene blue injection (**b**), before polypectomy

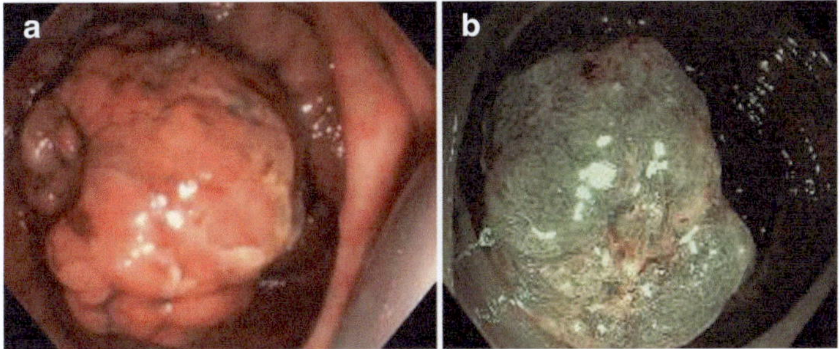

Fig. 34.10 JNET 2B colonic polyp, visualized in white-light mode (**a**) and NBI mode (**b**), with an irregular pit-pattern and tortuous vessels

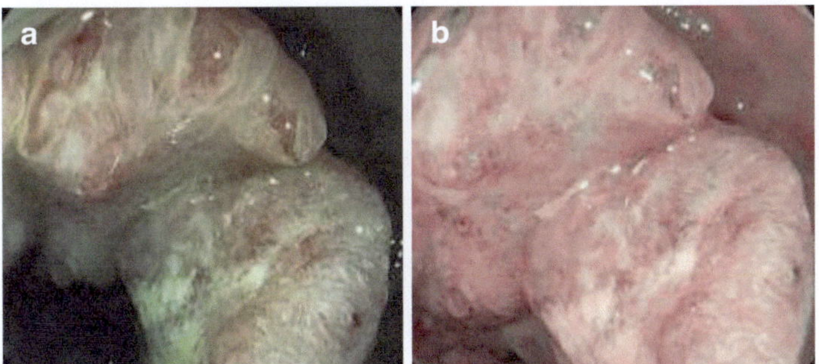

Fig. 34.11 JNET 3 colonic polyp, visualized in i-SCAN mode (**a**) and OE i-SCAN mode (**b**), with an absent pit-pattern (amorphous areas) and interrupted/irregular vessels

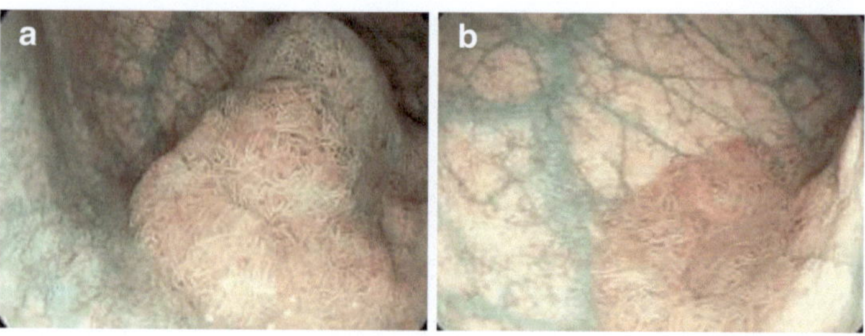

Fig. 34.12 Sessile Paris 0-IIa + Is, JNET 2A (regular surface and vascular pattern) rectal polyp, visualized in i-SCAN mode (**a**), with lateral extension (**b**) (LST-G with a dominant component)

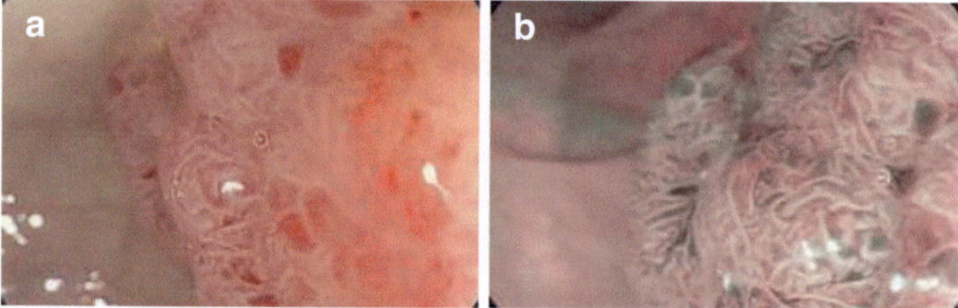

Fig. 34.13 Sessile Paris Is, JNET 2A (regular surface and vascular pattern) colonic polyp, visualized in white-light mode (**a**) and i-SCAN mode (**b**) using magnification endoscopy

34.7 Treatment

- Endoscopic resection is the treatment of choice for most lesions [4]
  - conventional polypectomy
    with clip placement (Fig. 34.14a, b)
    with elastic loop placement (Fig. 34.15a, b)
  - endoscopic mucosal resection
    one-fragment
    frequently in multiple fragments ("piecemeal") (Fig. 34.16a, b)

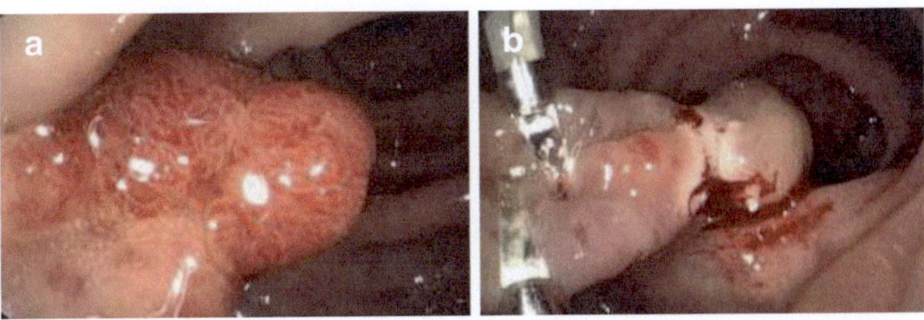

Fig. 34.14 Pedunculated Paris Ip JNET 2A (regular surface and vascular pattern) colonic polyp, with a 10-mm thick stalk (**a**) with two hemostatic clips placed at its base, before performing polypectomy at half of the stalk (**b**)

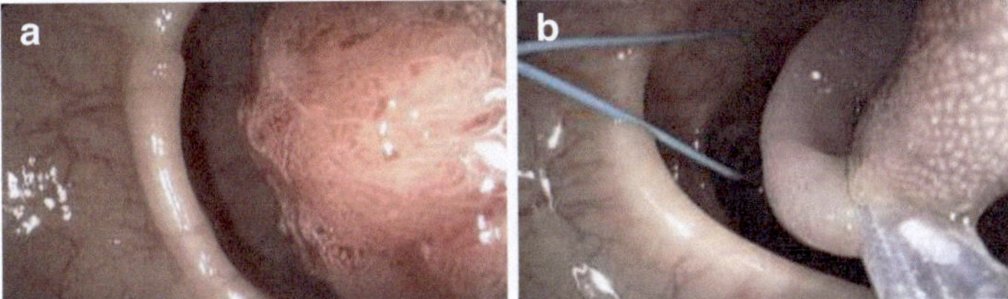

Fig. 34.15 Pedunculated Paris Ip, JNET 2A (regular surface and vascular pattern) large-sized (35 mm) colonic polyp, with a long, approximately 5-mm thick stalk (**a**) with an endoloop placed at its base, before performing polyp-ectomy at half of the stalk (**b**)

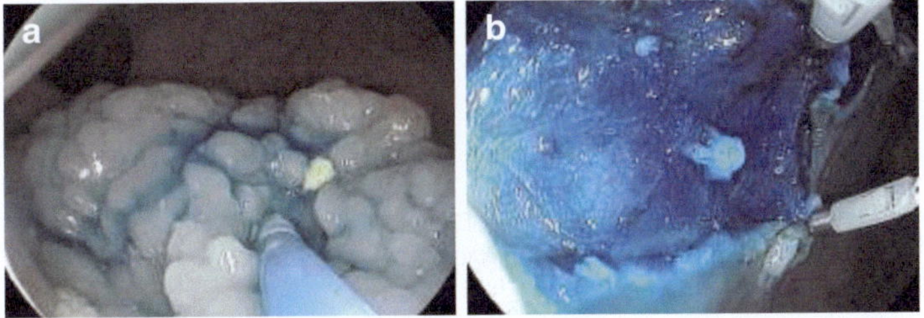

Fig. 34.16 Flat large-sized (35 mm) Paris 0-IIa, JNET 2A (regular surface and vascular pattern) polyp, injected with gelofusine + adrenaline 1:10,000 + methylene blue (**a**) and resected "piecemeal" (**b**), without complications

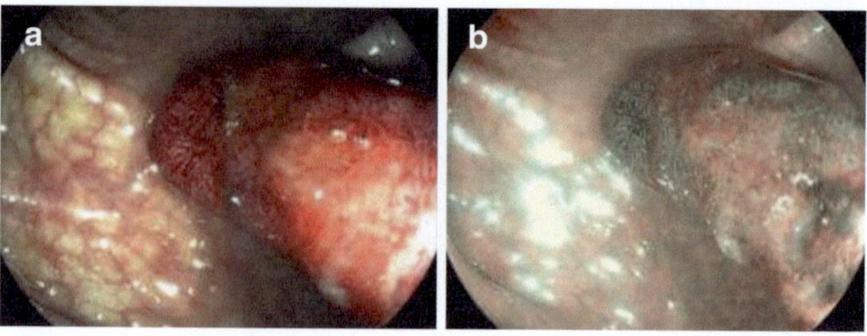

Fig. 34.17 Malignant pedunculated polyp (J-NET 2B). Images obtained with i-SCAN-2 (**a**) and i-SCAN OE (**b**) modes

- – endoscopic submucosal dissection
  - has the advantage of obtaining a single fragment
  - higher risk of perforation
- Malignant polyps may be resected in early stages [5], particularly if they are pedunculated (Fig. 34.17a, b)
  - – assessment of submucosal invasion is performed with:
    - Haggitt classification for pedunculated polyps
    - Kikuchi classification for sessile polyps
- Surgical resection is used when endoscopic resection is not possible/not feasible (advanced lesions with malignant risk) (Fig. 34.11a, b)

References

1. Mathews AA, Draganov PV, Yang D. Endoscopic management of colorectal polyps: from benign to malignant polyps. World J Gastrointest Endosc. 2021;13(9):356–70.
2. Shussman N, Wexner SD. Colorectal polyps and polyposis syndromes. Gastroenterol Rep. 2014;2(1):1–15.
3. Ribeiro MS, Wallace MB. Endoscopic treatment of early cancer of the colon. Gastroenterol Hepatol. 2015;11(7):445–52.

4. Tanaka S, Saitoh Y, Matsuda T, Igarashi M, Matsumoto T, Iwao Y, Suzuki Y, Nozaki R, Sugai T, Oka S, Itabashi M, Sugihara KI, Tsuruta O, Hirata I, Nishida H, Miwa H, Enomoto N, Shimosegawa T, Koike K. Evidence-based clinical practice guidelines for management of colorectal polyps. J Gastroenterol. 2021;56(4):323–35.
5. Ferlitsch M, Moss A, Hassan C, Bhandari P, Dumonceau JM, Paspatis G, Jover R, Langner C, Bronzwaer M, Nalankilli K, Fockens P, Hazzan R, Gralnek IM, Gschwantler M, Waldmann E, Jeschek P, Penz D, Heresbach D, Moons L, Lemmers A, Paraskeva K, Pohl J, Ponchon T, Regula J, Repici A, Rutter MD, Burgess NG, Bourke MJ. Colorectal polypectomy and endoscopic mucosal resection (EMR): European Society of Gastrointestinal Endoscopy (ESGE) Clinical Guideline. Endoscopy. 2017;49(3):270–97.

Colorectal Tumors 35

Vlad-Florin Iovănescu and Adrian Săftoiu

35.1 Epidemiology

- Colorectal cancer usually appears:
  - after 50 years
  - men > women
  - approximately 1 million new cases/year worldwide

35.2 Etiopathogenesis

- Known risk factors [1]:
  - advanced age
  - male gender
  - dietary factors (red meat consumption, high-fat, low-fiber diet)
  - alcohol consumption + smoking

V.-F. Iovănescu (✉)
University of Medicine and Pharmacy of Craiova, Craiova, Romania
e-mail: vlad.iovanescu@umfcv.ro

A. Săftoiu
Department of Gastroenterology and Hepatology, Elias Emergency
University Hospital, Carol Davila University of Medicine and Pharmacy,
Bucharest, Romania

© The Author(s), under exclusive license to Springer Nature
Switzerland AG 2023
A. Săftoiu (ed.), *Pocket Guide to Advanced Endoscopy in
Gastroenterology*, https://doi.org/10.1007/978-3-031-42076-4_35

- obesity + sedentarism
- acromegaly
- inflammatory bowel disease
- hereditary colorectal cancer syndromes (Lynch syndrome)
- personal/family history of
  colorectal cancer
  colorectal adenomas
  colonic polyposis syndromes
- Adenocarcinoma is the most common (90–95%); the rest are primary lymphomas, melanomas, or carcinoid tumors
- Located most commonly in distal colon (incidence of proximal tumors rising in past years)
- Pathogenic sequences involve the adenoma-carcinoma sequence in most cases
- Three molecular pathways associated with colorectal cancer
  - chromosomal instability
  - microsatellite instability
  - methylation pathway

35.3　Diagnosis

- Clinical signs
  - symptoms present in advanced stages
  - rectal bleeding
  - diarheea/constipation (constipation occurs in bowel obstruction, mostly in distal tumors due to reduced luminal diameter of the colon)/recent changes in bowel habit
  - abdominal pain
  - anorexia and weight loss
  - tenesmus (in rectal cancer)
  - symptoms related to complications/metastasis
- Physical exam
  - palpable abdominal mass
  - hepatomegaly (metastatic disease)
  - left supraclavicular adenopathy (Virchow)

- – angular cheilosis/koilonychia/pallor in tumors that induce iron-deficiency anemia
- – blood or palpable mass on rectal examination
- Laboratory studies
  - – hypocromic microcytic anemia (right-sided colon tumors)
  - – CEA tumor marker increased in postoperative recurrence (not useful in diagnosis)
  - – increased GGT, AP, ALT, AST, and sometimes total and conjugated bilirubin levels when liver metastases are present
- Imaging tests
  - – colonoscopy: diagnostic procedure of choice; allows identification and biopsy of the lesions
  - – CT colonography (virtual colonoscopy): when colonoscopy is not feasible/incomplete (to determine eventual synchronous lesions)
  - – abdominal ultrasound: useful for staging as it detects distant (liver) metastasis
  - – CT/MRI: used for assessing locoregional and distant extension and complications; pelvic MRI used in rectal cancer for assessing local tumour invasion and lymph node involvement (T and N stages)
  - – rectal EUS: used in rectal tumours for assessing local invasion and lymph node involvement (T and N stages)

35.4 Role of Endoscopy

- Colonoscopy is the diagnostic test of choice
  - – it allows direct visualization of the lesion + biopsies (Figs. 35.1a, b and 35.2a, b)
  - – identification of synchronous tumors
- Rectal EUS is used for rectal cancer staging (rectal wall invasion and nodal involvement—T and N stages) [2]
  - – superior accuracy for T staging (Figs. 35.3a, b and 35.4a, b)

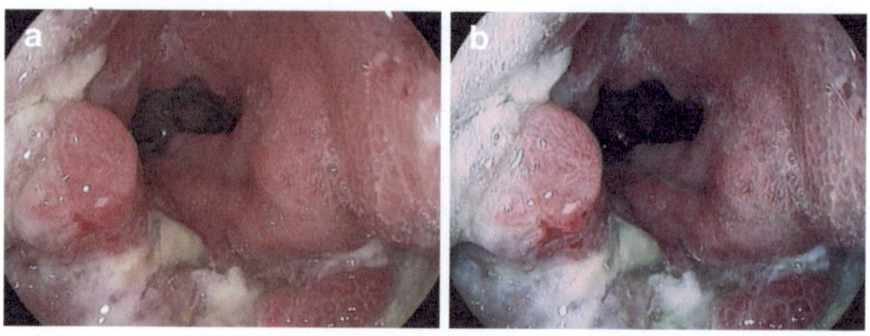

Fig. 35.1 Exophytic ulcerated nonobstructive colon adenocarcinoma visualized in white-light mode (**a**) and i-SCAN mode (**b**)

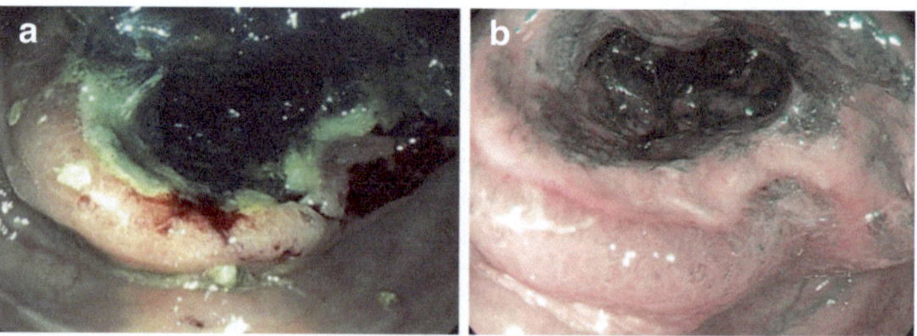

Fig. 35.2 Exophytic ulcerated stenosing (obstructive) colon adenocarcinoma visualized in i-SCAN mode (**a**) and i-SCAN OE (**b**)

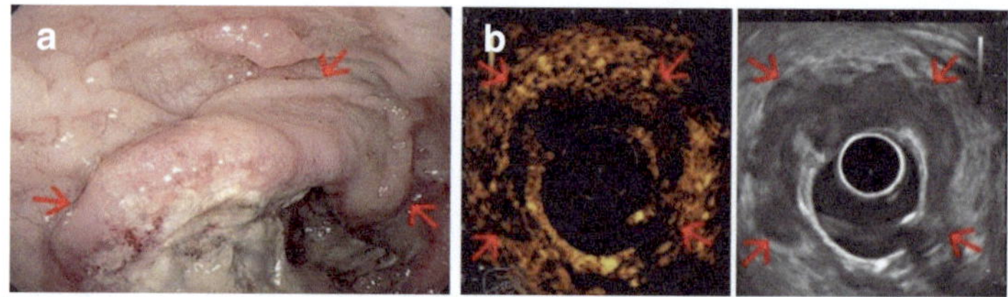

Fig. 35.3 Exophytic ulcerated stenosing rectal adenocarcinoma visualized in white-light mode (**a**) and during contrast-enhanced transrectal endoscopic ultrasound—T3N1Mx (**b**)

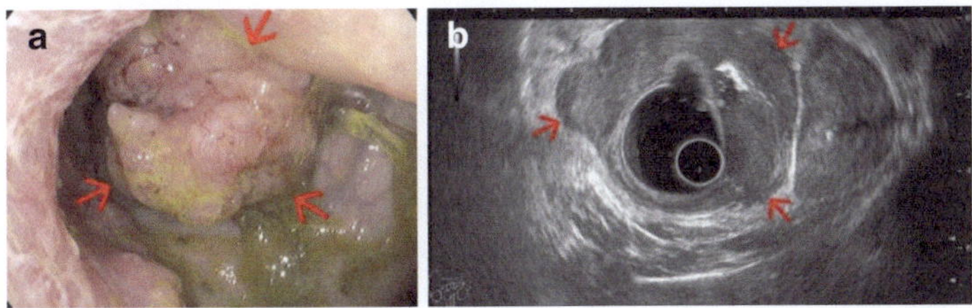

Fig. 35.4 Exophytic stenosing rectal adenocarcinoma visualized in white-light mode (**a**) and during transrectal endoscopic ultrasound in proximity of the prostate—T3NxMx (**b**)

35.5 Staging (8th AJCC) [3]

- **TX:** primary tumor cannot be assessed
- **T0:** no evidence of primary tumor
- **Tis:** carcinoma in situ, intramucosal carcinoma (involvement of lamina propria with no extension through muscularis mucosae)
- **T1:** tumor invades submucosa (through the muscularis mucosa but not into the muscularis propria)
- **T2:** tumor invades muscularis propria
- **T3:** tumor invades through the muscularis propria into the pericolorectal tissues
- **T4:**
  - **T4a:** tumor invades the visceral peritoneum (including gross perforation of the tumor through the bowel wall and continuous tumoral invasion of the surface of visceral peritoneum)
  - **T4b:** tumor directly invades or adheres to other adjacent organs or structures
- **NX:** regional lymph nodes cannot be assessed
- **N0:** no regional lymph node metastasis

- **N1:** metastasis in 1–3 regional lymph nodes
  - **N1a:** metastasis in 1 regional lymph node
  - **N1b:** metastasis in 2–3 regional lymph nodes
  - **N1c:** no regional lymph nodes metastasis but there are tumor deposits in the subserosa, mesentery or nonperitonealized pericolic or perirectal/mesorectal tissues
- **N2:** metastasis in 4 or more regional lymph nodes
  - **N2a:** metastasis in 4–6 regional lymph nodes
  - **N2b:** metastasis in 7 or more regional lymph nodes
- **M0:** no distant metastasis by imaging; no evidence of tumor presence in other sites or organs
- **M1:** distant metastasis
  - **M1a:** metastasis confined to 1 organ or site without peritoneal metastasis
  - **M1b:** metastasis to 2 or more sites or organs without peritoneal metastasis
  - **M1c:** metastasis to the peritoneal surface alone with/without other site or organ metastases

35.6 Treatment

Resectable colon cancer

- Endoscopic resection for malignant polyps (polyps with noninvasive cancer) without unfavorable prognostic histologic features
  - consider colectomy for sessile malignant polyps even if they lack unfavorable histology [4]
- Obstructing
  - colectomy + lymphadenectomy + anastomosis/resection + diversion/diversion (ileostomy/colostomy)
- Non-obstructing
  - right/left/transverse colectomy (depending on location) with lymphadenectomy + anastomosis for malignant polyps with unfavourable histologic features/advanced lesions

- consider neoadjuvant treatment with FOLFOX/CAPEOX in T4b
- Adjuvant treatment not usually indicated; may be considered in high-risk stage II and stage III disease
  - preferred adjuvant regimens
    capecitabine or 5-FU/leucovorin in T3N0M0
    capecitabine or 5-FU/leucovorin or FOLFOX or CAPEOX in high-risk T3N0M0 or T4N0M0
    CAPEOX or FOLFOX in nodal disease

Unresectable/metastatic colon cancer [4]

- Chemotherapy
  - preferred regimens
    FOLFOX ± bevacizumab/FOLFOX + cetuximab/panitumumab in KRAS/NRAS/BRAF wild type and left-sided tumor
    5-FU + leucovorin ± bevacizumab indicated in patients who cannot tolerate aggressive regimens [5]

Resectable rectal cancer

- Endoscopic resection for malignant polyps without unfavourable prognostic histologic features
  - consider transanal excision/transabdominal resection for sessile malignant polyps without unfavourable prognostic features
- Transanal excision for T1N0 [5]
- Transabdominal resection for more advanced lesions
  - neoadjuvant chemoradiotherapy in T3N (any)/T1-2N1-2/T4N (any)
    capecitabine + RT/5-FU + RT

Unresectable rectal cancer

- Neoadjuvant chemoradiotherapy
  - preferred regimens
    capecitabine + RT/5-FU + RT followed by restaging
- Transabdominal resection if restaging is favorable

Metastatic rectal cancer

- Resectable single liver/lung metastases
  - preferred regimens
    FOLFOX or CAPEOX
    short-course RT can be considered
- Unresectable single liver and/or lung only metastases
  - preferred regimens
    FOLFIRI/FOLFOX/CAPEOX/FOLFOXIRI± bevacizumab
    FOLFIRI/FOLFOX /FOLFOXIRI ± cetuximab or panitumumab (KRAS/NRAS/BRAF wild type only) [5]
- Unresectable metastases of other sites
  - similar to colon cancer

References

1. Hossain MS, Karuniawati H, Jairoun AA, Urbi Z, Ooi J, John A, Lim YC, Kibria KMK, Mohiuddin AKM, Ming LC, Goh KW, Hadi MA. Colorectal cancer: a review of carcinogenesis, global epidemiology, current challenges, risk factors, preventive and treatment strategies. Cancer. 2022;14(7):1732.
2. Van Cutsem E, Verheul HM, Flamen P, Rougier P, Beets-Tan R, Glynne-Jones R, Seufferlein T. Imaging in colorectal cancer: progress and challenges for the clinicians. Cancer. 2016;8(9):81.
3. Amin MB, Greene FL, Edge SB, Compton CC, Gershenwald JE, Brookland RK, Meyer L, Gress DM, Byrd DR, Winchester DP. The Eighth Edition AJCC Cancer Staging Manual: continuing to build a

bridge from a population-based to a more "personalized" approach to cancer staging. CA Cancer J Clin. 2017;67(2):93–9.

4. Van Cutsem E, Cervantes A, Nordlinger B, Arnold D, ESMO Guidelines Working Group. Metastatic colorectal cancer: ESMO Clinical Practice Guidelines for diagnosis, treatment and follow-up. Ann Oncol. 2014;25(Suppl 3):1–9.

5. Benson AB, Venook AP, Al-Hawary MM, Cederquist L, Chen YJ, Ciombor KK, Cohen S, Cooper HS, Deming D, Engstrom PF, Grem JL, Grothey A, Hochster HS, Hoffe S, Hunt S, Kamel A, Kirilcuk N, Krishnamurthi S, Messersmith WA, Meyerhardt J, Mulcahy MF, Murphy JD, Nurkin S, Saltz L, Sharma S, Shibata D, Skibber JM, Sofocleous CT, Stoffel EM, Stotsky-Himelfarb E, Willett CG, Wuthrick E, Gregory KM, Gurski L, Freedman-Cass DA. Rectal cancer, Version 2.2018, NCCN clinical practice guidelines in oncology. J Natl Compr Cancer Netw. 2018;16(7):874–901.

Lower Gastrointestinal Bleeding

36

Sevastița Iordache

36.1 Definition

- Bleeding from a source distal to the ligament of Treitz (small bowel, colon, and rectum)

36.2 Classification

- Severe bleeding
  - Hemodynamic instability
  - Hemoglobin level <7 g/dl
- Moderate bleeding
  - Hemodynamically stable
- Occult bleeding
  - Chronic iron-deficiency anemia

S. Iordache (✉)
Department of Gastroenterology, University of Medicine and Pharmacy Craiova, Craiova, Romania

© The Author(s), under exclusive license to Springer Nature Switzerland AG 2023

A. Săftoiu (ed.), *Pocket Guide to Advanced Endoscopy in Gastroenterology*, https://doi.org/10.1007/978-3-031-42076-4_36

36.3 Epidemiology

- Incidence of 33–87/100,000 [1].
- Male > female
- Elderly patients with comorbidities

36.4 Etiology

- Colonic diverticulosis (Fig. 36.1)
  - The most frequent cause of severe bleeding
- Anorectal lesions:
  - hemorrhoids (Fig. 36.2), fissures, and rectal ulcers (Fig. 36.3)
- Vascular lesions: angioectasias (Fig. 36.4) and Dieulafoy lesions (Fig. 36.5)

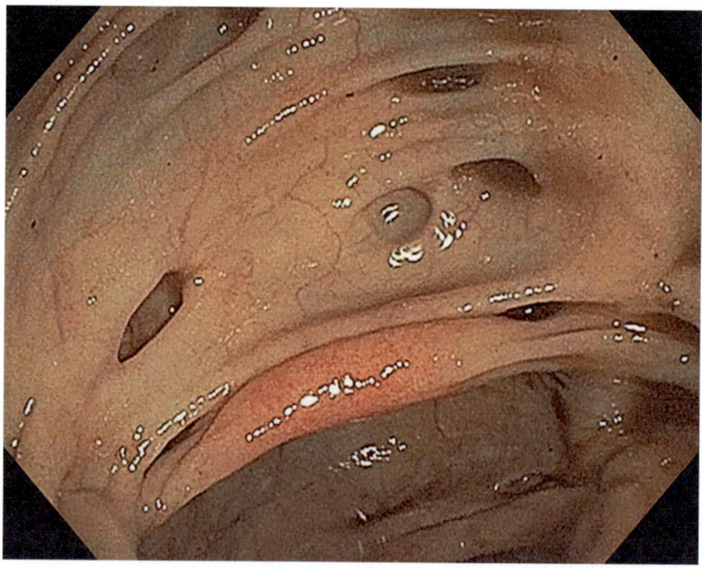

Fig. 36.1 Multiple diverticula in the descending colon, without bleeding stigmas

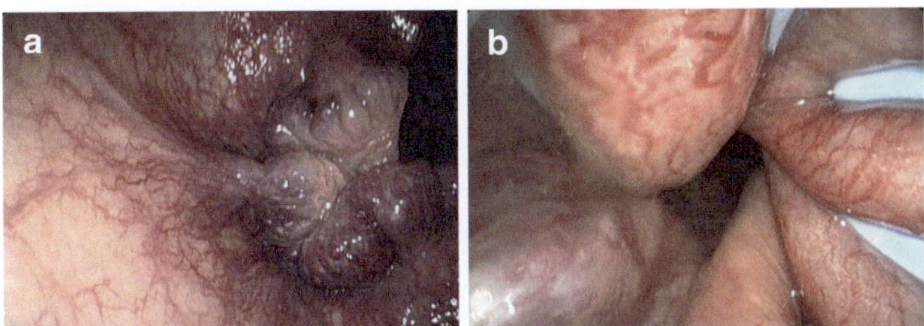

Fig. 36.2 Internal hemorrhoids viewed in retroflection (**a**) and in direct image, facilitated by an EndoCuff device (**b**)

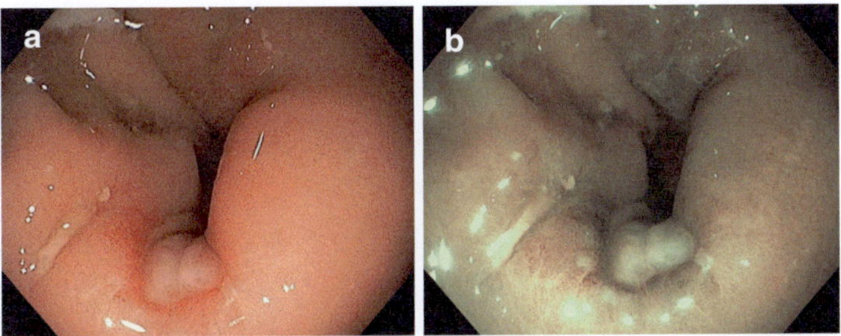

Fig. 36.3 Solitary rectal ulcer in a patient with chronic constipation, visualized in white light mode (**a**) and NBI mode (**b**)

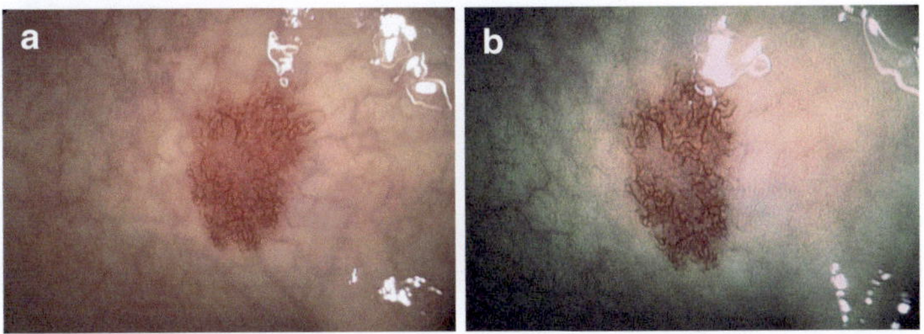

Fig. 36.4 Angiodysplasia in the cecum visualized in white light mode (**a**) and i-SCAN mode (**b**)

- Irradiation proctitis (Fig. 36.6)
- Inflammatory bowel disease (IBD) (see Chap. 28)

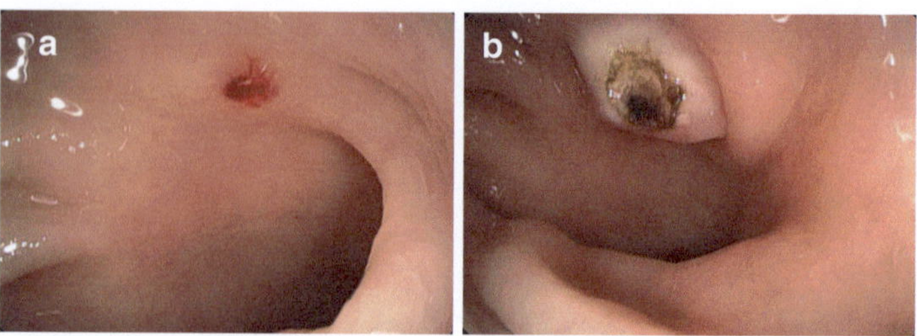

Fig. 36.5 Dieulafoy lesion in ascending colon (**a**), coagulated with gold probe (**b**)

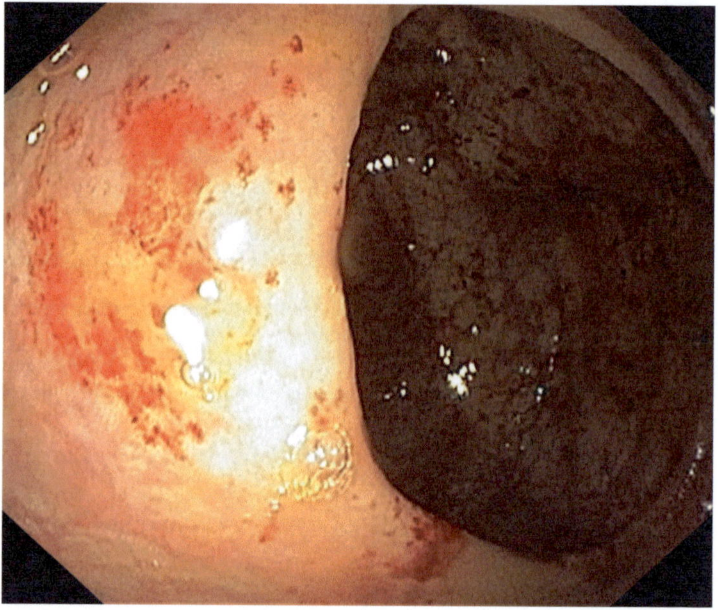

Fig. 36.6 Irradiation proctopathy

- Colorectal malignant tumors (Fig. 36.7)
- Polyps
  - Post-polypectomy bleeding (Fig. 36.8)
  - Ulcerated polyps
- Vascular diseases
  - Ischemic colitis (Fig. 36.9)—in elderly with cardiovascular risk factors
  - Vasculitis: rheumatoid arthritis, Henoch–Schönlein purpura, polyarteritis nodosa, Churg–Strauss syndrome, etc [2].
  - Rectal, or colonic varices (Fig. 36.10)
- Aortoenteric fistula
  - Severe bleeding with a high mortality rate

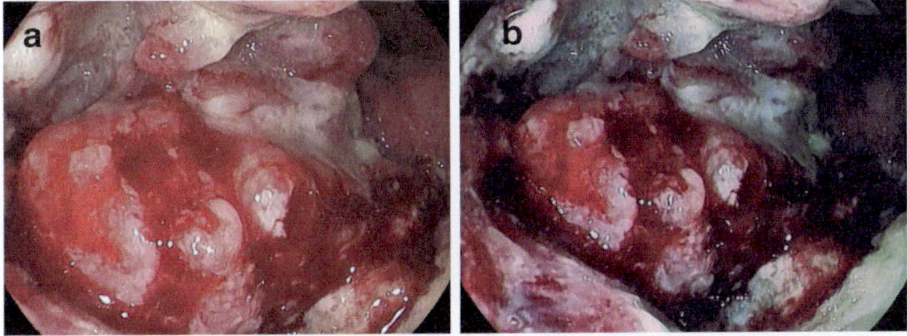

Fig. 36.7 Bleeding in a stenotic rectal tumour, visualized in white light (**a**) and i-SCAN (**b**)

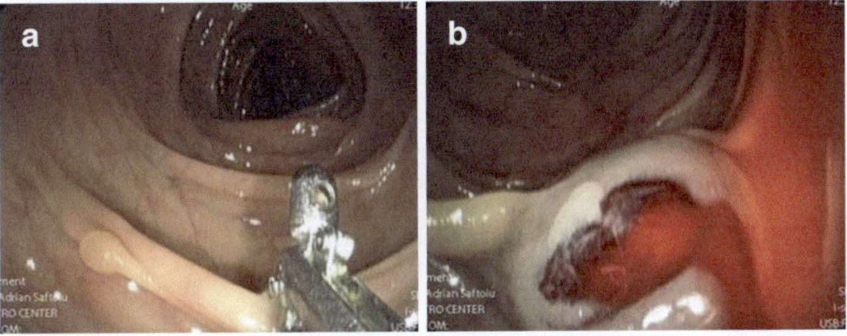

Fig. 36.8 Post-polypectomy bleeding in a diminutive polyp (3 mm) resected with biopsy forceps (**a**), stopped after placement of a hemostatic clip (**b**)

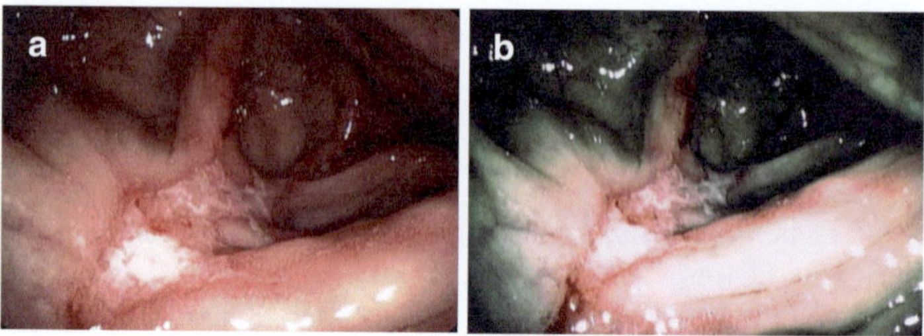

Fig. 36.9 Ischemic colitis, with edema, hyperemia, and longitudinal ulcerations, visualized in white light (**a**) and i-SCAN (**b**), respectively

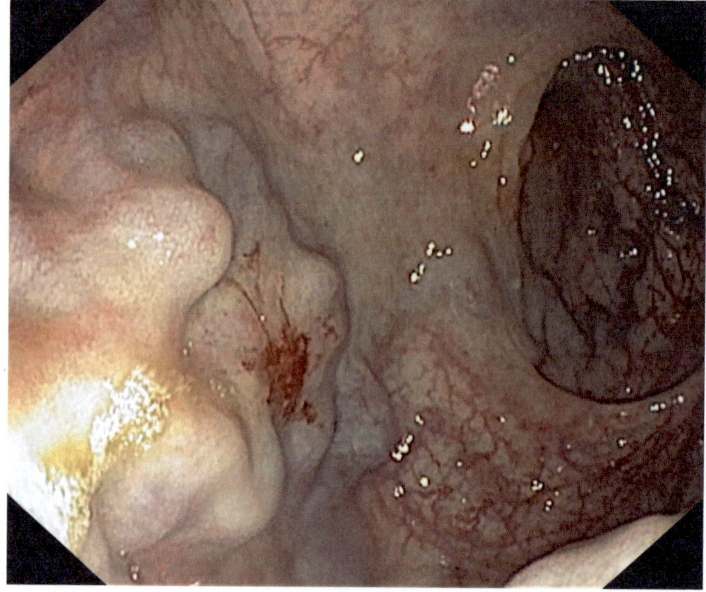

Fig. 36.10 Rectal varices with bleeding stigmas in a patient with cirrhosis and severe LGIB

36.5   Risk Factors

- Advanced ages
- Antithrombotic drugs
- NSAIDs
- Radiotherapy (cervical, or prostate cancer)
- Coagulopathy [3]

36.6   Initial Assessment [1, 3]

- Hemodynamic parameters
    - Shock index (SI) = heart rate (HR)/systolic blood pressure (SBP)
    - Stable patients (SI < 1) or unstable patients (SI > 1)
- Digital rectal examination (DRE)
- Nasogastric tube (to exclude UGIB)
- Risk factors assessment and comorbidities
- Blood parameters: hemoglobin level, platelets count, BUN, creatinine, and coagulation parameters
- Risk assessment
    - Oakland score (OS) for stable patients (Table 36.1)
        OS > 8 major bleeding → admission
        OS < 8 minor bleeding → discharged

Table 36.1 Oakland score for risk assessment [1]

Parameter		Score
Age (years)	<40	0
	40–69	1
	≥70	2
Gender	Female	0
	Male	1
Previous LGIB admission	No	0
	Yes	1
DRE	No blood	0
	Blood	1
HR	<70	0
	70–89	1
	90–109	2
	≥110	3
SBP	<90	5
	90–119	4
	120–129	3
	130–159	2
	≥160	0
Hemoglobin (g/dL)	<7	22
	7–8.9	17
	9–10.9	13
	11–12.9	8
	13–15.9	4
	≥16	0

36.7 Diagnosis

- For LGIB: stools aspect, DRE, nasogastric tube
- For source
  - CT angiography
  - Rectosigmoidoscopy
  - Colonoscopy
  - Red cells-labeled scintigraphy

36.8 Imaging Methods

- Rectosigmoidoscopy
  - A useful method for lesions of the rectum, and left colon, when the colonoscopy is not feasible
  - Retroflection is mandatory: hemorrhoidal disease and low rectal lesions assessment
- Colonoscopy [4–6]
  - First investigation
  - Safe procedure
  - After bowel preparation with PEG-based solutions—a nasogastric tube could be useful
  - An excellent tool for detecting bleeding sites located in the colon or distal ileum, with therapeutic possibilities
  - Timing:
      Early colonoscopy (<24 h) reduced hospitalization, and transfusions but important clinical outcomes such as mortality, rebleeding, and surgery are comparable to elective colonoscopy
      Elective colonoscopy (36–60 h)
      Delayed maximum 2 weeks in patients with minor bleeding
- CT angiography
  - In hemodynamically unstable patients
      After initial resuscitation
      In suspected active bleeding
  - Localize the site of blood loss before planning endoscopic or radiological therapy
- Catheter angiography (CTA)
  - First-line investigation in patients with an active LGIB (shock index of ≥ 1)
- Upper GI endoscopy
  - For differential diagnosis with upper GI bleeding
  - Should be performed prior to colonoscopy, in patients with active bleeding and unclear site of bleeding (upper or lower GI tract)

- This could be the first investigation of stable patients after initial resuscitation
- Nuclear scintigraphy (99mTc pertechnetate-labeled autologous red blood cell scan (TRBC scan) or indium-111 (111In)-labeled RBC scintigraphy)
  - Can detect hemorrhage at low rates
  - More sensitive than mesenteric angiography in detecting ongoing bleeding
  - The main disadvantage is the lack of therapeutic abilities
  - Rarely indicated because of delaying therapy
- Video capsule endoscopy
  - Indications
      Suspected hemorrhagic lesions in the small intestine
      Negative colonoscopy or upper GI endoscopy and unknown source of the bleeding
  - Limitations: no therapeutic method, poorly located lesion, delaying reading the images and getting the result [1, 3]

36.9 Treatment

- Antithrombotic therapy management [7]
  - *Oral anticoagulants* (warfarin or acenocoumarin) should be stopped at presentation in all patients
      In low thrombotic risk patients—could be restarted after 7 days
  - *In high thrombotic risk patients* (mechanical heart valve, cardiac assist device, CHA_2DS_2-VASc score ≥ 4)—replaced with low-molecular-weight therapy after 48 h. Oral anticoagulants could be restarted during first week in selected patients (efficient and durable hemostasis)
      In overdoses of oral anticoagulants, endoscopy should be delayed until the INR decreases < 5
  - *Aspirin*
      When used for primary prophylaxis—could be permanently stopped

When used for secondary prophylaxis—stopped until hemostasis is achieved
- *Dual antiplatelet therapy* for coronary stent: stop only P2Y12 receptor antagonist – advice from a cardiologist is necessary

  DOAC (direct oral anticoagulants) should be stopped at the presentation and restarted in 7–15 days after hemorrhage if hemostasis is achieved

  In the case of triple therapy (OAC and DAPT), downgrading to dual therapy (OAC and clopidogrel) should be considered
- Blood transfusions
  - Red blood cell transfusion is indicated at a Hb level <7 g/dl, target Hb is 8 g/dl. The target Hb is 9 g/dl in patients with cardiovascular disease
- Endoscopic therapy—options:
  - *Epinephrine injection* (1:10,000 dilution) in the submucosa, around the lesion. In the rectum low doses and dilution of 1:100,000 are recommended due to rich vascularization and the risk of spreading in the systemic circulation

    Indicated in association with other techniques (thermic, or mechanical)

    In post-polypectomy bleeding
  - *Thermocoagulation*: different approach as compared to UGIB: lower power, less pressure, and shorter pulses (due to risk of perforation). Is safer in rectal lesions approaching

    Indicated in selected cases after polypectomy
  - *Argon plasma coagulation* is recommended at lower power and gasflow

    Indicated in angioectasias and irradiation proctitis
  - *Mechanical methods* (hemoclips)

    Diverticular bleeding

    Post-polypectomy bleeding
  - *Hemostatic powders* in tumor bleeding:
- Radiologic treatment
  - Coils embolization

- N-butyl cyanoacrylate injection
- Risk: ischemia
- Surgery
  - When endoscopic or radiological interventional measures have failed
  - For the management of complications of endoscopic or radiological interventions

36.10 Prognosis

- Mortality varies between 3.6 and 3.9%
- High mortality rate:
  - Elderly
  - Male > female
  - Comorbid illness
  - Intestinal ischemia
  - Coagulopathy/hematological disorders
  - Bleeding during hospitalization
  - Hypovolemia or shock
  - High transfusion requirement [8, 9]
- Patients with colorectal polyps and perianal disease (hemorrhoids, or fissures) have a better prognosis.

References

1. Oakland K, Chadwick G, East JE, Guy R, Humphries A, Jairath V, et al. Diagnosis and management of acute lower gastrointestinal bleeding: guidelines from the British Society of Gastroenterology. Gut. 2019;68:776–89.
2. Geboes K, Dalle I. Vasculitis and the gastrointestinal tract. Acta Gastroenterol Belg. 2002;65:204–12.
3. Oakland K, Guy R, Uberoi R, Hogg R, Mortensen N, Murphy MF, Jairath V, UK Lower GI Bleeding Collaborative. Acute lower GI bleeding in the UK: patient charactaristics, interventions, and outcomes in the first nationwide audit. Gut. 2018;67:654–62.

4. Green BT, Rockey DC, Portwood G, et al. Urgent colonoscopy for evaluation and management of acute lower gastrointestinal hemorrhage: a randomized controlled trial. Am J Gastroenterol. 2005;100:2395–402.
5. Laine L, Shah A. Randomized trial of urgent vs. elective colonoscopy in patients hospitalized with lower GI bleeding. Am J Gastroenterol. 2010;105:2636–41.
6. Lim DS, Kim HG, Jeon R, et al. Comparison of clinical effectiveness of the emergent colonoscopy in patients with hematochezia according to the type of bowel preparation. J Gastroenterol Hepatol. 2013;28:1733–7.
7. Gimbel ME, Minderhoud SCS, ten Berg JM. A practical guide on how to handle patients with bleeding events while on oral antithrombotic treatment. Neth Hear J. 2018;26(6):341–51.
8. Strate L, Ayanian JZ, Kotler G, Syngal S. Risk factors for mortality in lower intestinal bleeding. Clin Gastroenterol Hepatol. 2008;6:1004–10.
9. Kwak MS, Cha JM, Han YJ, Yoon JY, Jeon JW, Shin HP, Joo KR, Lee JI. The clinical outcomes of lower gastrointestinal bleeding are not better than those of upper gastrointestinal bleeding. J Korean Med Sci. 2016;31:1611–6.

Obscure and Occult Gastrointestinal Bleeding

Sevastiţa Iordache and Ana-Maria Barbu

37.1 Occult Bleeding

37.1.1 Definition

- Gastrointestinal bleeding that is unknown to the patient, manifests as faecal occult blood and/or iron-deficiency anaemia (IDA)

37.1.2 Causes

Lesion from any segment of gastrointestinal tract

- Upper GI tract lesions
    - Angiodysplasia (Fig. 37.1a–c)
    - Duodenal ulcer (Fig. 37.2a, b)
    - Esophagitis (Fig. 37.3)

S. Iordache (✉)
Department of Gastroenterology, University of Medicine and Pharmacy Craiova, Craiova, Romania

A.-M. Barbu
University of Medicine and Pharmacy Craiova, Craiova, Romania

© The Author(s), under exclusive license to Springer Nature Switzerland AG 2023
A. Săftoiu (ed.), *Pocket Guide to Advanced Endoscopy in Gastroenterology*, https://doi.org/10.1007/978-3-031-42076-4_37

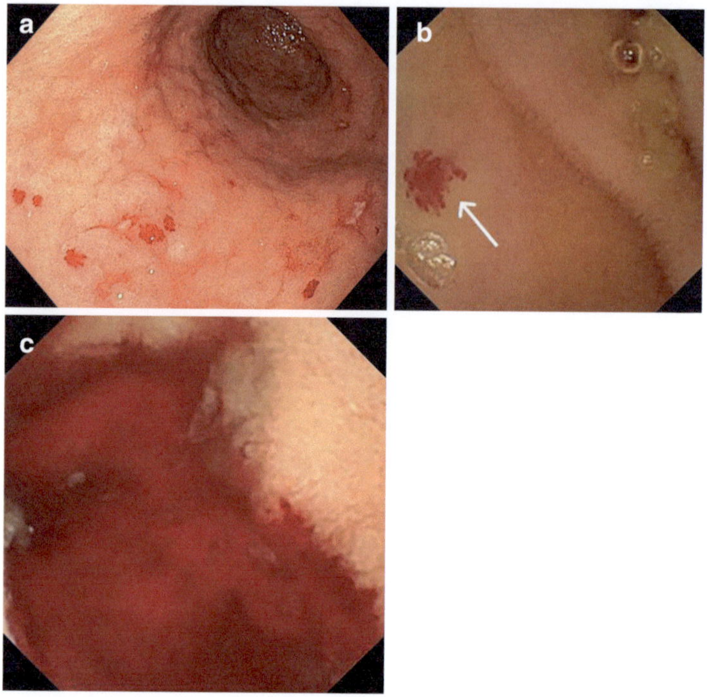

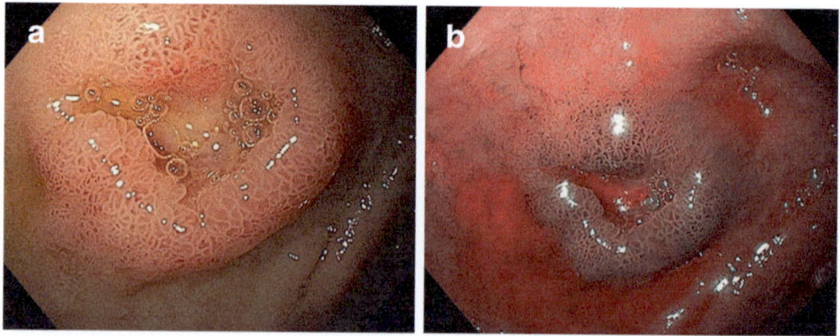

Fig. 37.1 Multiple ulcerations and angioectasias in a patient with IDA (**a**). Videocapsule endoscopy: angioectasia detected in a patient with obscure Gi bleeding (**b**); active bleeding from angiodysplasia (**c**)

Fig. 37.2 Duodenal ulcer—WLE (**a**) and NBI (**b**)

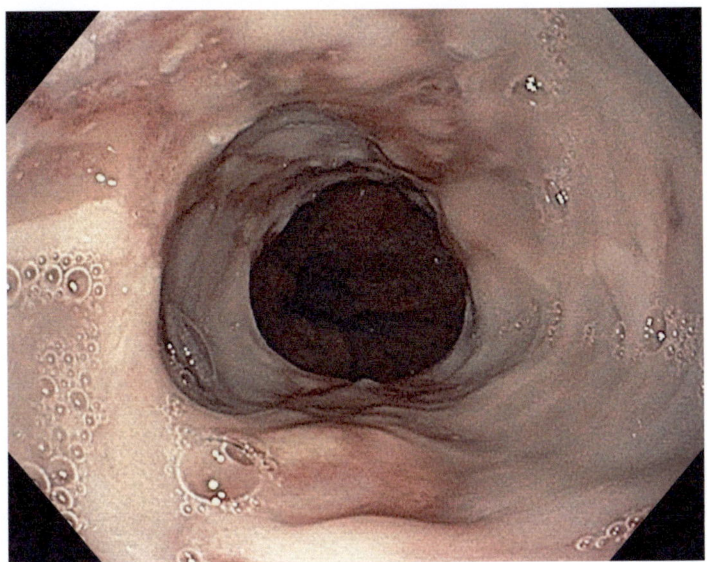

Fig. 37.3 Severe reflux esophagitis in patient with liver cirrhosis and oesophageal varices

- Gastric cancer (Fig. 37.4)
- Gastric ulcer (Fig. 37.5a, b)
- Gastritis (Fig. 37.6)
- Portal-hypertension gastropathy (Fig. 37.7)
- GAVE (Fig. 37.8)
- Cameron's erosions within a hiatal hernia
- Colorectal source
  - Angiodysplasia (Fig. 37.9)
  - Inflammatory bowel disease (Fig. 37.10)
  - Colon cancer (Fig. 37.11)
  - Large adenomas (>1.5 cm)—(Fig. 37.12a, b)
- Small bowel source
  - Crohn's disease (Fig. 37.13)
  - Meckel's diverticulum
  - Vascular diseases: Rendu–Osler syndrome (Fig. 37.14)
  - Celiac sprue and other causes of malabsorption

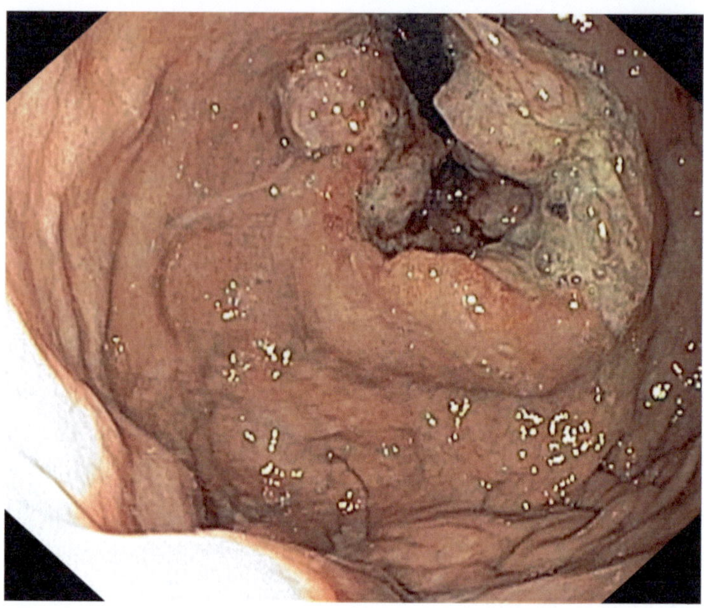

Fig. 37.4 Subcardial ulcerated tumour in a patient with chronic iron-deficiency anaemia

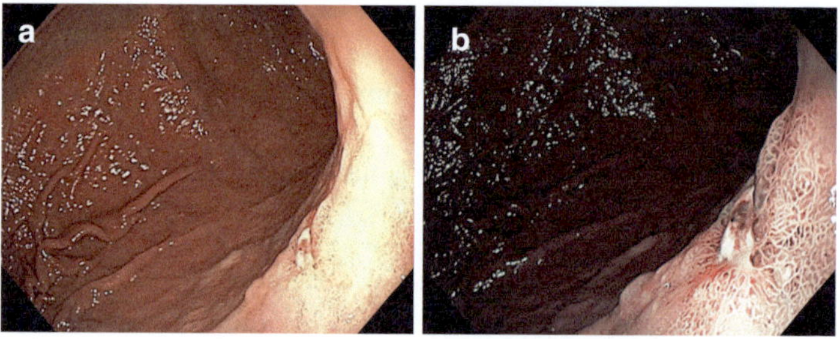

Fig. 37.5 Small curvature gastric ulcer undetected at first endoscopy during active bleeding. WLE (**a**) and NBI (**b**)

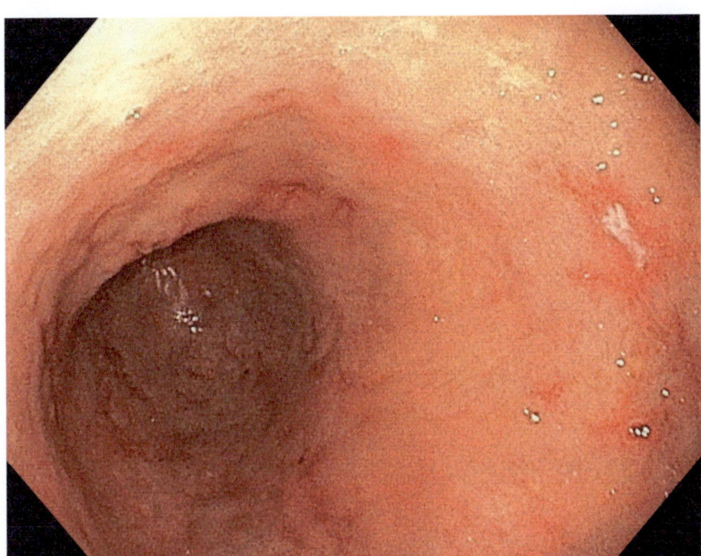

Fig. 37.6 Erosive gastritis in a patient with IDA in treatment with low-dose aspirin

37.1.3 Risk Factors

- Advanced age
- Comorbidities
    - Cardiovascular diseases
    - Cerebrovascular diseases
    - Chronic renal diseases
    - Chronic liver diseases
    - Chronic respiratory diseases
- Drugs
    - NSAIDs
    - Antithrombotic therapy (antiplatelet drugs/anticoagulants)

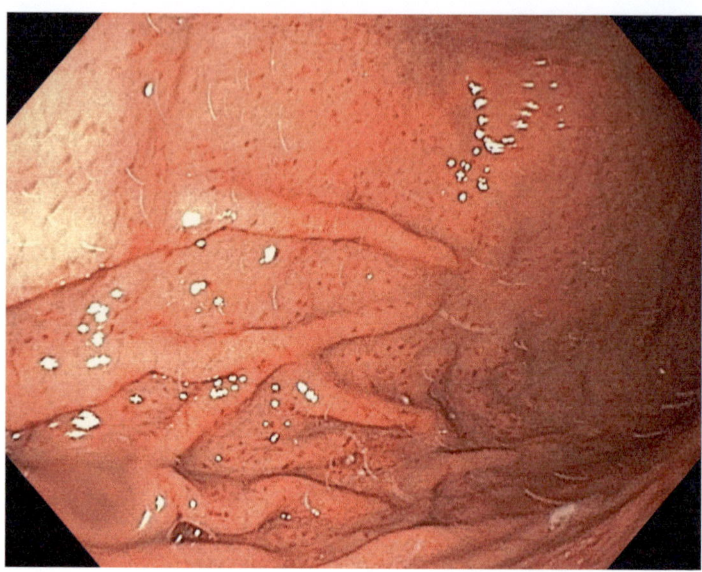

Fig. 37.7 Portal-hypertensive gastropathy: corporeal petechias in a patient with liver cirrhosis

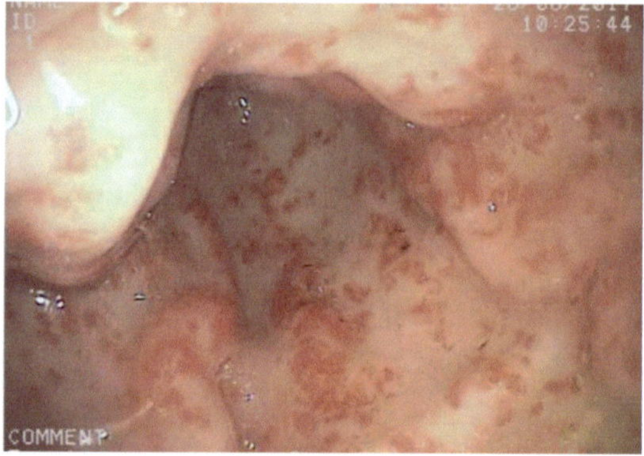

Fig. 37.8 Gastric antral vascular ectasia (GAVE)

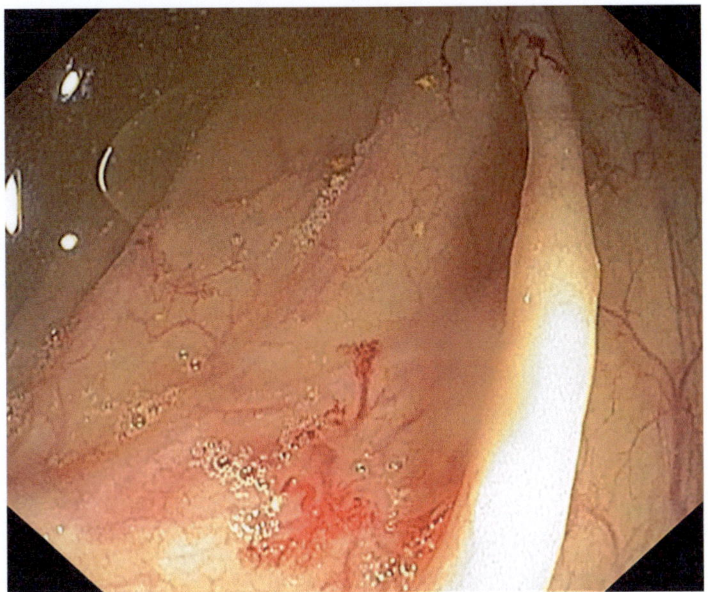

Fig. 37.9 Telangiectasia detected at colonoscopy in a patient with IDA

37.1.4 Diagnosis

- History and physical examination
  - Personal history of GI bleeding, surgery, or comorbidities, NSAIDs and antithrombotic therapy, gastric bypass surgery, history of diarrhoea, chronic liver disease
  - Family history of GI bleeding may suggest an inherited disease like hereditary haemorrhagic telangiectasia (Rendu–Osler)
- Differential diagnosis with extraintestinal causes of iron deficiency anaemia/bleeding: epistaxis, haematuria, haemoptysis, and gynaecologic bleeding

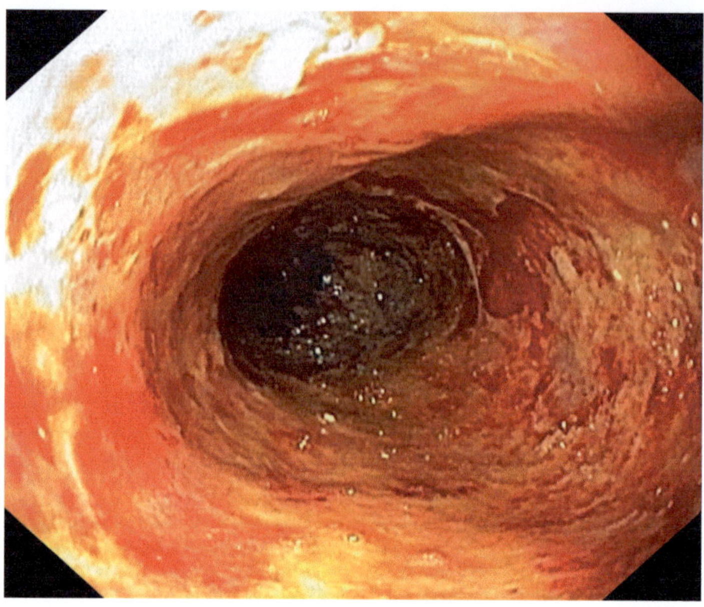

Fig. 37.10 Ulcerative colitis in a patient with mixed anaemia (post-haemorrhagic and IDA), chronic diarrhoea, and rectal bleeding. Ulcerated and fragile hyperaemic mucosa in a colon without haustral folds can be seen.

- Iron-deficiency anaemia
  - Low–haemoglobin level
  - Hypochromic and microcytic anaemia
  - Low serum of iron and ferritin level
  - Increased level of transferrin and total iron-binding capacity (TIBC)
- Faecal occult bleeding tests (FOBTs)
  - Detect occult bleeding that is not observed by the patient
  - The most valuable FOBTs are immunochemical tests (no special meal is needed prior testing, better sensitivity as compared to guaiac tests)

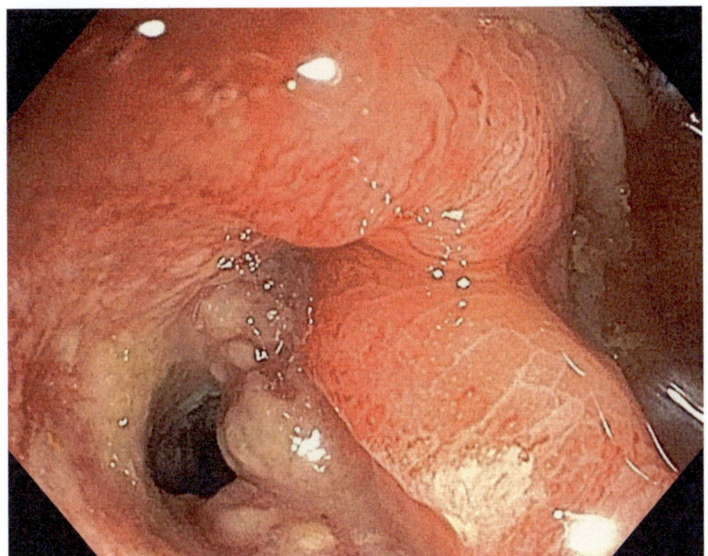

Fig. 37.11 Ulcerated and stricturing tumour of the colon

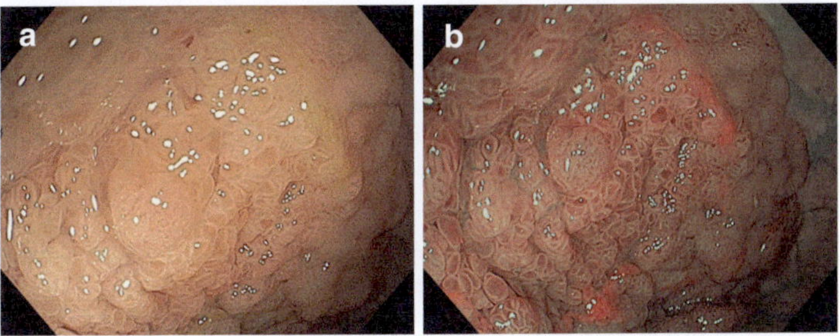

Fig. 37.12 Large flat villous adenoma of the rectum—WLE (**a**) and NBI (**b**)

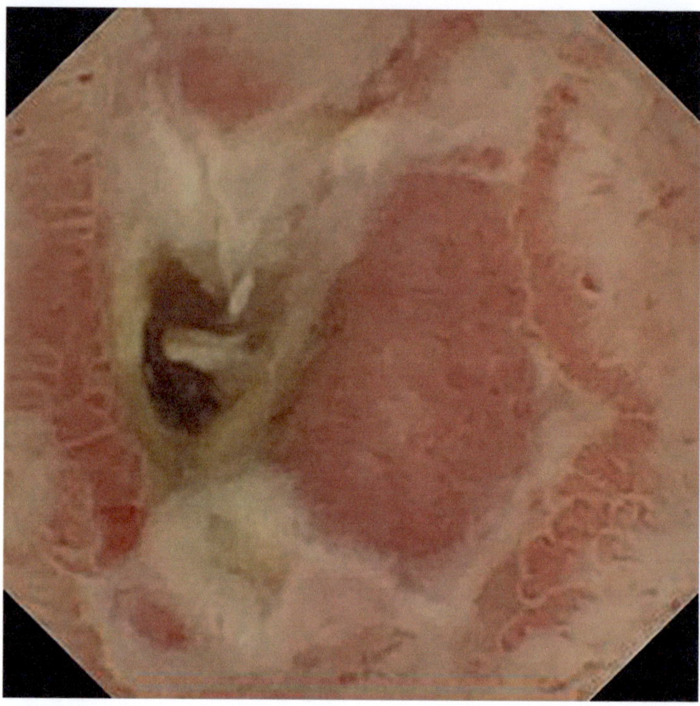

Fig. 37.13 Circumferential ulceration in the ileum in a patient with Crohn's disease detected at VCE in a patient with IDA, abdominal pain, and diarrhoea, after negative upper GI endoscopy and colonoscopy

- Endoscopy—the standard method to detect lesions, with important advantages: safe, allows biopsies and haemostasis
  - Upper GI endoscopy
  - Colonoscopy
  - Enteroscopy
- Small bowel biopsy—in patients with IDA and suspected celiac sprue
- CT scan—indicated in malignant tumours
- CT enterography in negative results in endoscopy

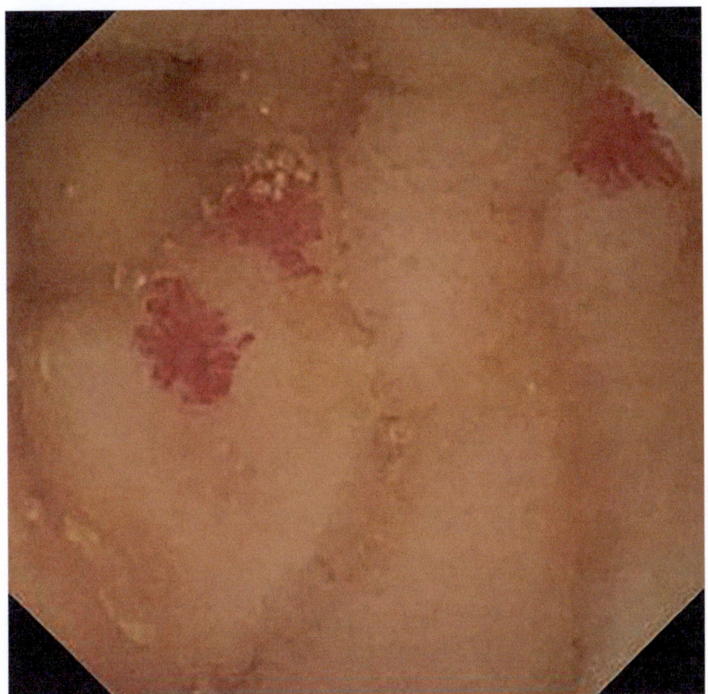

Fig. 37.14 Rendu–Osler syndrome: numerous angioectasia detected with VCE in a patient with IDA and recurrent digestive bleeding (melena)

37.1.5 Assessment

- Positive FOBT and/or iron-deficiency anaemia
  - Upper GI endoscopy and colonoscopy should be performed
  - If negative results: enteroscopy should be performed
  - CT enterography represents next step in negative result after endoscopic assessment

37.2 Obscure Bleeding

37.2.1 Definition

Bleeding from the gastrointestinal tract that persists or recurs after a negative initial evaluation (upper endoscopy and colonoscopy).

37.2.2 Causes

- Vascular
    - Angioectasias (Fig. 37.15)
    - Dieulafoy lesion (Fig. 37.16)
    - GAVE
    - Portal-hypertensive gastropathy

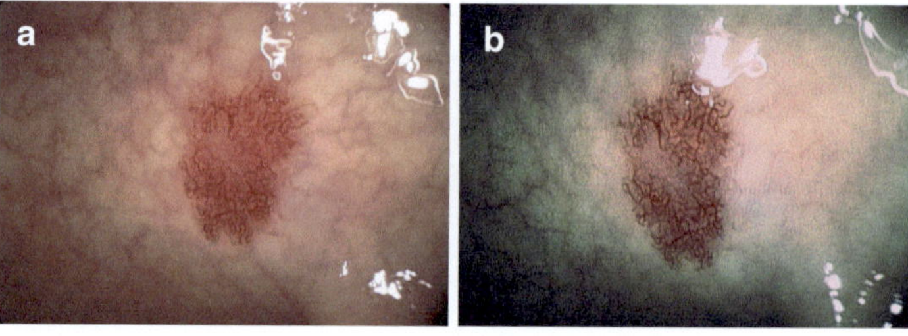

Fig. 37.15 Colonic angioectasia—WLE (**a**) and i-SCAN (**b**)

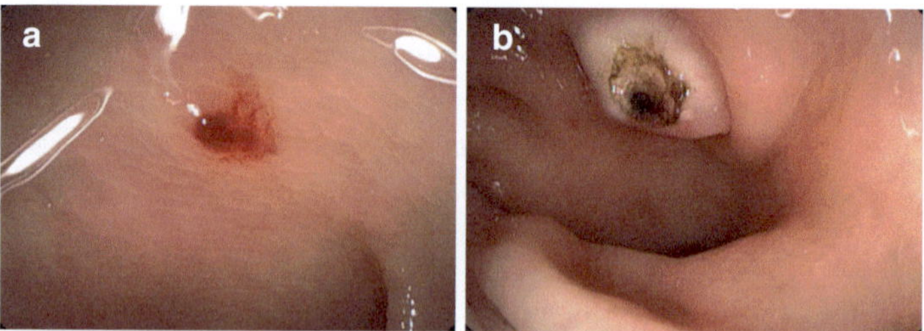

Fig. 37.16 Colonic Dieulafoy lesion with visible vessel (**a**) and the aspect immediately after coagulation (**b**)

- Varices (oesophageal, gastric, small bowel, and colonic) (Fig. 37.17)
- Haemorrhoids (Fig. 37.18)
- Radiation enteritis (Fig. 37.19)

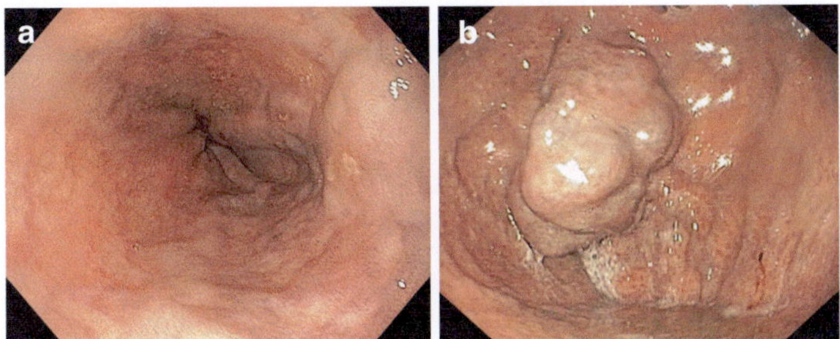

Fig. 37.17 Oesophageal varices with ulcerations on the surface (**a**) and isolated gastric varices (**b**)

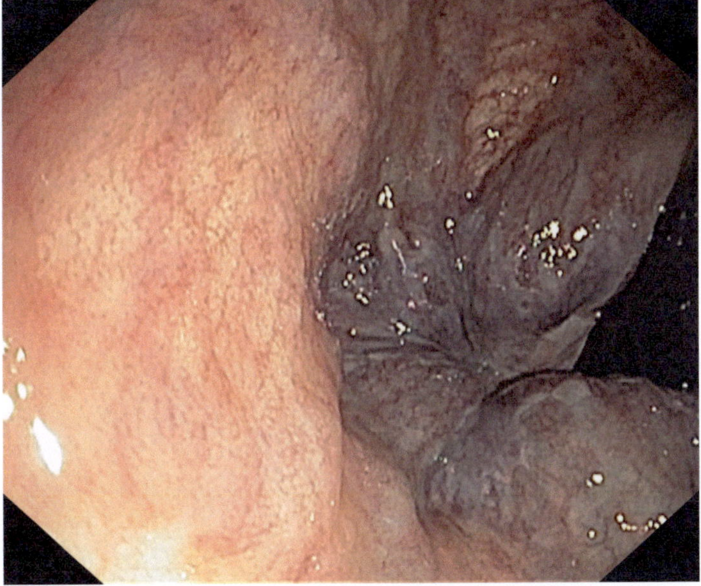

Fig. 37.18 Haemorrhoids in a patient with recurrent bleeding and previous colonoscopy without significant other source of bleeding

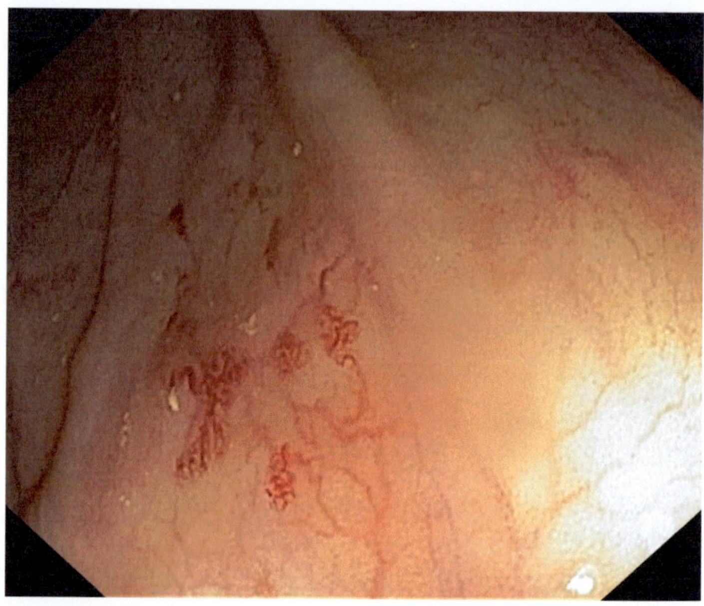

Fig. 37.19 Small angioectasias detected in the rectum at 1 year after radiotherapy for prostate cancer

- Inflammatory
  - Esophagitis
  - Peptic ulcer disease
  - Cameron erosions
  - Inflammatory bowel disease
- Meckel diverticulum
- NSAID-related pathology of digestive tract
- Neoplastic
  - Carcinoid
  - GIST (Fig. 37.20)
  - Adenocarcinoma
  - Lymphoma

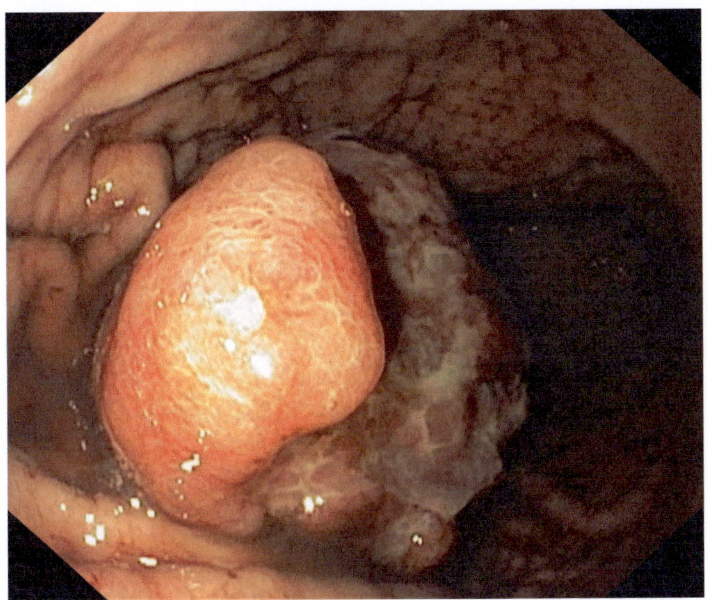

Fig. 37.20 Submucosal ulcerated tumour of the stomach. Immunohisto-chemistry revealed the GIST aspect

- – Ampullary adenoma/carcinoma
- – Metastases (melanoma)
- Extraluminal
  - – Haemobilia
  - – Wirsungorrhagia
- Vasculoenteric fistula
- Rare causes
  - – Hereditary haemorrhagic telangiectasia
  - – von Willebrand disease
  - – Pseudoxanthoma elasticum
  - – Amyloidosis
  - – Henoch–Schöenlein purpura

37.2.3 Diagnosis

In case of unidentified lesions at first endoscopic assessment, upper endoscopy and colonoscopy should be repeated. ESGE recommend routinely second-look endoscopy in selected patients. If no lesions are identified at the second examination, enteroscopy should be considered

- Endoscopy
  - Upper GI endoscopy
  - Colonoscopy
  - Enteroscopy:

    Videocapsule endoscopy (VCE) represents first-line investigation after negative standard endoscopy. It should be performed as soon as possible after the lower GI bleeding.

    Push enteroscopy. The main disadvantages are the looping of the enteroscope and patient discomfort. Development of capsule endoscopy and other enteroscopy techniques led to replacement of these technique.

    Single-balloon enteroscopy is a technique using an overtube with an inflatable balloon fixed to the distal tip.

    Double-balloon enteroscopy (DBE) has the advantage of assessment of entire small bowel using anterograde or the retrograde route.

    Spiral enteroscopy. The enteroscope can be locked in the overtube. Thus, the overtube advances using clockwise rotating. At withdrawal the spiral overtube is rotating counterclockwise.

    Balloon-guided endoscopy—the working channel of the scope allows the passage of balloon catheter for advancing into the small bowel.

    Intraoperative enteroscopy. The progression of the endoscope is facilitated by the manual external assistance.

- Radiological evaluation
  - Technetium 99m-labeled red blood cell nuclear scan (RBCS)

    Can detect gastrointestinal bleeding at a low rate 0.1–0.4 mL/min

    Disadvantages: low accuracy for localization of bleeding source; therapeutic measures are not possible during procedure
  - Angiography

    Useful for localization of active bleeding and diagnosis of nonbleeding vascular lesions and tumours

    Detect bleeding at a higher rate as compared to RBCS (>0.5 mL/min)

    Allow therapeutic manoeuvres: stenting, coil embolization, vasopressin infusion, etc.
  - CT enterography/enteroclysis
  - Angio CT

37.2.4 Management

- First assessment in emergency room
  - Risk factors
  - Type of bleeding (melena or haematochezia)
  - Severity of bleeding
  - Transfusions need
  - Presence of iron-deficiency anaemia
  - Associated clinical symptoms (abdominal pain and/or weight loss)
- Identification of bleeding lesion and proper treatment
  - Endoscopic interventions
  - Angiographic embolization
  - Surgical resection
- Medical management has not been shown to be effective in the long-term management of patients with OGIB

- Endoscopic treatment is possible in most cases with bleeding from upper GI tract and colon
- Radiological and surgical treatment represents second-line therapy after endoscopic treatment failure
- Endoscopic therapy
  - For angiodysplasias, gastric antral vascular ectasia, vascular malformations, and hereditary haemorrhagic telangiectasia: thermal contact probes, injection sclerotherapy, argon plasma coagulation (Fig. 37.21), neodymium: yttrium-aluminium-garnet (Nd:YAG) laser
- Angiographic therapy
  - Embolization of bleeding source
    Adverse events: intestinal infarction, fistulization, arterial thrombosis, etc.
  - Vasopressin infusion—effective for small bowel and colonic bleeding sources.
    Adverse events: cardiovascular—myocardial infarction, hypertension, arrhythmias
- Surgery is indicated for tumour bleeding and life-threatening bleeding.

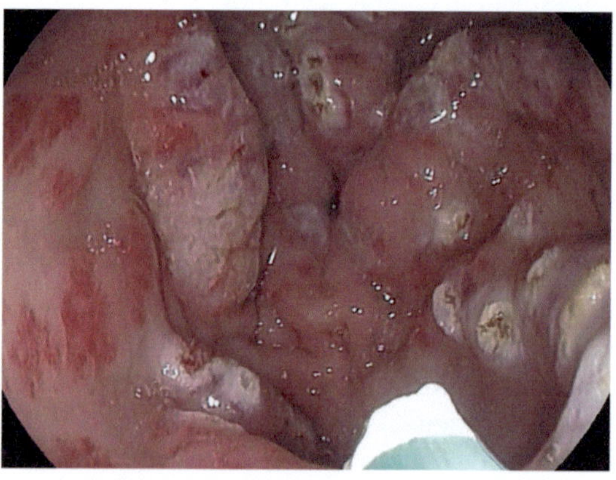

Fig. 37.21 Plasma Argon coagulation in a patient with occult beeding and gastric antral vascular ectasia (GAVE)

- – In case of failure of endoscopy or radiological techniques:
      Segmental resection
      Total colectomy—in massive bleeding
- Medical treatment—adjuvant or in case of failure of other techniques: endoscopy, surgery, or radiologic treatment.
- Drugs:
  - – Progesterone/oestrogen therapy
  - – Octreotide
  - – Other pharmacological agents: danazol, desmopressin, aminocaproic acid
- Other measures:
  - – Correction of coagulation disorders, platelets
  - – Transfusion
  - – Blood transfusions
  - – Treatment of IDA

References

1. Zuckerman GR, Prakash C, Askin MP, Lewis BS. AGA technical review on the evaluation and management of occult and obscure gastrointestinal bleeding. Gastroenterology. 2000;118(1):201–21.
2. Pasha SF, Hara AK, Leighton JA. Diagnostic evaluation and management of obscure gastrointestinal bleeding: a changing paradigm. Gastroenterol Hepatol. 2009;5(12):839–50.
3. Bull-Henry K, Al-Kawas FH. Evaluation of occult gastrointestinal bleeding. Am Fam Physician. 2013;87(6):430–6.
4. Pennazio M, Spada C, Eliakim R, et al. Small-bowel capsule endoscopy and device-assisted enteroscopy for diagnosis and treatment of small-bowel disorders: European Society of Gastrointestinal Endoscopy (ESGE) Clinical Guideline. Endoscopy. 2015;47(4):352–76.
5. van Cutsem E, Rutgeerts P, Vantrappen G. Treatment of bleeding gastrointestinal vascular malformations with oestrogen-progesterone. Lancet. 1990;335:953–5.
6. Leitman IM, Paull DE, Shires GT. Evaluation and management of massive lower gastrointestinal bleeding. Ann Surg. 1989;209:175–80.
7. Kunihara S, Oka S, Tanaka S. Management of occult obscure gastrointestinal bleeding patients based on long-term outcomes. Ther Adv Gastroenterol. 2018;11:1–9.

Part VIII

Pancreatico-Biliary Diseases

Acute Pancreatitis

38

Bogdan Silviu Ungureanu
and Adrian Săftoiu

38.1 Definition and Classification

Acute pancreatitis (AP) represents an inflammatory disorder of the pancreas associated with or without local or systemic inflammatory response.

- *Acute edematous pancreatitis*—mild form (85%), uncomplicated evolution, complete and fast recovery, low mortality rate (<3%)
- *Acute necrotizing pancreatitis*—severe form (15%), local or systemic complications associated, organ failure, high mortality rate (17%)

B. S. Ungureanu (✉)
Department of Gastroenterology, University of Medicine and Pharmacy Craiova, Craiova, Romania

A. Săftoiu
Department of Gastroenterology and Hepatology, Elias Emergency University Hospital, Carol Davila University of Medicine and Pharmacy, Bucharest, Romania

A. Săftoiu (ed.), *Pocket Guide to Advanced Endoscopy in Gastroenterology*, https://doi.org/10.1007/978-3-031-42076-4_38

38.2   Epidemiology

- AP is:
  - more common as people age
  - 5–80 cases/100,000 population/year
  - men = women
- Risk factors (Table 38.1)

Table 38.1   Etiology of AP

Causes of acute pancreatitis	
Alcohol	Genetic PRSS1; SPINK1; CFTR mutation
Obstructive gallstones Tumors Parasites Duodenal diverticula Annular pancreas choledochocele biliary microlithiasis	Drugs azathioprine/6-mercaptopurine Didanosine Pentamidine Sulfonamide l-asparaginase thiazide diuretics
Mechanical Sphyncter of Oddi dysfunction Pancreas divisum Trauma	Vascular Vasculitis Atherosclerosis Pancreatic vessel embolism hypotension/ ischemia
Postoperative/Post-ERCP Peptic ulcer Inflammatory bowel disease	Infectious viral bacterial parasitic
Metabolic Hypertriglyceridemia hypercalcemia Diabetes mellitus	Other Scorpion sting Idiopathic pancreatitis Cystic fibrosis Coronary bypass tropical pancreatitis oganophosphorus insecticides

38.3 Etiopathogenesis

- Trypsinogen is converted to its active form -trypsin-, which leads to further activation of other molecules of trysin and also other pancreatic enzymes that cause the autodigestion of the pancreas.
- Depending on acinar injury, local complications, systemic inflammatory response, and sepsis may occur [1].

38.4 Diagnosis

- Clinical history/signs:
    - characteristic upper abdominal pain that can sometimes radiate to the back
    - nausea and vomiting
    - pain eased/relieved by leaning forward
    - fever
- Physical examination
    - Painful sensitivity to palpation ± muscular defense
        decreased or absent bowel sounds (paralytic ileus)
        bruising in the subcutaneous fatty tissue of the umbilical area (Cullen's sign) or of the flanks (Turner's sign) or hemorrhagic discoloration of the umbilicus (Cullen's sign) or of the flanks (Grey–Turner's sign)
        jaundice (acute biliary pancreatitis, compression of the main billiary duct by enlarged pancreatic head or pancreatic fluid collections, alcohol-related liver disease)
        palpable abdominal mass (acute collections, tumors)
        tachycardia, hypotension
        dyspnea, tachypnea
- Biochemical
    - elevated serum amylase or lipase levels over three times normal
    - leukocytosis
    - elevated haematocrit (HTC)
    - hypocalcemia, hypoalbuminemia

- elevated AST, ALT, ALP, and bilirubin (biliary acute pancreatitis)
- elevated triglycerides (1000 mg/dL in hypertriglyceridemia-related acute pancreatitis)
- reactive C protein ≥150 mg/l (prognostic factor of severe acute pancreatitis)
- Imagistic investigation
  - Abdominal Ultrasound
    - is the first investigation performed on admission, being able to determine biliary etiology:
      - gallstones
      - IHBD and EHBD dilatation
      - biliary and sludge
      - aerocolia can make the investigation more difficult
      - choledocholitiasis usually passes unnoticed
        - ultrasound can detect:
      - enlarged, hypoechoic pancreas
      - local complications
      - typical aspects of chronic pancreatitis (intraductal/intrapancreatic calcifications, dilated Wirsung's duct)
- Computed tomography (CT)
  - is the preferred assessment tool to diagnose acute pancreatitis ± local complications, to determine the severity of AP (CT severity score), to exclude other abdominal pathology
    - should be performed at 72–96 h after symptom presentation
    - enlarged pancreas or pancreatic edema ± peripancreatic fat infiltration
    - to exclude pancreatic cancer in elderly patients/people
    - the presence of gas bubbles = pancreatic infection
- **MRI + magnetic resonance cholangiopancreatography (MRCP)**
  - similar to CT imaging for staging the severity of AP and detecting fluid collections
  - superior to CT imaging, similar to EUS and ERCP in detecting gallbladder stones

- Abdominal X-ray
  - shows hydroaeric levels
  - pancreatic and peripancreatic calcifications
  - excludes bowel obstruction and perforation
- Thoracic X-ray
  - emphasizes elevated diaphragm, pleural effusion (more frequently on the left side), atelectasis, and lung infiltrates
- *AP is diagnosed* when a patient presents with two of three findings, including:
  - abdominal pain suggestive of pancreatitis
  - serum amylase and/or lipase levels at least three times the normal level
  - characteristic findings on imaging (CT or MRI) [2]

38.5 The Role of Endoscopic Ultrasonography (EUS)

- EUS (linear or radial)/(radial scanning or linear array)
  - highly accurate in detecting microlithiasis, biliary sludge, or choledocholithiasis (Fig. 38.1a, b)
  - shows cystic or solid tumors of the pancreas (Figs. 38.2a, b and 38.3a, b)/small size ampullary cancers, pancreas divisum, or chronic pancreatitis

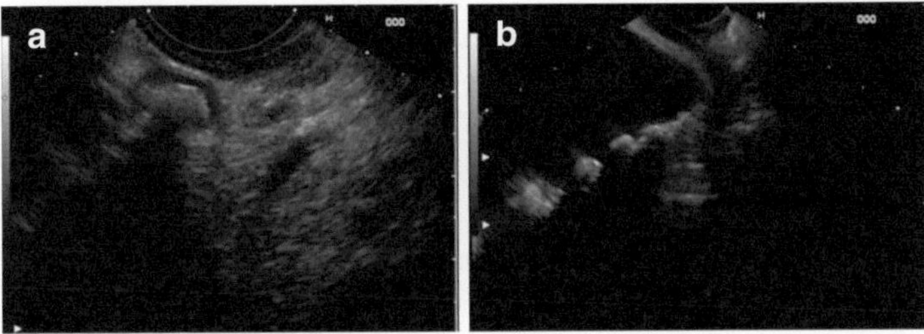

Fig. 38.1 EUS (duodenal view) showing choledocholithiasis with a single stone measuring 10 mm (posterior acoustic shadowing) (**a**), EUS (antrum view) showing multiple gallstones (**b**)

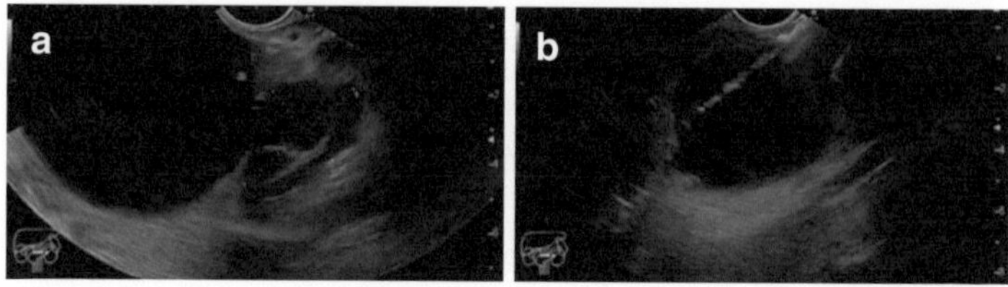

Fig. 38.2 Pseudocyst in the body of the pancreas, situated near a cystic tumor of the pancreas (**a**), EUS-guided drainage into the stomach (**b**)

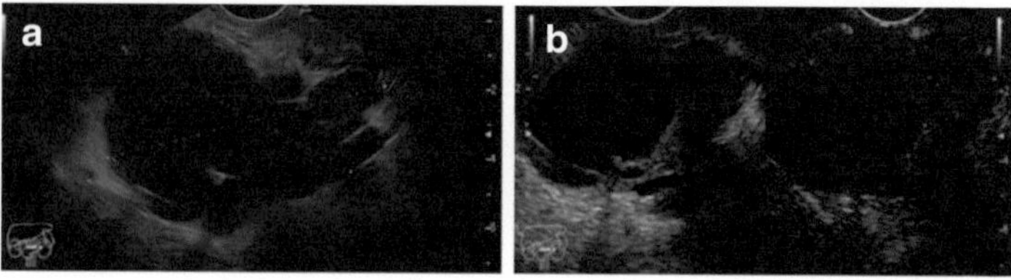

Fig. 38.3 Pseudocyst in the body of the pancreas (**a**), caused by obstructive acute pancreatitis due to pancreatic head adenocarcinoma, detected using contrast agent, with hypocaptant wall (**b**)

- – EUS fine-needle aspiration biopsy in patients with suspected pancreatic/peripancreatic infection (Fig. 38.4)
- EUS-guided drainage
  - – EUS-guided drainage of large, symptomatic pseudocysts can be performed preferably transgastric (Fig. 38.5a, c)/ transduodenal (Fig. 38.6a, c)/rarely transesophageal (Fig. 38.7a, d)
  - – pancreatic necrosectomy of WON (walled off necrosis) or pancreatic/peripancreatic necrosis, after expandable stent placement (Fig. 38.8a, b)
- ERCP has therapeutic role:
  - – Sphincterotomy and CBD stone extraction in the cases of biliary acute pancreatitis associated with cholangitis or persistant bile duct stone/obstructive jaundice

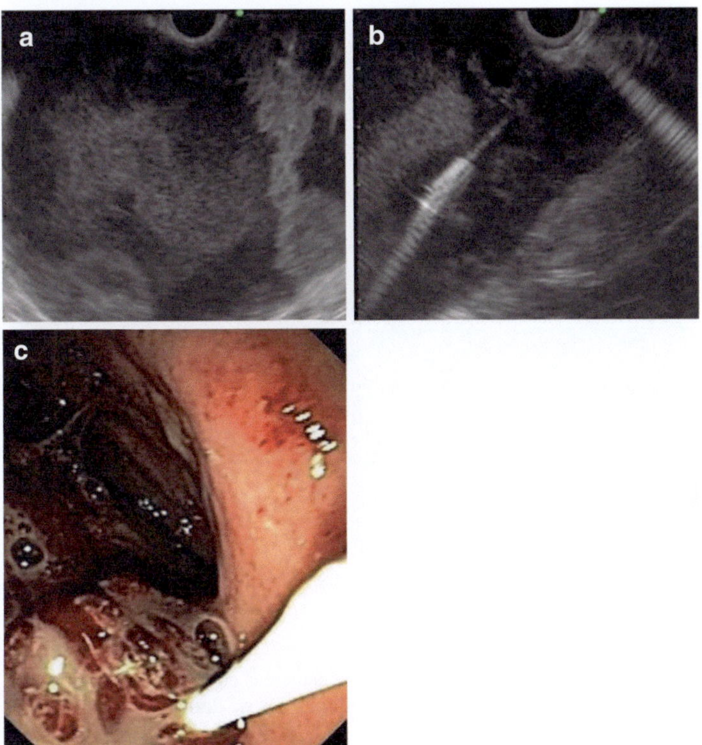

Fig. 38.4 Pseudocyst in the body of the pancreas with highly heterogeneous content, suggestive for infection (**a**), punctured using a 19 G needle and drained under EUS guidance (**b**)

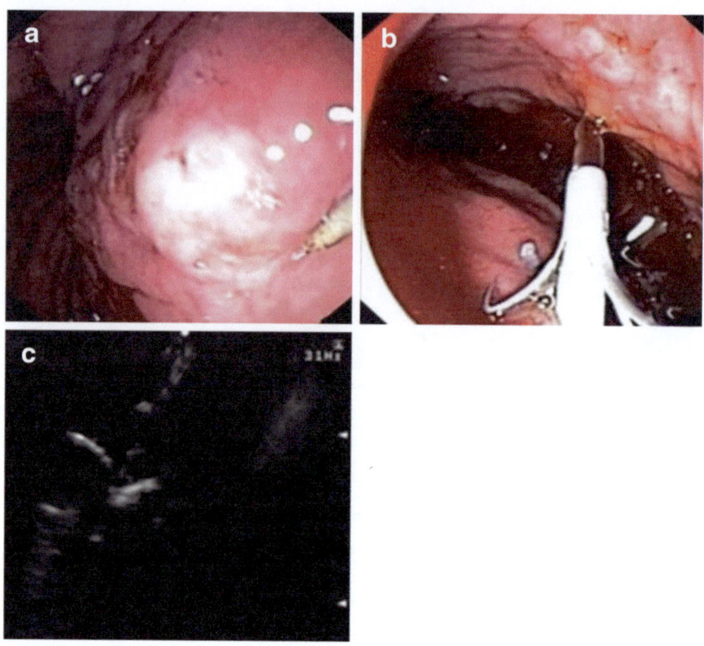

Fig. 38.5 Pseudocyst in the head of the pancreas compressing the posterior surface of the stomach (**a**), EUS-guided transgastric drainage (**b, c**)

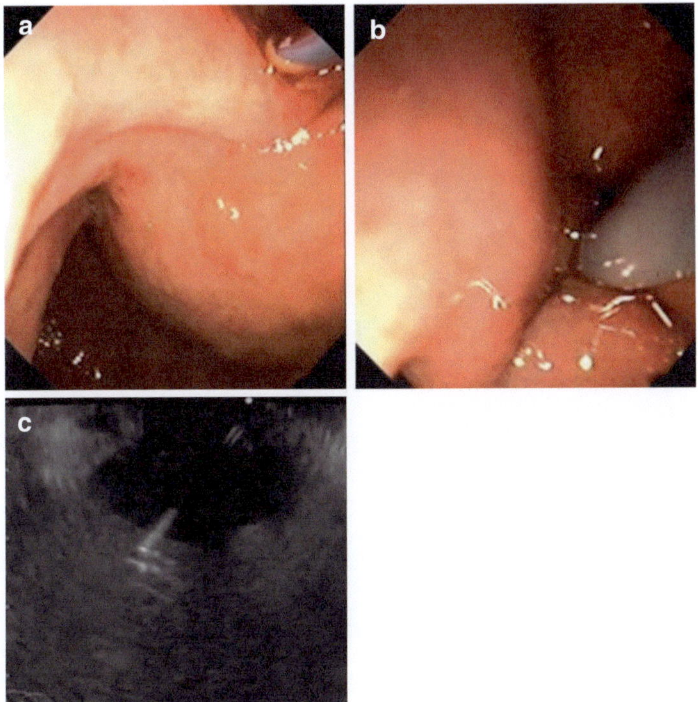

Fig. 38.6 Pseudocyst in the head of the pancreas compressing the duodenal bulb (**a**), EUS-guided transduodenal drainage (**b**, **c**)

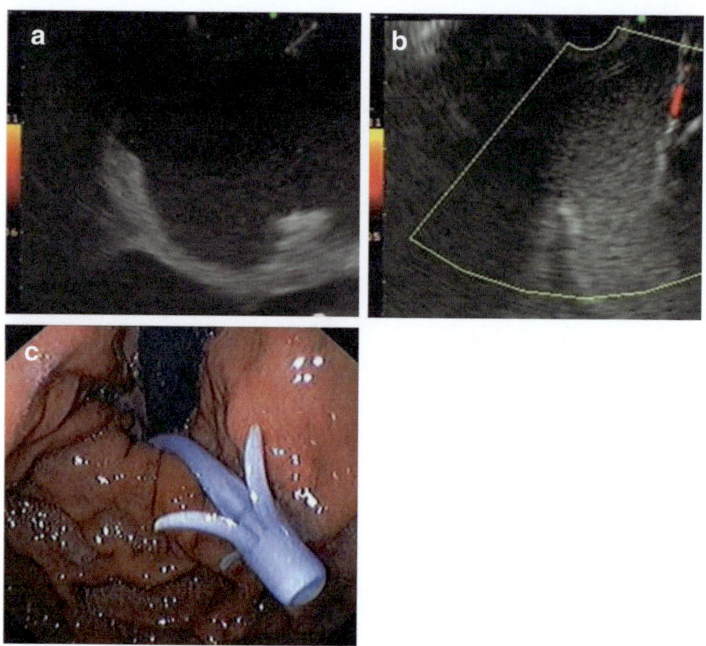

Fig. 38.7 Pseudocyst in the body of the pancreas extending into the mediastinum through the diaphragm hiatus (**a**), EUS-guided transesophageal drainage (**b**, **c**)

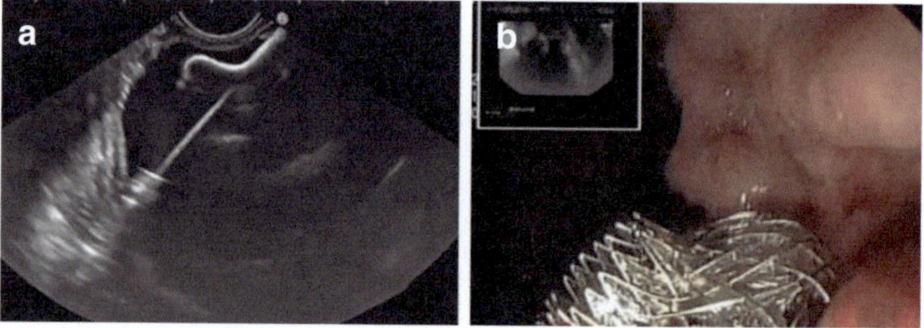

Fig. 38.8 Pseudocyst in the body of the pancreas, drained under EUS guidance using an expandable stent, firstly through the distal part of WOPN (**a**), then through stomach (**b**, **c**)

38.6 Differential Diagnosis

- Other digestive diseases
  - acute cholecystitis
  - perforated duodenal ulcer
  - biliary colic
  - bowel perforation
  - mesenteric ischemia or infarction
  - myocardial infarction
  - aortic aneurysm and aortic dissection
  - ectopic pregnancy
  - other causes of hyperamylasemia

38.7 Complications

- Local
  - *acute peripancreatic fluid collections (APC)* ‹4 weeks—interstitial edematous pancreatitis—fluid collections, with homogenous fluid content, non-encapsulated, located near pancreas
  - *acute necrotic collections (ANC)* ‹4 weeks—necrotizing pancreatitis—heterogeneous, non-encapsulated, intra- or extra-pancreatic
  - *pseudocyst* >4 weeks, fluid collection, with homogenous fluid content, surrounded by a well-defined wall, located near the pancreas
  - *walled-off necrosis (WON)* >4 weeks—necrotizing pancreatitis—heterogeneous, well-defined wall, intra- or extra-pancreatic

    all collections can get infected!
  - other local complications: splenic vein thrombosis, gastric varices, pseudoaneurysm, ascites, pleural effusion
- Systemic
  - SIRS, systemic infection, organ failure (respiratory, heart, or kidney failure), coagulopathy, stress gastritis, metabolic disorders, delirium, pannculitis, gastrointestinal bleeding, abdominal compartment syndrome [3]

38.8 Prognosis

- Scoring systems in predincting the severity and prognosis of AP
  - Revised Atlanta Classification
  - CT severity index
  - APACHE II score
  - Ranson score (Tables 38.2, 38.3, and 38.4) [4, 5]

Table 38.2 Revised Atlanta classification for acute pancreatitis

Revised Atlanta classification	
Mild acute pancreatitis	• No organ failure • No local or systemic complications
Moderately severe acute pancreatitis	• Transient organ failure (<48 h) and/or • Local or systemic complications without persistent organ failure
Severe acute pancreatitis	• Persistent organ failure (>48 h); single or multiple organ failure

Table 38.3 APACHE II score

APACHE II score[a]	
Clinical parameters	• Temperature • Heart rate • Respiratory rate • Mean arterial pressure • Glasgow coma scale • Kidney injury • Age • Organ failure • Imunocompromised state
Laboratory parameters	• Oxigenation (FiO_2) • Arterial pH-ul • Serum parameters: sodium • Potasium creatininehematocrit • White blood cells

[a] Increasing score corresponds to a severe pathology and it is associated with increasing risk of mortality

Table 38.4 Ranson's criteria for acute pancreatitis

Ranson's criteria	
Criteria	Score
On admission	
Age	>55 years
White blood cells	>16 × 100/mm³ (16,000/mm³)
Glucose	>11 mmol/L (>200 mg/dl)
Serum lactic dehydrogenase	>600 U/L
Serum transaminase	>250 U/L
Within 48 h of admission	
Decrease in hematocrit	>10%
Serum transaminase	>200 U/L
Serum calcium	<2 mmol/L (<8 mg/dL)
Increase in BUN	>1.8 mmol/L (>5 mg/dL)
Base deficit	>4 mEq/L
FiO_2	<8.0 kPa (60 mmHg)

38.9 Treatment

- Supportive therapy
  - aggressive hydration (lactated ringer solution/saline solution) in the first 24 h
  - analgesics
  - nasogastric tube in case nausea, vomiting, or gastric stasis persist
  - oral refeeding when it is tolerated (decreases the risk of infectious complications)
- Management of complications
  - signs of organ failure—transfer to the intensive care unit
  - antibiotics are only indicated when infection is suspected (imipenem, meropenem, fluoroquinolones, metronidazole)
  - biliary pancreatitis associated with cholangitis/persistent common bile duct stones—emergency ERCP with sphincterotomy and stone extraction

- laparoscopic cholecystectomy should be performed in patients who present with biliary acute pancreatitis
- asymptomatic pseudocyst: echographic monitoring
- sterile necrotic pancreatic collections
    supportive treatment
    in case symptoms occur: percutaneous, endoscopic, or surgical draingage
- infected necrotic collections
    percutaneous drainage
    endoscopic drainage
    + antibiotics
- infected pancreatic/peripancreatic necrosis
    endoscopic or surgical necrosectomy
    video-assisted retroperitoneal debridement (VARD) [6]

References

1. Leppäniemi A, Tolonen M, Tarasconi A, et al. 2019 WSES guidelines for the management of severe acute pancreatitis. World J Emerg Surg. 2019;14:27.
2. Greenberg JA, Hsu J, Bawazeer M, et al. Clinical practice guideline: management of acute pancreatitis. Can J Surg. 2016;59:128–40.
3. Banks PA, Bollen TL, Dervenis C, et al. Classification of acute pancreatitis - 2012: revision of the Atlanta classification and definitions by international consensus. Gut. 2013;62:102–11.
4. Inadomi JM, Bhattacharya R, Hwang JH, Ko C. Yamada's handbook of gastroenterology, vol. 31. 4th ed. Hoboken: Wiley; 2020. p. 335–47.
5. Feldman M, Friedman LS, Brandt LJ. Sleisenger and Fordtran's gastrointestinal and liver disease, vol. 58. 10th ed. Amsterdam: Elsevier; 2016. p. 969–93.
6. Feather A, Randall D, Waterhouse M. Kumar and Clark's clinical medicine, vol. 35. 10th ed. Amsterdam: Elsevier; 2020. p. 1323–37.

Chronic Pancreatitis

39

Sergiu Cazacu and Adrian Săftoiu

39.1 Definition and Classification

- Replacement of the pancreatic normal parenchyma with fibrotic connective tissue as a result of recurrent inflammatory episodes [1–3].
- Exocrine and endocrine progressive pancreatic insufficiency [1–3].
- Classification [3]:
    - Calcifying pancreatitis,
    - Obstructive pancreatitis,
    - Autoimmune pancreatitis,
    - Pseudotumoral pancreatitis.

39.2 Epidemiology

S. Cazacu (✉)
Gastroenterology Department, University of Medicine and Pharmacy Craiova, Craiova, Romania

A. Săftoiu
Department of Gastroenterology and Hepatology, Elias Emergency University Hospital, Carol Davila University of Medicine and Pharmacy, Bucharest, Romania

- 1.6–23 cases/100,000 [3], predominantly in men [1]
- Risk factors [1–4, 6]:
    - Alcohol abuse (2–3% of consumers >5 drinks/day over 6–12 years),
    - Smoking,
    - Genetic factors,
    - Autoimmune pancreatitis,
    - Pancreas divisum (possible),
    - Hyperparathyroidism.

39.3 Etiology and Pathogenesis (TIGAR-O) [3]

- Toxic-metabolic.
    - Alcohol consumption (50–80%),
    - Hypercalcemia,
    - Hyperlipidemia,
    - Chronic renal failure.
- Idiopathic, tropical.
- Genetics (mutations, genetic variants).
    - PRSS1 (p.N29I, p.R122H) – cationic trypsinogen gene.
    - SPINK1 (serine protease inhibitor).
    - CPA1 (carboxypeptidase A1).
    - CTRC (chymotrypsinogen C).
    - CEL (carboxyesterlipase).
    - CFTR (cystic fibrosis transmembrane conductance regulator).
- Autoimmune.
- Recurrent.
- Obstructive:
    - Pancreas divisum,
    - Ductal obstruction,
    - Duodenal wall cyst,
    - Oddi sphincter dysfunction (possible).

Pathogenesis: Double-strike theory (in patients with genetic, metabolic, and environmental risk factors, an episode of acute pancreatitis initiates or activates the immune system with progression to PC)

- Genetic abnormalities: premature activation of trypsinogen (PRSS1), loss of inhibition of trypsin activation (SPINK1, CTRC), alteration of the flow of pancreatic enzymes in the duodenum (CTFR).
- Stellate pancreatic cells can play a critical role in activating and producing collagen [4].

39.4 Pathological Anatomy

- Fibrosis, later calcifications (advanced).
- Ductal abnormalities (dilations, strictures, lithiasis).
- Initially hypertrophy, late atrophy.

39.5 Diagnosis

- Symptoms [3–5].
- Epigastric/abdominal pain (50–85%),
      Recurrent or continuous,
      May decrease in advanced stages,
- Exocrine pancreatic insufficiency (when 90% of exocrine function is lost),
    - Steatorrhea,
    - Weight loss (50% of patients, causes: pain, alcohol, malabsorption),
- Endocrine pancreatic insufficiency,
    - Diabetes (type 3c, 50% of patients),
- Jaundice in some patients,

- Laboratory tests [1–4].
  - Amylase, serum lipase: normal/minimally elevated/ decreased late,
  - Some patients: increase in total and conjugated BR, AP, GGT (CBP compression),
  - AST/ALT normal/minimum increased.
  - Increased IgG4 in type 1 autoimmune pancreatitis,
  - Circulating biomarkers? TGF-β, MMP-9,TNF-α.

39.5.1 Imaging Tests [2–4]

- Transabdominal echo: advanced forms (calcifications, ductal dilations), low sensitivity.
- CT: calcifications, ductal dilations, atrophy.
- MRCP can use i.v. secretin.
- EUS is useful for early pancreatitis and may be positive even for CT or normal MRI, with overdiagnosis (> 60 years, alcohol consumption) [3].
  - Rosemont criteria: parenchymal abnormalities – foci and hyperechoic bands (Fig. 39.1a), lobular contour, cysts, stones (Fig. 39.1b).
  - Ductal abnormalities: Wirsung dilation, irregular duct, hyperechoic margins (Fig. 39.2), visible secondary branches, intraductal/intraparenchymal lithiasis,

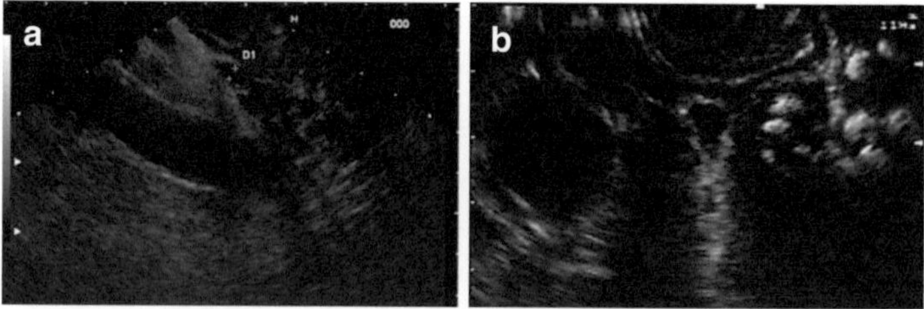

Fig. 39.1 Endoscopic ultrasound showed a lobular aspect with hyperechoic bands (**a**), multiple calcifications in the pancreatic head (**b**)

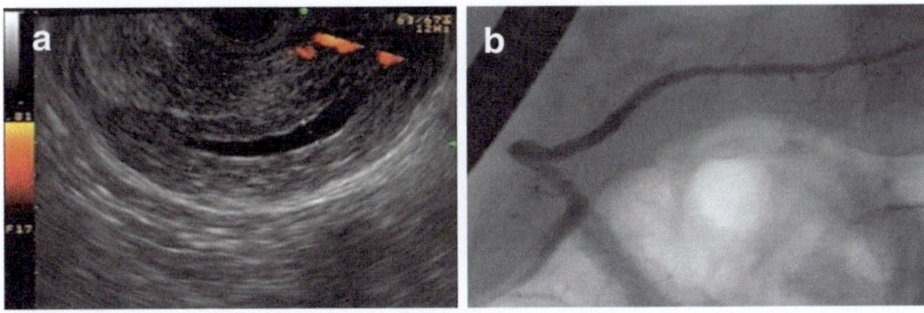

Fig. 39.2 Endoscopic ultrasound showed a dilated pancreatic duct, with irregular hyperechoic margins (**a**), which correspond to those obtained by ERCP pancreatography (**b**)

- Elastography [3, 4] can obtain complementary information: mixed blue-green frequent aspect (Fig. 39.3a, b),
  Strain ratio/strain histogram scores intermediate between normal and carcinoma,
- Contrast-enhanced EUS can help [3].
  Hyperenhancement = hypervascular in pseudotumoral pancreatitis (Fig. 39.4a, b)/autoimmune.
  Rich collaterals, in cases with stenosis/splenic vein thrombosis, and splenic infarction, respectively (Fig. 39.5a,b).
- Three-dimensional (3D) endoscopic ultrasound examinations allow spatial evaluation of the pancreas, and characterization of relation with adjacent vascular structures (Fig. 39.6a, b).

ERCP detects only ductal abnormalities, useful in cases with inconclusive CT/RM/EUS, and can help treat ductal lesions.

39.5.2 Functional Tests

- May be useful in cases of uncertain imaging diagnosis [4].
  - Most are positive only in advanced forms,
  - Measurement of fecal fat/72 h (positive also in mucosal diseases of the small intestine),

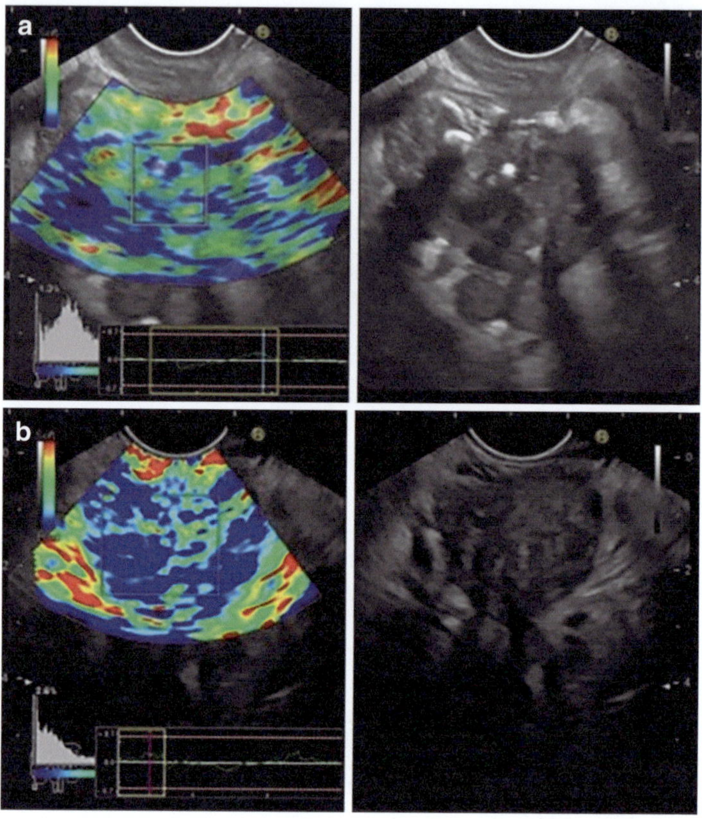

Fig. 39.3 Endoscopic ultrasound elastography with mixed aspect in chronic calcifying pancreatitis (**a**), hard aspect in pancreatic adenocarcinoma, respectively (**b**), with different values of strain histogram

- Fecal elastase (<100–200 μg/g stool) and fecal chymotrypsin,
- Serum trypsinogen <20 ng/mL,
- Respiratory tests (mixed triglyceride respiratory test),
- Direct pancreatic functional tests using secretagogues.

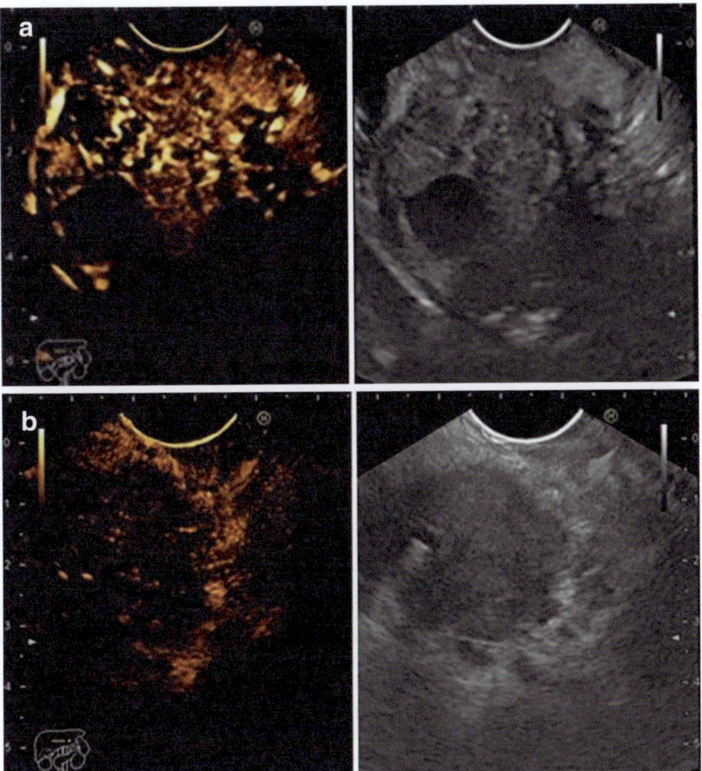

Fig. 39.4 EUS with contrast (low mechanical index mode), with hyperenhanced aspect (except for two cystic lesions), in chronic pseudotumoral pancreatitis (**a**), and hypo-enhanced aspect in pancreatic adenocarcinoma, respectively (**b**)

39.5.3 Genetic Testing

- Early onset/childhood, family history, recurrent acute idiopathic pancreatitis [2].

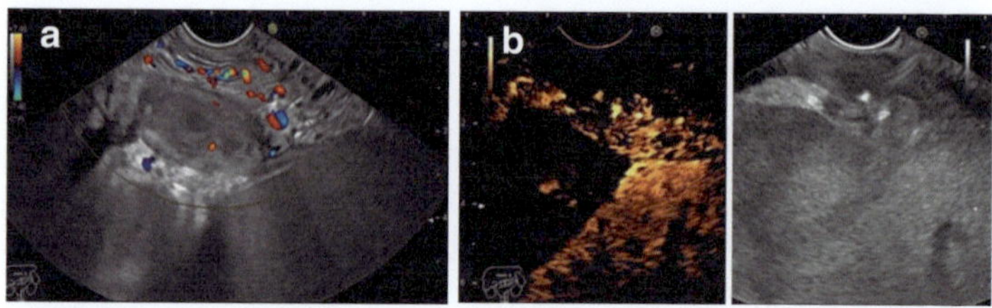

Fig. 39.5 Chronic pseudotumoral pancreatitis, with collateral peripancreatic circulation, visualized in color Doppler mode (**a**), and splenic infarction visible during contrast examination (**b**)

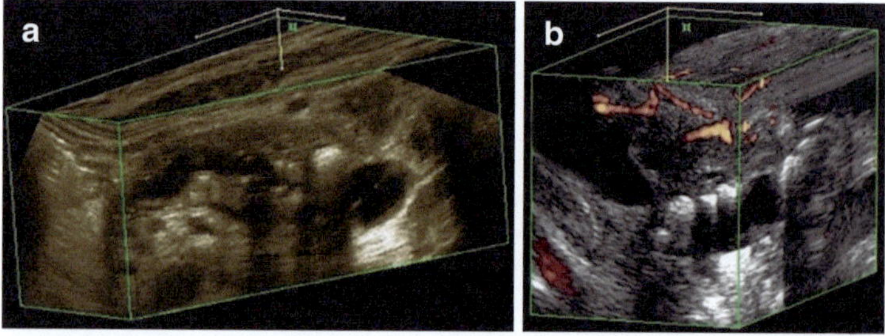

Fig. 39.6 Endoscopic ultrasound 3D aspect with the examination of the common bile duct and main pancreatic duct which are both dilated, blocked intraductal stone (**a**), and multiple intraductal stones (**b**)

39.6 Diagnosis

- Difficult in early stages (preferably EUS, 2–3 criteria, lobularity, "honeycomb" appearance, hyperechoic foci, stranding, cysts, secondary branch dilatations, Wirsung hyperechoic edges).

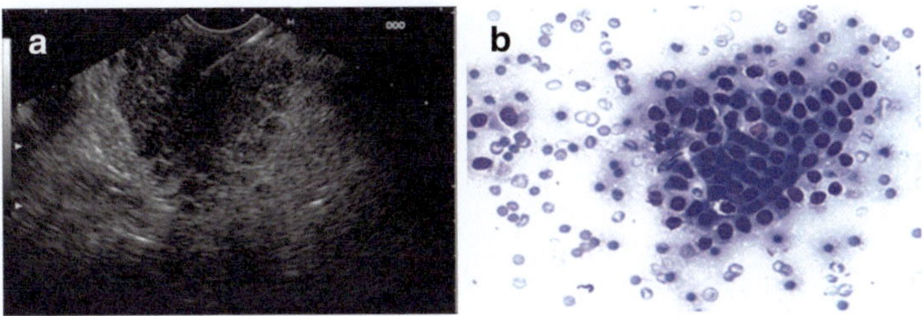

Fig. 39.7 Endoscopic ultrasound with fine needle aspiration in chronic pseudotumoral pancreatitis (**a**), with a suggestive aspect of benign canalicular cells on smear slides. (courtesy of Dr. Carmen Popescu) (**b**)

39.7 Differential Diagnosis

- Pancreatic carcinoma versus pseudotumoral pancreatitis (contrast EUS, EUS elastography, EUS-FNA/EUS-FNB, tumor markers) [3].
  - Tissue diagnosis of malignancy is essential ("tissue is still the issue") (Fig. 39.7a, b).

39.8 Complications [5]

- Exocrine insufficiency: malabsorption, steatorrhea, weight loss.
- Endocrine insufficiency: diabetes.
- Pseudocysts (Fig. 39.8a, b): pain, infection, vascular compression, bleeding, biliary stenosis.
- Splenic vein thrombosis, segmentary portal hypertension, and gastric varices (Fig. 39.9a,b),
- Risk of pancreatic carcinoma 13.3× [5].

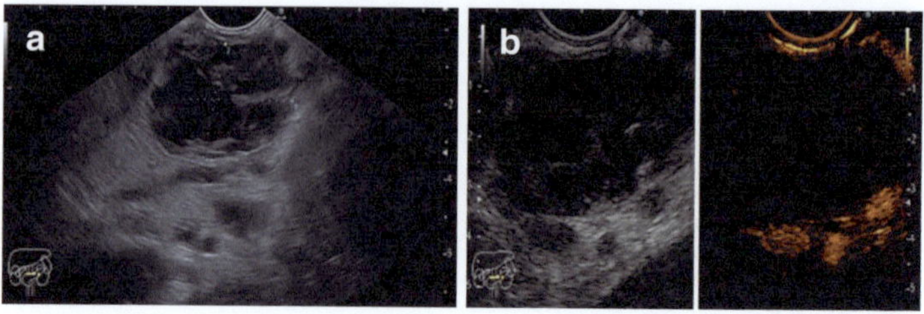

Fig. 39.8 Contrast-enhanced endoscopic ultrasound in a case of chronic pancreatitis, with visualization of a pseudocyst with its own wall and detritus (**a**), both hypo-enhanced during examination with contrast, in both arterial and venous phase, respectively (**b**)

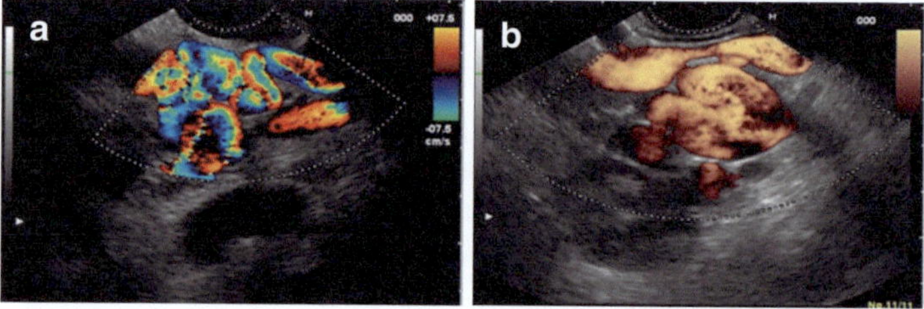

Fig. 39.9 Gastric varices and perigastric collateral vessels visualized in Doppler color mode (**a**) and power Doppler (**b**), in a patient with advanced chronic pancreatitis and splenic vein thrombosis

39.9 Prognosis

- 50% mortality in 20–25 years [4].

39.10 Treatment [2–4, 6]

- Diet: abstinence from alcohol, smoking cessation [4].
- Statins may lower the risk (some studies) [4].
- Pain treatment (medical) [3, 4].
  - Analgesics: usual, opioids, pregabalin,
  - Antidepressants,

- – Pancreatic enzymes,
- – Antioxidants: Se, vitamin C, A, E, Met.
- Pain treatment (endoscopic) [2, 3] – effective in 2/3.
  - – Sphincterotomy, stenting in obstructive stones, strictures,
  - – Temporarily effective EUS-guided celiac blockade in some cases,
  - – EUS/ERCP drainage in bulky/complicated pseudocysts.
  - – ESWL (extracorporeal lithotripsy).
- Pain treatment (surgical) [3, 4].
  - – Decompression in cases with refractory pain and ductal dilation, more effective than endoscopy,
  - – Resection in case of inflammatory mass, damage to small ducts,
  - – Ductal/pseudocyst drainage,
- Exocrine insufficiency: pancreatic enzymes (40,000 lipase units/meal) [2, 6], vitamin supplements.
- Endocrine failure: treatment of diabetes (risk of hypoglycemia due to impaired glucagon secretion!) [4, 6]
- Corticotherapy, immunosuppressive treatment in autoimmune pancreatitis.

References

1. Weiss FU, Laemmerhirt F, Lerch MM. Etiology and risk factors of acute and chronic pancreatitis. Visc Med. 2019;35:73–81.
2. Kwon CI, Cho JH, Choi SH, Ko KH, Tirkes T, Gromski MA, Lehman GA. Recent advances in the diagnosis and management of chronic pancreatitis. Korean J Intern Med. 2019;34:242–60.
3. Löhr JM, Dominguez-Munoz E, Rosendahl J, Besselink M, Mayerle J, Lerch MM, Haas S, et al. United European gastroenterology evidence-based guidelines for the diagnosis and therapy of chronic pancreatitis (HaPanEU). United European Gastroenterol J. 2017;5:153–99.
4. Lew D, Afghani E, Pandol S. Chronic pancreatitis: current status and challenges for prevention and treatment. Dig Dis Sci. 2017;62:1702–12.
5. Ramsey ML, Conwell DL, Hart PA. Complications of chronic pancreatitis. Dig Dis Sci. 2017;62:1745–50.
6. Waldthaler A, Valente R, Arnelo U, Löhr JM. Endoscopic and conservative Management of Chronic Pancreatitis and its Complications. Visc Med. 2019;35:98–108.

Irina F. Cherciu Harbiyeli
and Ioana Streață

40.1 Definition [1, 2]

- **Hereditary pancreatitis (HP).**
  - Rare autosomal-dominant genetic disorder,
  - Characterized by personal history of acute (AP), recurrent acute (RAP) and chronic pancreatitis (CP) that runs in family,
  - Pancreatitis diagnosed in two first-degree relatives or in three second-degree relatives crossing at least two generations.

I. F. Cherciu Harbiyeli (✉)
Research Center of Gastroenterology and Hepatology Craiova,
University of Medicine and Pharmacy Craiova, Craiova, Romania

I. Streață
Human Genomics Laboratory, University of Medicine and Pharmacy
Craiova, Craiova, Romania

A. Săftoiu (ed.), *Pocket Guide to Advanced Endoscopy in
Gastroenterology*, https://doi.org/10.1007/978-3-031-42076-4_40

40.2 Epidemiology [1]

- The frequency varies widely by geographic region.
  - HP is rare and primarily a disease of Caucasians, with an estimated prevalence of 3 in 1,000,000 people in Western countries.
- Recurrent episodes of pancreatitis begin at age < 40 years, with CP developing in 50% of cases.
- Near 80% of patients with HP have pathogenic variants in PRSS1.

40.3 Etiology and Pathogenesis [1, 3]

- The mechanism of disease induction by genetic mutations is complex and only partially understood.
  - Frequently, the interaction between mutations and environmental factors leads to clinical pancreatitis,
  - The genetic mutations are all primarily linked to the trypsin pathway.
- Mutations in PRSS1 or SPINK1.
  - Increase autocatalytic conversion of trypsinogen to active trypsin,
  - disrupt the intrapancreatic equilibrium of proteases and their inhibitors,
  - prematurely activate intrapancreatic trypsin,
  - Activated trypsin cannot be degraded and/or activation of trypsinogen into trypsin is stimulated, hence the excess enzyme production, leading to autodigestion and pancreatitis.
- The role of CFTR is until now poorly understood.

40.4 Diagnosis [1–3]

- **Clinical presentation.**

- With the exception of young age (when symptoms typically begin with attacks of AP that become more and more frequent) and the slow progression,
- Clinical evolution, morphological features, laboratory findings and treatment of HP do not differ from those of patients with CP of other causes (see Chapter 39).
- **The workup for HP diagnosis typically involves:**
  - A detailed personal history to look for the clinical symptoms,
  - An extended family history to identify possible inheritance patterns,
  - imaging techniques to evaluate for signs of AP or CP.
- **Differential diagnosis**.
  - Cystic fibrosis (one of the most important differential diagnoses),
  - hyperlipidemia type I,
  - Familiar (hypocalciuric) hypercalcemia,
  - Hereditary hyperparathyroidism,
  - Autoimmune pancreatitis,
- **The final diagnosis** is established by gene sequencing.

40.5 Genetic Testing [2, 4]

- Medically indicated to establish a diagnosis and to define a management plan.
  - Commercial genetic tests are presently available for PRSS1, SPINK1, CFTR, and CTRC.
- **Symptomatic patients** should be referred for a PRSS1 mutation testing when fulfilling at least one of the subsequent conditions:
  - ≥ 2 episodes of acute pancreatitis (documented outbursts with hyper-amylasemia) of unidentified etiology (in the absence of anatomical anomalies, trauma, gallstones, alcohol, drugs intake, ampullary or main pancreatic strictures, viral infection, hyperlipidemia, etc.)

- idiopathic chronic pancreatitis, in particular if the age of the onset is <25 years,
  - One first-degree (parent, sibling, child) or one second-degree (aunt, uncle, grandparent) relative with pancreatitis,
  - Inexplicable episode of childhood pancreatitis that called for hospitalization,
  - Patients with pancreatitis eligible for the inclusion in a research protocol.
- **Asymptomatic individuals** should be tested for A PRSS1 mutation when having one first-degree relative known with causative HP gene mutations.
  - **A negative genetic test** result in the affected proband does not exclude the diagnosis of HP.
- **SPINK1, CFTR, and CTRC mutation analysis** requires:
  - No previous genetic testing of requested gene,
  - AND.
  - Previous PRSS1 sequence analysis was performed and no mutations were found.
- **CASR, CLDN2, and CPA1 analysis.**
  - These tests are considered investigational and/or experimental.
- Mutations continue to be discovered since the advent and increasing use of next-generation sequencing.

40.6 Management and Treatment

- Once the diagnosis is established, the goal is minimizing recurrence and complications.
- Standard management for acute and chronic pancreatitis of other etiologies applies (see Chaps. 38 and 39).

40.7 Complications

- Similar as patients with other forms of CP.

40.8 Pancreatic Cancer (PC), Cancer Risk, Cancer Screening [5–8]

- **HP-associated risks.**
  - HP acts as the greatest risk factor for PC.
  - It is estimated that 30% to 40% of HP affected individuals will develop PC by the age of 70,
  - The increased risks for PC are associated with prolonged pancreatic exposure to chronic inflammation, particularly in HP patients with disease onset in adolescence,
  - The risk does not strongly correlate with the severity of pancreatic inflammation and fibrosis,
  - The relative risk is estimated to be 26-fold to up to 87-fold while cumulative risk varies between 7.2% to 53.5%,
  - Risk is further increased by smoking and diabetes mellitus.
- **Screening for pancreatic cancer in HP.**

Who should be screened

- Candidates should carry a > ten-fold increased risk for developing cancer, category which includes all individuals diagnosed with HP.

When to begin screening

- Most experts recommend age 40 or 20 years after the first pancreatitis attack, regardless of gene status.

How to screen

- Screening is best performed within research protocols or registries involving multidisciplinary teams with expertise in genetics, gastroenterology, radiology, surgery, and pathology.

What tests should be used for pancreatic surveillance

– The consensus among experts is that MRI/MRCP and EUS should be the first-line tests for pancreatic surveillance,
– EUS and MRI detect pancreatic asymptomatic precursor lesions and invasive malignant pancreatic neoplasms better than CT. Both imaging techniques are complementary.
– Pancreatic-protocol CT is reserved for individuals unable to undergo MRI or EUS.
– Patients' surveillance should include clinical examinations and laboratory testing (CEA, CA 19–9, serum glucose/HbA1c, amylase, lipase, bilirubin, alkaline phosphatase).

How frequently should screening be performed

– Yearly screening is recommended.
  In case a suspicious lesion is observed, control EUS with FNA (if necessary) after 6 weeks.

40.9   Role of Endoscopy [3, 9]

• Endoscopy and endoscopic pancreatic function testing.
  – Can be used to establish the diagnosis of CP,
  – Can be extremely valuable in managing sequelae of HP.
• Upper gastrointestinal endoscopy is useful.
  – For biopsy of tumors infiltrating the duodenum,
  – For palliative decompression of the duodenum and/or bile duct,
• EUS and ERCP are the two most common endoscopic procedures used to evaluate the pancreas.
• EUS.
  – The HP changes can be nonspecific, with similar abnormalities detected in patients with pancreatitis of other etiology (see Chap. 39 for the Rosemont criteria),
  – It can reveal subtle changes of the pancreatic ductal structures and parenchymal, even prior to traditional imaging methods and laboratory tests reveal any anomaly,

- It is an important complementary examination regarding the diagnosis and staging of PC as it permits:
    Examining the primary tumors,
    Evaluating the relationship with neighboring structures,
    Obtaining tissue for pathological diagnoses.
- The sensitivity and specificity of EUS and EUS-FNA are 90% and 98%, respectively,
- ERCP.
    - Can highlight structural anomalies such as irregular ducts, poor filling, narrowing, or dilatation of ducts,
    - Endoscopic decompression of obstructed pancreatic ducts (caused by strictures or stones) determined in patients with HP a long-term pain relief, decreased narcotic use and hospitalizations, avoidance of surgical intervention,
    - In pancreatic cancer, ERCP is limited to cases with obstruction of the bile duct as it is associated with important adverse effects and has low effectiveness in attaining a histological diagnosis,
- Choosing endoscopic management versus surgical therapy in PE.
    - Therapeutic endoscopy should be considered as an important initial treatment option for patients with HP but must be individualized to the patient and performed by expert endoscopists,
    - For children with HP a step-ups strategy is recommended, starting with early ERCP and progressing to surgery if ERCP was unsuccessful,
    - Surgical intervention is superior to endoscopic intervention, pain-free intervals between procedures being longer after surgical therapy,
    - Choosing one intervention over the other is a complex decision and it should take into consideration the age, comorbidities, safety profiles, the focal aspect of the pancreatic lesion,

40.10 Prognosis [7]

- The course of disease and prognosis is unpredictable,
  - Significantly reduced quality of life due to the symptoms and the frequent need for interventions and hospitalizations,
  - HP patients without pancreatic cancer do not have increased mortality rates compared to the general population.
- If a HP patient develops pancreatic cancer, it usually occurs 20 years earlier than in the general population, hence being associated with an earlier and increased mortality.

References

1. Raphael KL, Willingham FF. Hereditary pancreatitis: current perspectives. Clin Exp Gastroenterol. 2016;9:197–207.
2. Ellis I, Lerch MM, Whitcomb DC. Genetic testing for hereditary pancreatitis: guidelines for indications, counselling, consent and privacy issues. Pancreatology. 2001;1:405–15.
3. Conwell DL, Lee LS, Yadav D, et al. American pancreatic association practice guidelines in chronic pancreatitis: evidence-based report on diagnostic guidelines. Pancreas. 2014;43:1143–62.
4. Rosendahl J, Bödeker H, Mössner J, Teich N. Hereditary chronic pancreatitis. Orphanet J Rare Dis. 2007;2:1.
5. Goggins M, Overbeek KA, Brand R International Cancer of the Pancreas Screening (CAPS) Consortium, et al. Management of patients with increased risk for familial pancreatic cancer: updated recommendations from the international cancer of the pancreas screening (CAPS) Consortium. Gut. 2020;69:7–17.
6. Weiss FU. Pancreatic cancer risk in hereditary pancreatitis. Front Physiol. 2014;5:70.
7. Brand RE, Lerch MM, Rubinstein WS, et al. Advances in counselling and surveillance of patients at risk for pancreatic cancer. Gut. 2007;56:1460–9.
8. Langer P, Kann PH, Fendrich V, et al. Five years of prospective screening of high-risk individuals from families with familial pancreatic cancer. Gut. 2009;58:1410–8.
9. Ge QC, Dietrich CF, Bhutani MS, Zhang BZ, Zhang Y, Wang YD, Zhang JJ, Wu YF, Sun SY, Guo JT. Comprehensive review of diagnostic modalities for early chronic pancreatitis. World J Gastroenterol. 2021;27(27):4342–57.

Irina Mihaela Cazacu and Adrian Săftoiu

41.1 Definition and Classification [1]

- **Malignant tumors.**
  Origin:
  - Ductal cells.
    - Ductal adenocarcinoma—75–90%.
    - Giant-cell carcinoma—5%.
    - Cystadenocarcinoma—rare.
    - Mucinous carcinoma—rare.
    - Small-cell carcinoma—rare.
    - Anaplastic carcinoma—rare.
  - Acinar cells:
    - Acinar cell carcinoma.
    - Acinar cell cystadenocarcinoma.

I. M. Cazacu (✉)
Department of Oncology, Fundeni Clinical Institute, Bucharest, Romania

Faculty of Medicine, Carol Davila University of Medicine and
Pharmacy, Bucharest, Romania

A. Săftoiu
Department of Gastroenterology and Hepatology, Elias Emergency
University Hospital, Carol Davila University of Medicine and Pharmacy,
Bucharest, Romania

© The Author(s), under exclusive license to Springer Nature
Switzerland AG 2023
A. Săftoiu (ed.), *Pocket Guide to Advanced Endoscopy in
Gastroenterology*, https://doi.org/10.1007/978-3-031-42076-4_41

- Conjunctive tissue.
    Sarcoma—rare.
    Lymphoma—rare.
- Pancreatic metastasis (more frequently from breast carcinoma, lung carcinoma, melanoma, or non-Hodgkin lymphoma).
- **Tumors with malignant potential.**
  - Solid pseudopapillary tumors.
  - Intraductal papillary mucinous neoplasia (IPMN).
- **Benign tumors.**
  - Serous cystadenoma.
  - Mucinous cystadenoma.
  - Solid serous adenoma.
  - Lymphoepithelial cyst.
  - Hamartoma.

41.2 Pancreatic Ductal Adenocarcinoma

41.2.1 Epidemiology [2]

- Aggressive, 5-year survival rate < 10%,
- Rare before the age of 45, incidence rises sharply thereafter,
- Men > women,
- Risk factors [2, 3]:
  - Cigarette smoking,
  - Obesity,
  - Diabetes mellitus, metabolic syndrome,
  - Family history (>2 first-degree relatives),
  - Familial pancreatitis (PRSS1),
  - Peutz–Jeghers syndrome (STK11).
  - familial atypical multiple mole melanoma syndrome FAMMM (P16),
  - Lynch syndrome (MLH1, MSH2, MSH6, or PMS2).
  - Ataxia-telangiectasia (ATM),
  - Hereditary ovarian and breast cancer (BRCA1, BRCA2),
  - PALB2, CHECK2 mutations.

41.2.2 Pathogenesis [4]

– Precursor lesions: pancreatic intraepithelial neoplasia (PanIN).
   PanIN-1: flat/papillary without atypia.
   PanIN-2: papillary with atypia.
   PanIN-3: severe architectural and cytonuclear abnormalities, but invasion through the basement membrane is absent.
– The most frequent genetic abnormalities in invasive pancreatic adenocarcinoma:
   Mutational activation of Kras oncogene,
   Inactivation of tumor suppressor genes: CDKN2A/p16, TP53 si SMAD4.

41.2.3 Diagnostic [4, 5]

- Clinical signs.
  - Asthenia.
  - Weight loss.
  - Abdominal/epigastric/back pain.
  - Nausea, vomiting.
  - Steatorrhea.
- Physical exam.
  - Hepatomegaly or epigastric mass.
  - Jaundice,
  - Courvoisier's sign (nontender but palpable distended gallbladder at the right costal margin).
  - Cachexia.
  - Ascites.
- Laboratory tests:
  - Increased total and conjugated (direct) bilirubin, alkaline phosphatase (AP), GGT (obstructive jaundice—pancreatic head tumors),
  - CA 19–9 usually elevated.
  - Mild normochromic anemia, thrombocytosis,
  - Increased liver enzymes and AP (liver metastasis).

- Imaging tests:
  - Transabdominal ultrasound: indicates presence and level of obstruction, rarely the tumor (lesions smaller than 3 cm are usually missed).
  - CT with pancreatic protocol: preferred imaging tool for staging and resectability status [3].
  - MRCP: provides supplementary information; noninvasive method for imaging the biliary tree and pancreatic duct [3].
  - PET-CT: in high-risk patients to detect metastasis.

41.2.4 Role of Endoscopy

- EUS significantly improved PDAC diagnosis, especially for small-size tumors [3, 6–8].
  - Identifies dilated biliary ducts (Fig. 41.1) and the level of obstruction (Fig. 41.2).
  - Allows for the characterization of pancreatic lesions (using EUS-elastography and contrast-enhanced EUS) (Fig. 41.2).
  - EUS can be used for staging as it allows for the identification of liver metastasis (Fig. 41.3).
- EUS-FNA/FNB is preferable to a CT-guided FNA in patients with resectable disease because of better diagnostic yield, safety, and lower risk of peritoneal seeding (Fig. 41.4) [3, 6].

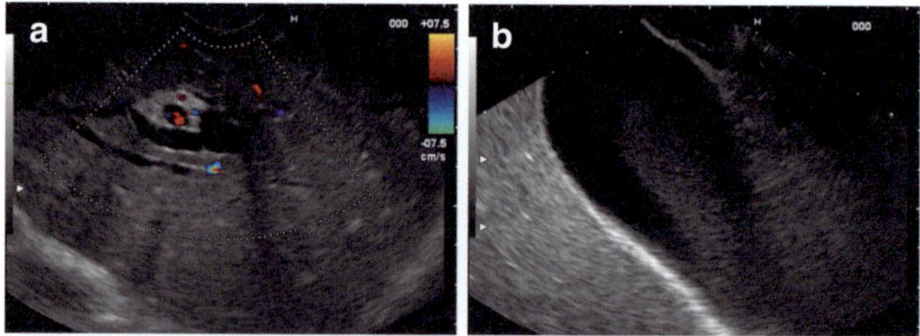

Fig. 41.1 EUS showing dilated intrahepatic biliary ducts in the left liver lobe (**a**) and a distended gallbladder with sludge (**b**) in a patient with pancreatic ductal adenocarcinoma

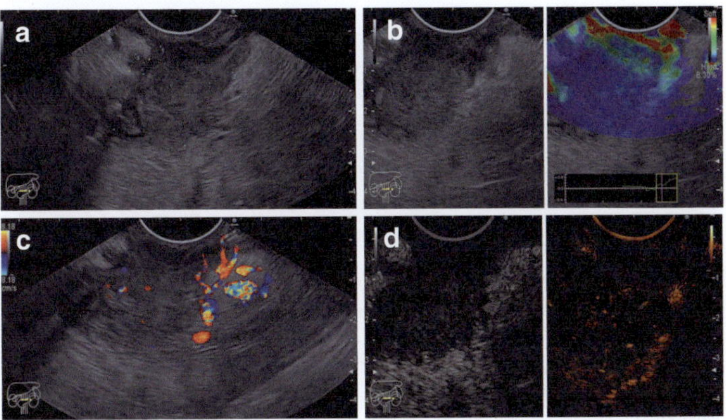

Fig. 41.2 EUS showing a hypoechogenic, irregular pancreatic tumor (**a**) with a "hard" appearance on EUS-elastography (**b**) with a poor Doppler signal and collateral circulation (**c**), hypoenhanced in the arterial and venous phase on contrast-enhanced EUS (**d**)

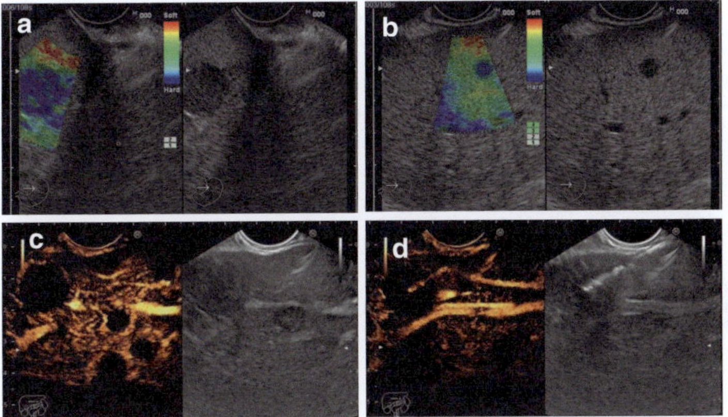

Fig. 41.3 EUS elastography showing liver metastasis (lesions with "hard" appearance on elastography) in left liver lobe in patient with pancreatic ductal adenocarcinoma (**a**, **b**); contrast-enhanced EUS showing liver metastasis with hypoenhancement in the arterial phase (**c**) and allows for guidance of EUS-FNA (**d**)

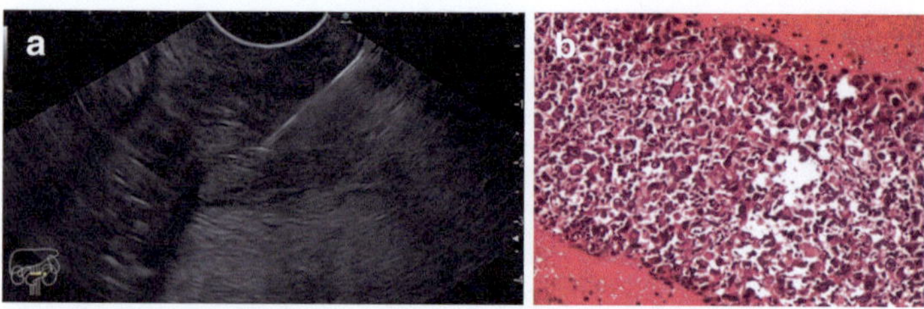

Fig. 41.4 EUS-guided fine-needle biopsy of a pancreatic tumor (**a**) with a histopathology examination showing pancreatic ductal adenocarcinoma (**b**)

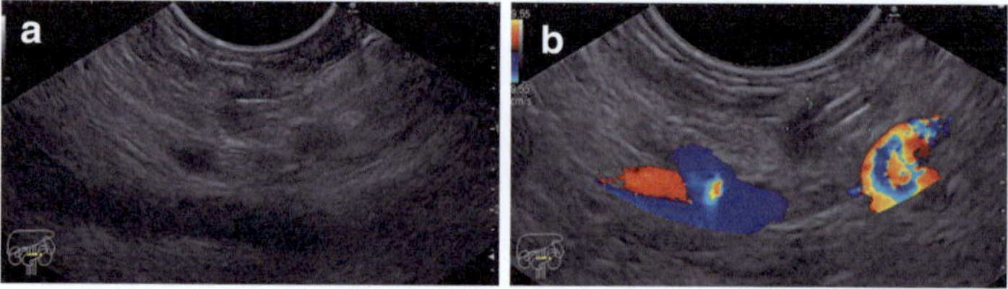

Fig. 41.5 EUS-guided fiducial marker placement (**b**) inside a pancreatic tumor (**a**) for guidance of radiotherapy

- EUS-FNA can be used for interventional procedures such as celiac plexus neurolysis, fiducial markers placement for guidance of radiotherapy (Fig. 41.5), or biliary drainage with metallic stents [9].
- A pathologic diagnosis is not required for resectable tumors before surgery [3].
- ERCP is used for confirmation of diagnosis (by brush cytology/direct biopsies) and for drainage with plastic stents or SEMS.

41.2.5 Staging [3]

2.5.1 TNM Staging
- **Tumor (T).**
  - TX—Primary tumor cannot be assessed.
  - T0—No evidence of primary tumor.

- Tis—Carcinoma in situ.
- T1—Tumor limited to the pancreas, 2 cm or smaller in greatest dimension.
- T2—Tumor limited to the pancreas, larger than 2 cm in greatest dimension.
- T3—Tumor extension beyond the pancreas (duodenum, bile duct, portal or superior mesenteric vein) but not involving the celiac axis or superior mesenteric artery.
- T4—Tumor involves the celiac axis or superior mesenteric arteries.
- **Regional lymph nodes (N).**
  - NX—Regional lymph nodes cannot be assessed.
  - N0—No regional lymph node metastasis.
  - N1—Regional lymph node metastasis.
- **Distant metastasis (M).**
  - MX—Distant metastasis cannot be assessed.
  - M0—No distant metastasis.
  - M1—Distant metastasis.

41.2.6 Criteria Defining Resectability Status at Diagnosis [3]

1. **Resectable.**
   (a) No arterial tumor contact with celiac axis (CA), superior mesenteric artery (SMA), common hepatic artery (CHA).
   (b) No tumor contact with the superior mesenteric vein (SMV) or portal vein (PV) or ≤ 180 vein contact.
2. **Borderline resectable.**
   (a) Tumor contact with CHA without extension with CA allowing for safe and complete resection and reconstruction.
   (b) Tumor contact with the CA or SMA $\leq 180°$.
   (c) Tumor contact with the SMV or PV $> 180°$, allowing for safe and complete resection and reconstruction (Fig. 41.6).

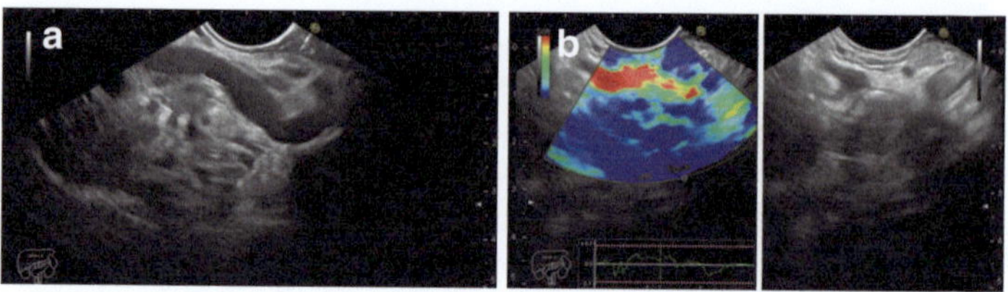

Fig. 41.6 EUS showing a ductal pancreatic adenocarcinoma with 180° tumor contact with SMV (**a**) with a hard appearance of the tumor on EUS elastography (**b**)

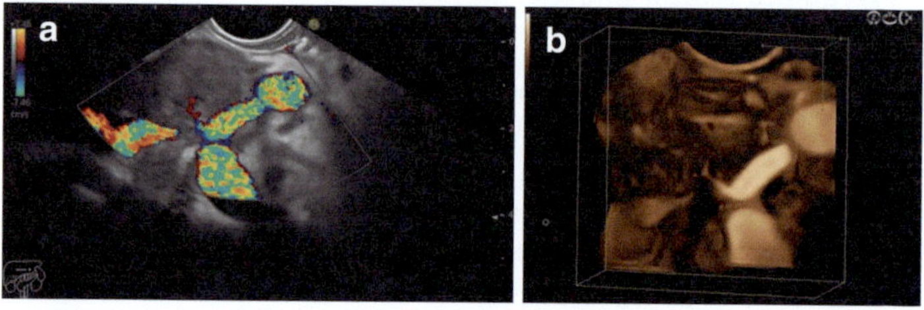

Fig. 41.7 Contrast-enhanced EUS showing a pancreatic ductal adenocarcinoma with circumferential invasion of the celiac axis and the hepatic artery visible on Doppler (**a**), with 3D reconstruction in harmonic mood with low mechanical index (**b**)

3. **Locally advanced, unresectable.**
    (a) Tumor contact with CA or SMA > 180° (Fig. 41.7).
    (b) Unreconstructible SMV/PV due to tumor involvement or occlusion.

41.2.7 Treatment [3, 10, 11]

- **Resectable disease (<20%).**
- Complete resection with negative margins (R0) is the only curative treatment.
- Surgical procedures:
    Pancreatoduodenectomy Whipple (or modified Whipple with pylorus preservation)—for tumors of the pancreatic head and uncinate.

Distal pancreatectomy with en-bloc splenectomy—for tumors of the pancreatic body and tail.
- Adjuvant therapy: mFOLFIRINOX* (fit patients, good performance status, and no important comorbidities); capecitabine + gemcitabine; fluorouracil/folinic acid.
- **Borderline disease.**
- Neoadjuvant chemotherapy (FOLFIRINOX or gemcitabine), followed by chemoradiation (with capecitabine).
- **Locally advanced disease.**
- Obstructive jaundice: stent placement (ERCP) or bypass surgical interventions (cholecystic-jejunostomy/choledochal-jejunostomy).
- Palliative chemotherapy: gemcitabine, 6 months.
- Chemoradiation improves local control.
- **Metastatic/recurrent disease.**
  - **First line.**

    FOLFIRINOX (European standard)/gemcitabine + nab-paclitaxel (American standard)—for patients with performance status 0–1.

    Gemcitabine monotherapy—for patients with performance status 2.

    BRCA1/BRCA 2 mutations: maintenance therapy with Olaparib after minimum 16 weeks of platinum-based chemotherapy.
- **Second line.**

  Performance status 0–1: fluoropyrimidine in combination with oxaliplatin, irinotecan, or nanoliposomal irinotecan (after gemcitabine +/− nab-paclitaxel in first line); gemcitabine +/− nab-paclitaxel (after FOLFIRINOX in first line).

  Performance status 2: monotherapy with a fluoropyrimidine (after gemcitabine in first line) or gemcitabine (after FOLFIRINOX in first line).

**FOLFIRINOX:5-fluorouracil + folinic acid + irinotecan + oxaliplatin.*

41.3   Pancreatic Cystic Neoplasms

41.3.1 Classification [1, 12]

- Benign.
    - Serous cystadenoma,
    - Lymphangioma/hemangioma/teratoma.
- Premalignant/malignant.
    - Mucinous cystadenoma,
    - Intraductal papillary mucinous neoplasms (**IPMN**),
    - Mucinous cystadenocarcinoma,
    - Cystic neuroendocrine tumors.

41.3.2 Epidemiology [12]

- Detected in approximately 10–15% of general population,
    - Without history of pancreatitis,
    - Discovered incidentally on IRM/CT scans.
- Represent 1–2% of malignant pancreatic tumors,
    - Better prognosis than pancreatic ductal adenocarcinoma.

41.3.3 Serous Cystadenoma [13]

- Almost always benign and occur more commonly in women,
- Classified into serous microcystic adenomas and serous macrocystic adenomas,
- Unifocal, round, well-demarcated, and often honeycombed,
- Contain serous fluid that is mucin-free,
- Characteristic aspect on EUS as described in Fig. 41.8.

41.3.4 Mucinous Cystadenoma [12]

- Premalignant lesions.
    - Frequent in women, incidentally discovered, commonly located in the pancreatic head/body.

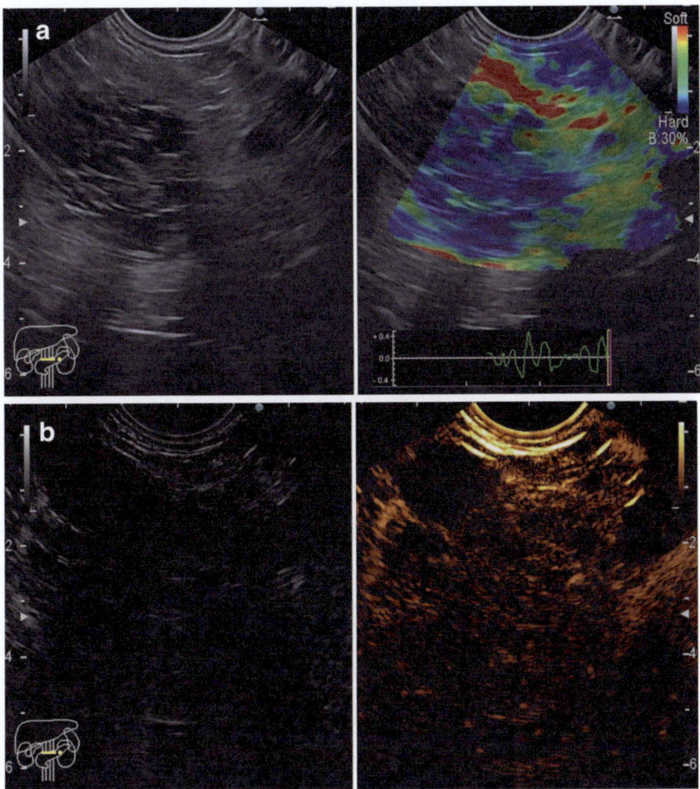

Fig. 41.8 Serous microcystic adenoma with pseudo- "hard" appearance on EUS elastography due to artifacts induced by microcysts and blood vessels located on the septations (a), with hypoenhanced septations on contrast-enhanced EUS (b)

- – Survival >60% for resected mucinous cystadenoma.
- – Survival <5% pentru resected mucinous cystadenocarcinoma.
- EUS aspect in described in Fig. 41.9.
  - – EUS-FNA with fluid aspiration (amylase, CEA, CA 19–9) + cytological examination.
  - – Risk factors for malignancy.
    - Mural nodules and thick wall.
    - Size >3 cm.

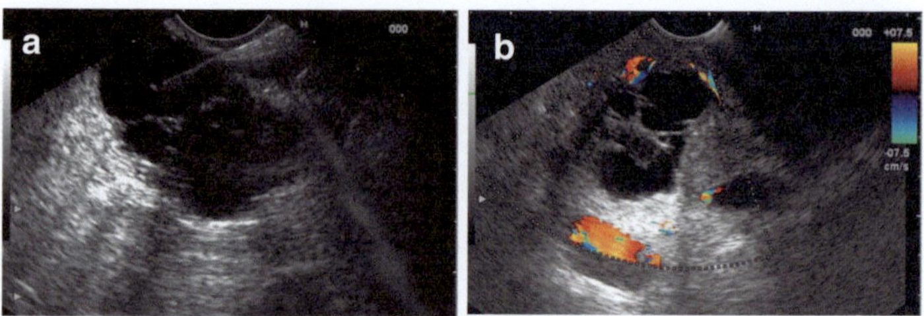

Fig. 41.9 Mucinous macrocystic adenoma with thick wall (**a**) and mural nodules (**b**) that requires EUS-FNA for diagnosis confirmation

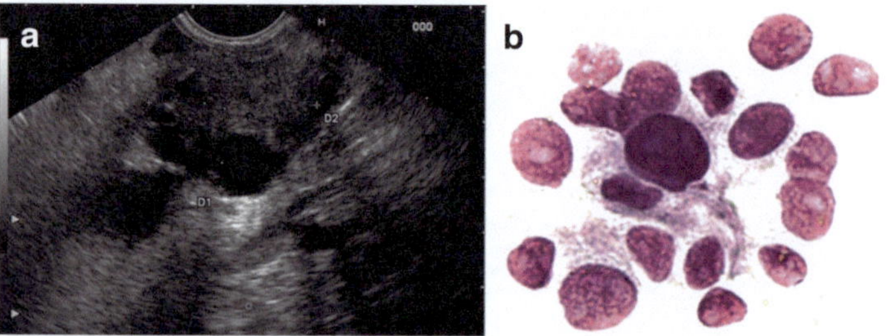

Fig. 41.10 Mucinous cystadenocarcinoma with hypoechogenic solid component (**a**), with EUS-FNA and cytological examination showing hyperchromatic nuclei, with decreased nuclei-cytoplasm ratio (**b**)

41.3.5 Mucinous Cystadenocarcinoma [12]

- Arises from mucinous cystadenoma.
- Characteristic EUS aspect as described in Fig. 41.10.
  - Irregular cystic lesions with solid areas and thick wall.
  - requires aspiration of the cystic lesions and EUS-FNA from the solid component.

41.3.6 Intraductal Papillary Mucinous Neoplasms (IPMN) [12]

- Premalignant lesions,

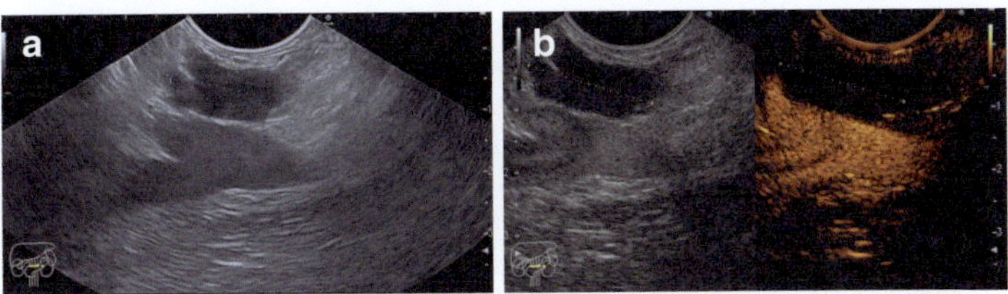

Fig. 41.11 Side branch IPMN located in the pancreatic isthmus, closed to the spleno-mesenteric confluent (**a**) without enhancement in the arterial and venous phase on contrast-enhanced EUS (**b**)

- EUS/EUS-FNA superior to CT and IRM.
  - Allows for the detection of mural nodules and differential diagnosis with mucus plugs using contrast enhanced EUS,
  - Identifies the communication with the pancreatic duct,
  - EUS-FNA enables the aspiration of the cystic fluid (positive "string sign").
  - Depicts concomitant pancreatitis changes.
- Types of IPMN:
  - Branch duct (Fig. 41.11), incidentally discovered, incidence increases with age,
  - Main duct, frequently located in the pancreatic head, symptomatic (weight loss, abdominal pain, jaundice).

References

1. Nagtegaal ID, Odze RD, Klimstra D, Paradis V, Rugge M, Schirmacher P, et al. The 2019 WHO classification of tumours of the digestive system. Histopathology. 2020;76(2):182.
2. Rawla P, Sunkara T, Gaduputi V. Epidemiology of pancreatic cancer: global trends, etiology and risk factors. World J Oncol. 2019;10(1):10.
3. Tempero MA. NCCN guidelines updates: pancreatic cancer. J Natl Compr Cancer Netw. 2019;17(5.5):605.
4. DeVita VT, Lawrence TS, Rosenberg SA. Cancer: principles & practice of oncology: primer of the molecular biology of cancer. Philadelphia, PA: Lippincott Williams & Wilkins; 2012.

5. Casciato DA, Territo MC. Manual of clinical oncology. Philadelphia, PA: Lippincott Williams & Wilkins; 2009.
6. Cazacu IM, Chavez AAL, Saftoiu A, Vilmann P, Bhutani MS. A quarter century of EUS-FNA: progress, milestones, and future directions. Endosc Ultrasound. 2018;7(3):141.
7. Kitano M, Yoshida T, Itonaga M, Tamura T, Hatamaru K, Yamashita Y. Impact of endoscopic ultrasonography on diagnosis of pancreatic cancer. J Gastroenterol. 2019;54(1):19–32.
8. Yamashita Y, Shimokawa T, Napoléon B, Fusaroli P, Gincul R, Kudo M, et al. Value of contrast-enhanced harmonic endoscopic ultrasonography with enhancement pattern for diagnosis of pancreatic cancer: a meta-analysis. Dig Endosc. 2019;31(2):125–33.
9. Matsubara S, Nakagawa K, Suda K, Otsuka T, Oka M, Nagoshi S. Interventional EUS for pancreatic cancer and cholangiocarcinoma. Management of pancreatic cancer and cholangiocarcinoma. Cham: Springer; 2021. p. 265–84.
10. Ducreux M, Cuhna AS, Caramella C, Hollebecque A, Burtin P, Goéré D, et al. Cancer of the pancreas: ESMO clinical practice guidelines for diagnosis, treatment and follow-up. Ann Oncol. 2015;26:v56–68.
11. Conroy T, Hammel P, Hebbar M, Ben Abdelghani M, Wei AC, Raoul J-L, et al. FOLFIRINOX or gemcitabine as adjuvant therapy for pancreatic cancer. N Engl J Med. 2018;379(25):2395–406.
12. van Huijgevoort N, Del Chiaro M, Wolfgang CL, van Hooft JE, Besselink MG. Diagnosis and management of pancreatic cystic neoplasms: current evidence and guidelines. Nat Rev Gastroenterol Hepatol. 2019;16(11):676–89.
13. Charville GW, Kao C-S. Serous neoplasms of the pancreas: a comprehensive review. Arch Pathol Lab Med. 2018;142(9):1134–40.

Pancreatic Neuroendocrine Tumors

42

Elena Codruța Gheorghe
and Adrian Săftoiu

42.1 Definitions and Classification

Neuroendocrine tumors are a group of tumors originating in neuroendocrine cells, with different anatomical locations (gastrointestinal tract, pancreas, lungs, thymus, endocrine glands). Pancreatic neuroendocrine tumors (NEN) can be classified as:

- Well-differentiated pancreatic neuroendocrine tumors = neuroendocrine tumors (**pNET**),
- Poorly-differentiated pancreatic neuroendocrine tumors = carcinoma neuroendocrine (**pNEC**) (Table 42.1).

Supplementary Information The online version contains supplementary material available at https://doi.org/10.1007/978-3-031-42076-4_42. The videos can be accessed individually by clicking the DOI link in the accompanying figure caption or by scanning this link with the SN More Media App.

E. C. Gheorghe (✉)
University of Medicine and Pharmacy Craiova, Craiova, Romania

A. Săftoiu
Department of Gastroenterology and Hepatology, Elias Emergency University Hospital, Carol Davila University of Medicine and Pharmacy, Bucharest, Romania

A. Săftoiu (ed.), *Pocket Guide to Advanced Endoscopy in Gastroenterology*, https://doi.org/10.1007/978-3-031-42076-4_42

Table 42.1 WHO classification of gastroenteropancreatic neuroendocrine tumors (2017)

	Mitotic count	Ki-67 index (%)
Well-differentiated pNEN		
NET G1	<2	<3
NET G2	2–20	3–20
NET G3	>20	>20
Poorly differentiated pNEN		
NEC G3	>20	>20
Mixed neuroendocrine-non-neuroendocrine neoplasm (MINEN)		

Classification according to the clinical picture and secretory status [1]:

- **Nonfunctional tumors (NFT).**
- **Functional tumors (FT).**
    - Gastrinoma.
    - Insulinoma.
    - VIPoma.
    - Glucagonoma.
    - Somatostatinoma.
    - hGH/ACTH/PTH secreting tumors,
    - Carcinoid tumors.

42.2   Epidemiology

- Incidence around 1:100,000, increases with age.
- Represents 1–2% of pancreatic neoplasms.
- 5-year survival rate of 55% for localized and resectable tumors and 15% for unresectable tumors
- Men > women.
- They occur sporadically more frequently, but also associated with genetic syndromes (<10%):
    - Multiple endocrine neoplasia (MEN) type 1.
    - Neurofibromatosis type 1.
    - Von Hippel–Lindau syndrome.
    - Tuberous sclerosis.

- NFT twice more frequent (70–90% of all pancreatic NENs) than FT.

42.3 Diagnostic

- Signs and symptoms.
    - Asymptomatic *or,*
    - Anorexia, weight loss,
    - Abdominal pain,
    - Jaundice,
    - Specific functional syndromes depending on the secreted hormone (functional tumors),
    - Carcinoid syndrome: severe diarrhea, abdominal pain, flushing.
- Laboratory tests.
    - Specific biomarkers: insulin, proinsulin, and peptide C for insulinoma, gastrin for Zollinger–Ellison syndrome, vasoactive intestinal peptide for VIPoma, glucagon for glucagonoma,
    - For nonfunctional tumors: serum levels of chromogranin A, neuron-specific enolase, pancreatic polypeptide, and/or pancreastatin.
- Imaging tests.
    - Endoscopic ultrasound-guided fine-needle aspiration (EUS-FNA),

        Confirmation of the diagnosis by microhistological examination,
    - Contrast-enhanced ultrasound (CEUS), CT scan, or MRI

        Evaluation of the extension of the primary tumor and TNM staging,
    - Scintigraphy with radiolabeled somatostatin analogues (octreoscan),

        Especially useful for the detection of gastrinomas, glucagonomas, VIPomas,
    - 18F-FDG and 68Ga-somatostatin analogs PET/CT

        Imaging methods with greater specificity,

        Useful for the identification of poorly differentiated tumors.

42.4   The Role of Endoscopy

- EUS has improved the diagnosis of NEN, becoming a routine diagnostic tool.
  - High sensitivity (83–94%) for detecting and diagnosing pancreatic NENs and locoregional lymph node metastases (Figs. 42.1 and 42.2; Video 42.1a, b),
  - Investigation of choice in case of negative results using other imaging tests,
  - Characterization of the pancreatic mass (color Doppler, elastography, and CE-EUS) (Figs. 42.3 and 42.4; Video 42.2a, b).
  - Establishing the cytological/histological diagnosis by fine-needle aspiration/biospy (EUS-FNA/FNB) (Fig. 42.5).
  - Precise localization during the laparoscopic/robotic surgery by performing EUS-guided preoperative tattoos,
  - Can be used for local ablative therapies such as EUS-guided radiofrequency ablation (EUS-RFA) for patients who are not candidates for surgical resection.

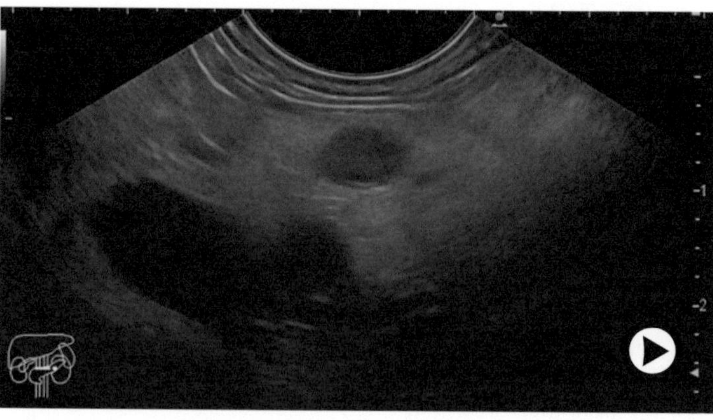

Fig. 42.1 Linear EUS showing a 7 mm hypoechoic mass at the level of the pancreatic body. (▶ https://doi.org/10.1007/000-b6h)

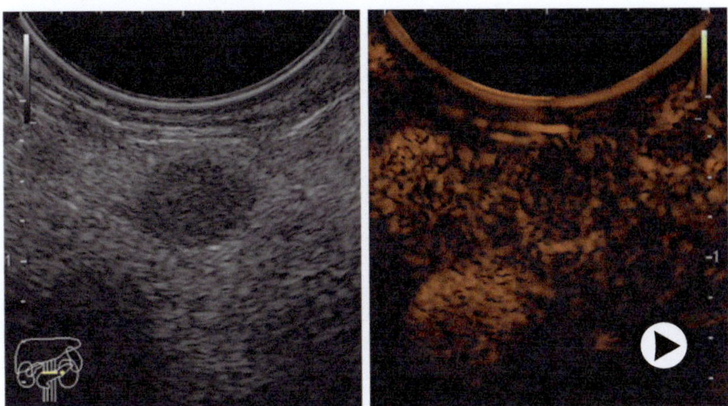

Fig. 42.2 Enhancement similar to the pancreatic parenchyma upon administration of the contrast substance, confirmed by EUS-FNA with microhistological examination (pNET G1). (▶ https://doi.org/10.1007/000-b6g)

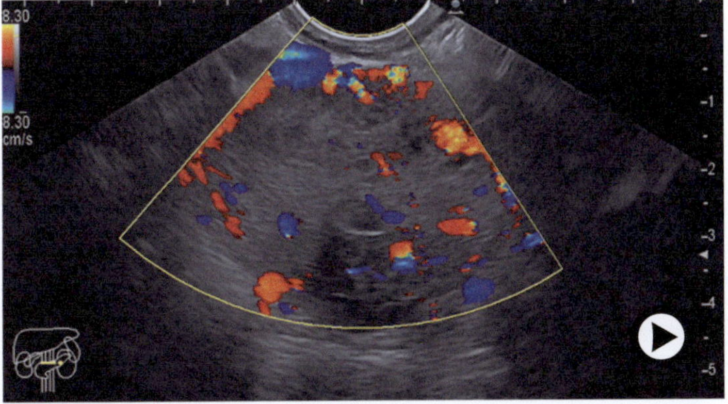

Fig. 42.3 Linear EUS showing a hypoechoic mass, with an intense color Doppler signal. (▶ https://doi.org/10.1007/000-b6f)

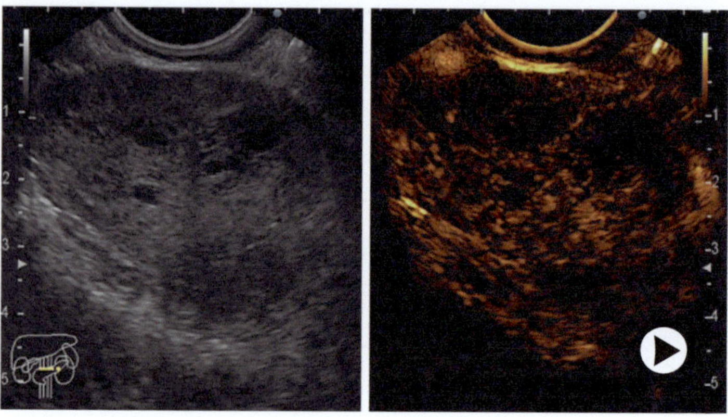

Fig. 42.4 Hyperenhancing inhomogeneous upon the administration of the contrast substance, confirmed by microhistological examination (pNEC). (▶ https://doi.org/10.1007/000-b6j)

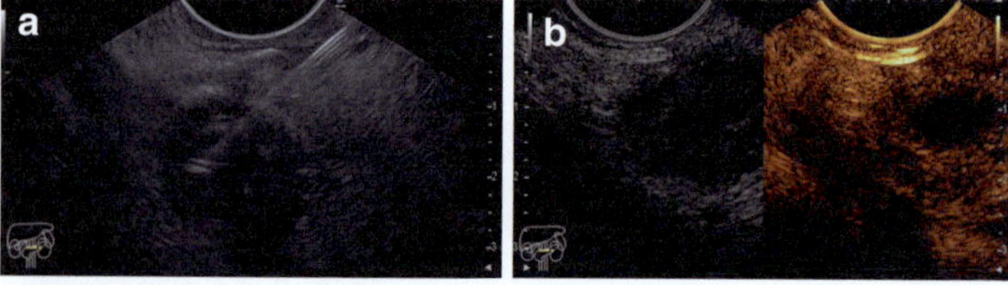

Fig. 42.5 Linear EUS showing a hypoechoic mass (**a**), hyperenhancing when contrast is administered, with a central necrosis area (**b**), confirmed by microhistological examination (pNET G1)

42.5 Staging

42.5.1 TNM Staging

- **Tumor (T).**
    - Tx: the primary tumor cannot be evaluated.
    - T1: the tumor is limited to the pancreas, < 2 cm.
    - T2: the tumor is limited to the pancreas, 2–4 cm.

- T3: the tumor is limited to the pancreas, >4 cm or the tumor is invading the duodenum or bile duct.
- T4: the tumor has grown into the stomach, spleen, colon, or adrenal gland, or the wall of the celiac axis or the superior mesenteric artery.
- **Regional lymph nodes (N).**
  - Nx: regional lymph nodes cannot be evaluated.
  - N0: no regional lymph node metastases.
  - N1: regional lymph node metastases.
- **Metastasis (M).**
  - M0: there is no distant spread.
  - M1: there is distant spread.

    M1a: metastases limited to the liver.

    M1b: metastases present in at least one extrahepatic location (lung, ovary, peritoneum, bone, distant lymph node) [1].

42.6   Treatment

- Surgical resection of the primary tumor.

    The only potentially curative treatment for well-differentiated NENs (G1/G2),

    The type of surgical intervention depends on the tumor stage, its location and the functional status of the tumor; it can vary from enucleation to pancreaticoduodenectomy,

    For NFT < 1.5 cm diagnosed incidentally, initial monitoring is recommended,
- Locoregional treatment of metastases: surgery, hepatic artery embolization/chemoembolization, radiofrequency ablation (RFA), selective internal radiotherapy (SIRT), external radiotherapy (bone and cerebral metastases).
- Medical treatment with somatostatin analogs (SSA) – octreotide, lanreotide.

    Useful for symptom control,

    Can also control tumor growth,

- Radiotherapy with radioactive analogs of somatostatin.
- Newer therapies:

  L-tryptophan hydroxylase inhibitors (teloristat ethyl, Xermelo®) for the treatment of carcinoid syndrome diarrhea in patients who are not adequately controlled with SSA. Radionuclides with peptide receptors (lutetium Lu 177 dotatate, Lutathera®) for patients with unresectable/metastatic tumors, well differentiated (G1 and G2), positive for somatostatin receptors [2–6].

References

1. Amin MB, Edge S, Greene F, et al. AJCC cancer staging manual. 8th ed. Cham: Springer; 2017. American Joint Commission on Cancer.
2. Kunz PL, Reidy-Lagunes D, Anthony LB, et al. Consensus guidelines for the management and treatment of neuroendocrine tumors. Pancreas. 2013;42:557–77.
3. Ramage JK, Ahmed A, Ardill J, et al. Guidelines for the management of gastroenteropancreatic neuroendocrine (including carcinoid) tumours (NETs). Gut. 2012;61:6–32.
4. Falconi M, Eriksson B, Kaltsas G, et al. ENETS consensus guidelines update for the Management of Patients with functional pancreatic neuroendocrine tumors and non-functional pancreatic neuroendocrine tumors. Neuroendocrinology. 2016;103:153–71.
5. Pavel M, Öberg K, Falconi M, et al. Gastroenteropancreatic neuroendocrine neoplasms: ESMO clinical practice guidelines for diagnosis, treatment and follow-up. Ann Oncol. 2020;31:844–60.
6. Ma ZY, Gong YF, Zhuang HK, et al. Pancreatic neuroendocrine tumors: a review of serum biomarkers, staging, and management. World J Gastroenterol. 2020;26:2305–22.

Common Bile Duct Stones

43

Vlad-Florin Iovănescu

43.1 Definition and Classification

- Primary bile duct stones.
  - Stones that develop inside the common bile duct (rare),
- Secondary bile duct stones.
  - Gallbladder stones migrated to the common bile duct (usually stones <5 mm).

43.2 Pathogenesis

- Primary bile duct stones.
  - Pigmented (exclusively): most often brown pigmented stones, in biliary obstruction/stasis and subsequent infection,
  - Rarely, black pigmented stones in chronic hemolysis/ileal Crohn's disease or extended ileal resections (high colonic concentrations of bile acids that increase the solubilization of unconjugated bilirubin and its secretion in bile).

V.-F. Iovănescu (✉)
Department of Gastroenterology, University of Medicine and Pharmacy Craiova, Craiova, Romania
e-mail: vlad.iovanescu@umfcv.ro

- Secondary bile duct stones.
  - Cholesterol gallstones (most common, exclusively developed in the gallbladder),
  - Black pigmented stones.

43.3 Diagnostic

- Clinical signs.
  - Colicky pain in the upper right quadrant,
  - jaundice,
  - Acholic stools (rare, because stones frequently cause incomplete obstruction) + dark urine (bilirubinuria) + pruritus,
  - Chills + fever (in acute bacterial cholangitis),
  - Charcot triad (biliary pain + jaundice + fever) in one-third of patients with cholangitis.
- Physical exam.
  - Pain in upper right quadrant on palpation,
  - Hepatomegaly (in persistent obstruction).
- Laboratory tests.
  - Increased total and conjugated (direct) bilirubin (total bilirubin usually <10 mg/dL, higher levels suggest malignant obstruction),
  - Increased AP, GGT,
  - Marked increased ALT, AST (sometimes >10 × N).
- Imaging tests.
  - Transabdominal ultrasound,
    - Initial imaging modality,
    - Low sensitivity because of proximity of distal CBD to the gas-filled duodenum,
    - May show indirect signs of obstruction (dilation of bile ducts proximal to the obstruction) [1].
  - MRCP.
    - High sensitivity and specificity,
    - Allows imaging of bile ducts without contrast media,
    - Noninvasive.

  – EUS.

  High sensitivity and specificity for detecting CBD stones,

  Invasive procedure.

  – ERCP.

  Highly sensitive and specific, associated with risk of complications (acute pancreatitis, bleeding, perforation, etc.) [2],

  used mainly as therapeutic procedure for stone extraction [3].

43.4 Role of Endoscopy

- EUS.
  - Excellent for imaging the distal CBD and establishing the diagnosis (Fig. 43.1a, b),
  - Superior to abdominal ultrasound and CT scan [4].
- ERCP.
  - Used mainly as a therapeutic procedure (endoscopic sphincterotomy and stone retrieval with extraction balloon or Dormia basket) (Figs. 43.2a, b and 43.3a, b),
  - Electrohydraulic/laser cholangioscopy-assisted lithotripsy in stones that are difficult to extract.

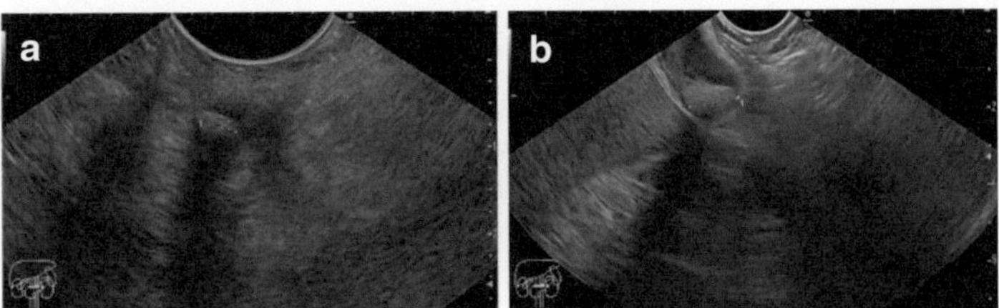

Fig. 43.1 Choledocholithiasis with solitary 5 mm stone (with posterior acoustic shadowing) visualized by EUS from the second part of the duodenum (**a**) and a solitary 15 mm stone (with posterior acoustic shadowing) and sludge in the CBD visualized by EUS from the duodenal bulb (**b**)

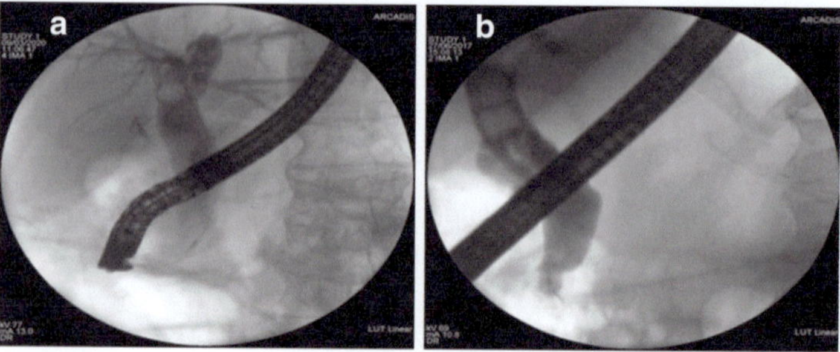

Fig. 43.2 Cholangiographic images of choledocholithiasis visualized during ERCP as contrast medium filling defects in the proximity of the hilum (solitary stone) (**a**) and in the middle portion of the choledocus (multiple faceted stones) (**b**)

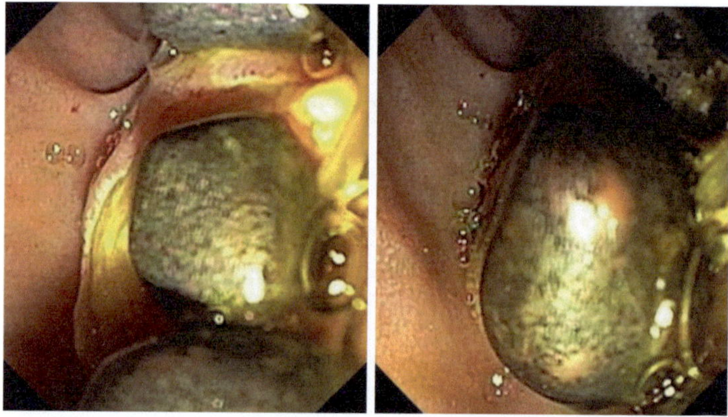

Fig. 43.3 Choledocholithiasis extracted during ERCP, visualized by endoscopy in DII at the level of the major duodenal papilla

43.5 Complications

- Acute pancreatitis: particularly for stones <5 mm,
- Acute cholangitis: frequent in choledocholithiasis because of incomplete obstruction and potential for ascending of bacteria with subsequent bile infection [5],

– Common bile duct strictures: induced by repeated trauma and chronic inflammation,
– Secondary biliary cirrhosis: in prolonged obstructions, typically longer than 5 years.

43.6 Treatment

– Analgesics/antispasmodics in case of pain,
– Antibiotics (in associated acute cholangitis),
– ERCP with extraction of stones/ERCP with laser/electrohydraulic cholangioscopy-assisted intraluminal lithotripsy in case of failed extraction.
– Surgery for stones extraction if endoscopic extraction fails,
– Laparoscopic cholecystectomy for associated gallbladder stones.

References

1. Molvar C, Glaenzer B. Choledocholithiasis: evaluation, treatment, and outcomes. Semin Intervent Radiol. 2016;33(4):268–76.
2. Manes G, Paspatis G, Aabakken L, et al. Endoscopic management of common bile duct stones: European Society of Gastrointestinal Endoscopy (ESGE) guideline. Endoscopy. 2019;51(5):472–49.
3. Buxbaum JL, Abbas Fehmi SM, Sultan S, et al. ASGE guideline on the role of endoscopy in the evaluation and management of choledocholithiasis. Gastrointest Endosc. 2019;89(6):1075–105.
4. Sonnenberg A, Enestvedt BK, Bakis G. Management of Suspected Choledocholithiasis: a decision analysis for choosing the optimal imaging modality. Dig Dis Sci. 2016;61(2):603–9.
5. Narula VK, Fung EC, Overby DW, et al. Clinical spotlight review for the management of choledocholithiasis. Surg Endosc. 2020;34(4):1482–91.

Bile Duct Tumors

44

Adrian Săftoiu and Irina Mihaela Cazacu

44.1 Definition and Classification [1]

- Malignant.
  - Cholangiocarcinoma (CCC),
  - Non-Hodgkin/MALT lymphoma,
  - Carcinoid tumor,
  - Metastases.
- Benign.
  - Biliary papillomatosis,
  - Biliary cystadenoma,
  - Adenoma or adenomyoma.

A. Săftoiu
Department of Gastroenterology and Hepatology, Elias Emergency
University Hospital, Carol Davila University of Medicine and Pharmacy,
Bucharest, Romania

I. M. Cazacu (✉)
Faculty of Medicine, Carol Davila University of Medicine and
Pharmacy, Bucharest, Romania

Department of Oncology, Fundeni Clinical Institute, Bucharest, Romania

437

A. Săftoiu (ed.), *Pocket Guide to Advanced Endoscopy in
Gastroenterology*, https://doi.org/10.1007/978-3-031-42076-4_44

44.2 Cholangiocarcinoma

44.2.1 Epidemiology [2, 3]

- CCC usually appears:
  - After the age of 60 years,
  - Men < women,
  - Around 1 in 100,000 per year.
- Known risk factors [2–4]:
  - Primary sclerosing cholangitis,
  - Chronic hepatolithiasis,
  - Choledochal cysts,
  - Intrahepatic lithiasis (Caroli disease),
  - Liver fluke infections (Clonorchis sinesis and Opisthorchis viverrini) and oriental cholangiohepatitis,
  - Chronic liver disease (HBV, HCV, liver cirrhosis regardless of etiology),
  - Genetic syndromes (Lynch syndrome, Multiple biliary papillomatosis),
  - Toxins (Dioxins, nitrosamines, and polychlorinated biphenyls).

44.2.2 Etiology and Pathogenesis [3]

- Location in the intra- or extrahepatic biliary ducts.
- Intrahepatic CCC (iCCC)
  - Located within the hepatic parenchyma, increasing incidence.
- Extrahepatic CCC (eCCC)
  - Located anywhere from the junction of the right and left hepatic ducts to the common bile duct;
  - Distal and hilar (bifurcation of the common hepatic duct – Klatskin tumors).
- Adenocarcinoma is the most common (>95%), the rest are squamous cell carcinoma.
- Hepatocholangiocarcinoma

- – Mixed form (CCC and hepatocellular carcinoma).
  - – Staging and treatment similar to CCC.
- – Pathogenic sequence involves chronic inflammation followed by mutations: Kras, TP53, IDH 1/2, FGFR2 gene fusions.

44.2.3 Diagnosis [4]

- Clinical signs.
  - – Jaundice + pale (clay-colored) stools + dark urine (bilirubinuria) + pruritus,
  - – Pain in the upper right quadrant,
  - – Weight loss.
- Physical exam.
  - – Palpable gallbladder (Courvoisier sign) if distal to the cystic duct,
  - – Hepatomegaly or palpable mass,
- Laboratory studies.
  - – Increased total & conjugated (direct) bilirubin, alkaline phosphatase, GGT,
  - – Normal/minimally increased AST/ALT,
  - – Increased prothrombin time (vitamin K malabsorbtion),
  - – CEA & CA 19–9 usually elevated.
- Imaging tests [2].
  - – Transabdominal ultrasound is the initial test: indicates the presence and level of obstruction, rarely the tumor (small/distal lesions are difficult to visualize).
  - – CT indicates the level of obstruction (intrahepatic or extrahepatic), with limited ability for staging and resectability (it should be supplemented by PET).
  - – MRCP provides supplementary information.

44.2.4 Role of Endoscopy [5]

- EUS enhances diagnosis, including confirmation by cytology/histopathology based on EUS-guided FNA/FNB (Fig. 44.1), with better accuracy as compared to brush cytology or direct biopsies under X-ray control.

- ERCP is used for confirmation of diagnosis (by brush cytology/direct biopsies) and for drainage with plastic stents (Figs. 44.2 and 44.3) or self-expanding metallic stents (Fig. 44.4) [5, 6].

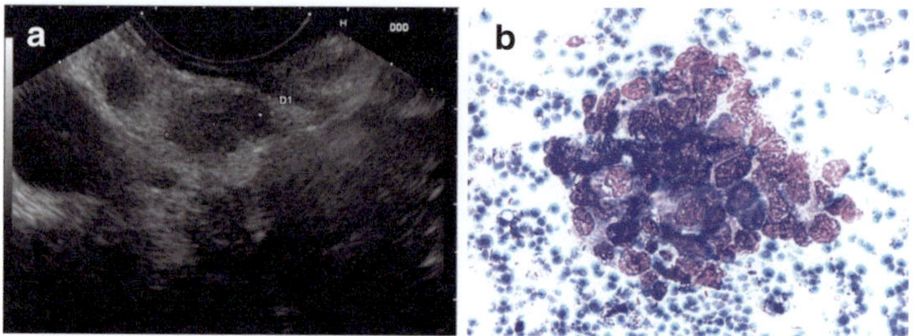

Fig. 44.1 Proximal CCC (Klatskin tumor) visible on EUS as a hypoechogenic lesion located in the proximity of portal vein and hepatic artery (**a**); diagnosis was confirmed by EUS-FNA and cytological examinations showing multiple cells with hyperchromatic nuclei and inverted nuclear-cytoplasmic ratio (**b**)

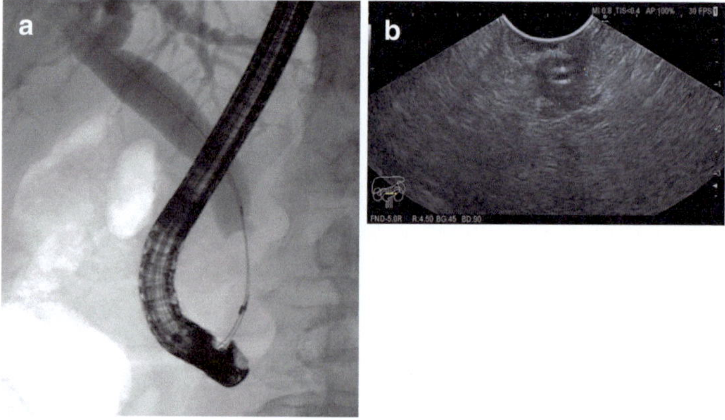

Fig. 44.2 Distal cholangiocarcinoma with ERCP showing complete blockage of the contrast substance (**a**); placement of a plastic stent which can be visualized on EUS inside the hypoechogenic tumor (**b**)

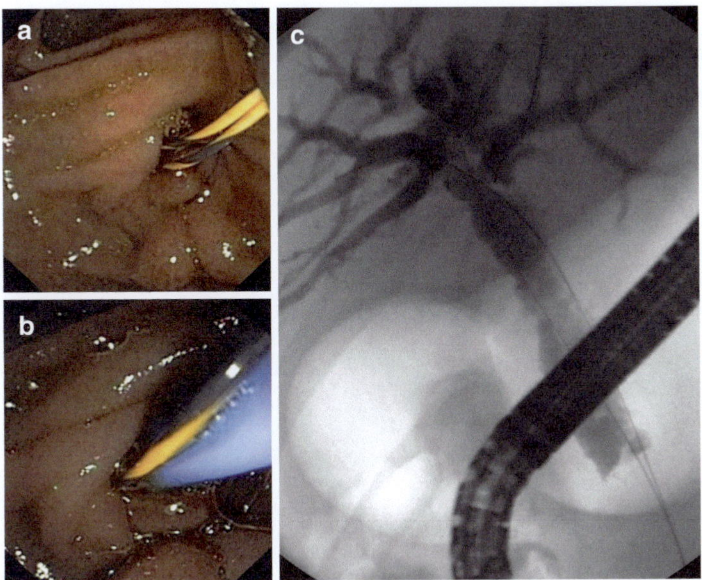

Fig. 44.3 Distal cholangiocarcinoma drained with two guide wires inserted into in the right and left hepatic duct (**a**, **b**), with simultaneous placement of two plastic stents (**c**)

- EUS can be used for drainage if ERCP is not possible (altered anatomy, technical inability, etc.)
- New intraductal techniques: cholangioscopy (spyglass)/intraductal ultrasound/confocal laser endomicroscopy, used for clinical research or selected cases [7, 8].

44.2.5 Staging (Eighth AJCC) [2]

- Intrahepatic CCC (iCCC).
    - T1a/b: solitary tumor $\leq$5/>5 cm without vascular invasion.
    - T2: solitary tumor with intrahepatic vascular invasion/multiple tumors.
    - T3: perforation of visceral peritoneum.

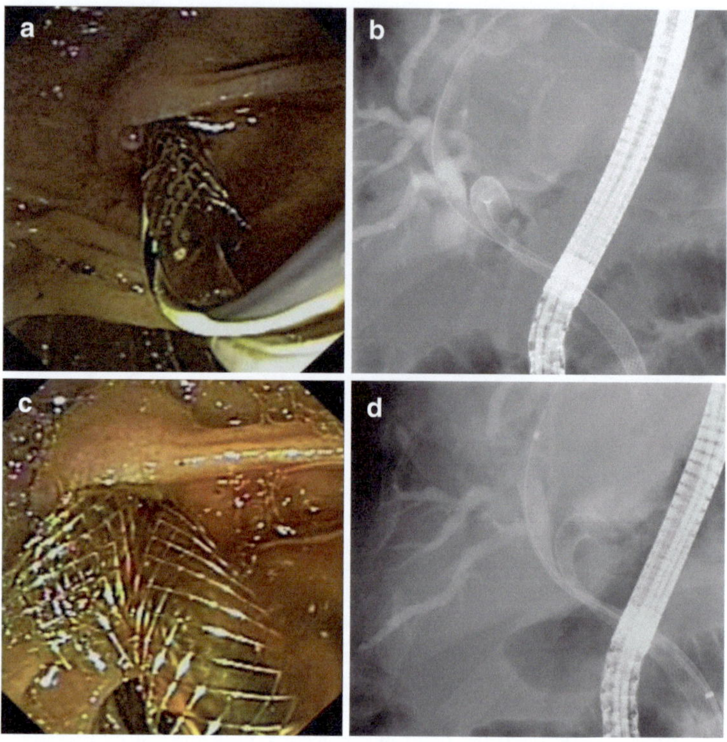

Fig. 44.4 Proximal cholangiocarcinoma (Klatskin tumor) drained with two guide wires inserted into the right and left hepatic duct (**b, d**) with sequential placement of two self-expanding metallic stents (**a, c**). (Courtesy of Vasile Sandru, MD)

- T4: tumor involving local extrahepatic structures by direct invasion.
- N0/1: without/with regional lymph node metastasis present.
- Extrahepatic—distal CCC.
  - T1: invades bile duct wall with a depth < 5 mm.
  - T2: invades bile duct wall with a depth 5–12 mm.
  - T3: invades bile duct wall with a depth > 12 mm.

- T4: involves the celiac axis, superior mesenteric artery, and/or common hepatic artery.
  - N0: no regional lymph node metastasis present.
  - N1: metastasis in 1–3 regional lymph nodes.
  - N2: metastasis in >3regional lymph nodes.
- Extrahepatic—perihilar CCC.
  - T1: confined to the bile duct.
  - T2a/b: invades beyond bile duct wall to surrounding adipose tissue/invades adjacent hepatic parenchyma.
  - T3: invades unilateral branches of portal vein or hepatic artery.
  - T4: involves main portal vein or its branches bilaterally; or the common hepatic artery.
  - N0: no regional lymph node metastasis present.
  - N1: metastasis in 1–3 regional lymph nodes.
  - N2: metastasis in >3 regional lymph nodes.

44.2.6 Treatment [2]

- **Resectable CCC.**
  - Complete resection with R0 is the only currative treatment.
  - Biopsy is not usually necessary for resectable tumors.
  - Transperitoneal biopsy contraindicated for potential transplant patients.
  - Type of surgery depending on location.
    - Bile duct excision and partial duodenopancreatectomy (Whipple) for distal CCC,
    - Resection of the involved biliary tract and en bloc resection for hilar CCC,
    - Hepatic resection for iCCC,
  - R0 resection: observation/chemo with fluoropyrimidine/gemcitabine; radiation is not recommended.
  - R1 resection/N+: fluropyrimidine or gemcitabine chemo; followed by fluoropyrimidine-based radiation.
  - Preferred adjuvant regimen: capecitabine,

- **Unresectable/metastatic CCC.**
  - Preferred regimen: durvalumab + gemcitabine + cisplatin (new standard of care),
  - Other regimes: gemcitabine + cisplatin, gemcitabine + oxaliplatin (GEMOX); gemcitabine monotherapy; 5FU + leucovorin.

References

1. Nagtegaal ID, Odze RD, Klimstra D, Paradis V, Rugge M, Schirmacher P, et al. The 2019 WHO classification of tumours of the digestive system. Histopathology. 2020;76(2):182.
2. Benson AB, D'Angelica MI, Abbott DE, Anaya DA, Anders R, Are C, et al. Hepatobiliary cancers, version 2.2021, NCCN clinical practice guidelines in oncology. J Natl Compr Cancer Netw. 2021;19(5):541–65.
3. DeVita VT, Lawrence TS, Rosenberg SA. Cancer: principles & practice of oncology: primer of the molecular biology of cancer. Philadelphia, PA: Lippincott Williams & Wilkins; 2012.
4. Casciato DA, Territo MC. Manual of clinical oncology. Philadelphia, PA: Lippincott Williams & Wilkins; 2009.
5. Urban O, Vanek P, Zoundjiekpon V, Falt P. Endoscopic perspective in cholangiocarcinoma diagnostic process. Gastroenterol Res Pract. 2019;2019:1.
6. Viesca MFY, Arvanitakis M. Early diagnosis and management of malignant distal biliary obstruction: a review on current recommendations and guidelines. Clin Exp Gastroenterol. 2019;12:415.
7. Rizvi S, Eaton J, Yang JD, Chandrasekhara V, Gores GJ. Emerging technologies for the diagnosis of perihilar cholangiocarcinoma. Semin Liver Dis. 2018;38(2):160.
8. Ayoub F, Yang D, Draganov PV. Cholangioscopy in the digital era. Translational Gastroenterol Hepatol. 2018;3:3.

Gallbladder Diseases

45

Irina F. Cherciu Harbiyeli and Valeriu Şurlin

45.1 Gallbladder Pathology [1]

- A common cause of upper abdominal pain.
- Prevalence increases with age, and is more common in women than men.
- It covers several types of conditions.
  - Gallstones,
  - Cholecystitis,
  - Biliary dyskinesia,
  - Gallbladder polyps,
  - Gallbladder cancer.
- Differential diagnosis:
  - Acute cholangitis,
  - Acute hepatitis,
  - Acute pancreatitis,
  - Appendicitis,

I. F. Cherciu Harbiyeli (✉)
Research Center of Gastroenterology and Hepatology Craiova,
University of Medicine and Pharmacy Craiova, Craiova, Romania

V. Şurlin
Department of Surgery, University of Medicine and Pharmacy Craiova,
Craiova, Romania

A. Săftoiu (ed.), *Pocket Guide to Advanced Endoscopy in
Gastroenterology*, https://doi.org/10.1007/978-3-031-42076-4_45

- Cardiac ischemia,
- Fitz-Hugh–Curtis syndrome.
- Irritable bowel disease,
- Non-ulcer dyspepsia,
- Peptic ulcer disease,
- Perforated viscus,
- Right-sided pneumonia,
- Subhepatic or intra-abdominal abscess.

45.2   Congenital Gallbladder Abnormalities

- Are not uncommon.
- Anomalies in number, size, and shape (agenesis of the gallbladder, duplications, rudimentary or oversized "giant" gallbladders, diverticula).
- Anomalies of position or suspension (left-sided/intrahepatic gallbladder/retro-displaced/"floating" gallbladder).

45.3   Gallstones [2]

- Affect up to 20% of the population.
- The most common gastrointestinal disorder for which patients are admitted to hospitals in European countries.
- The prevalence of gallstones is 10% to 15% in adults.
  - 80% of gallstones remain asymptomatic, with the risk of pain or complications of 1%–4% per year
  - Cholesterol gallstones account for 90–95% of all gallstones.
- **Risk factors.**
  - Female gender,
  - Age 60 or older,
  - Family history of gallstones,
  - High-calorie and low-fiber diets,
  - Being overweight or obese,
  - Rapid weight loss,
  - Low physical activity,

- Diabetes/metabolic syndrome,
- Estrogen medications,
- Crohn's disease and other conditions that affect how nutrients are absorbed.
- Cirrhosis or other liver diseases.
- **Clinical aspects.**
  - Episodic attacks of severe pain in the right upper abdominal quadrant or epigastrium for at least 15–30 min,
  - Radiation to the right back or shoulder,
  - A positive reaction to analgesics.
- **Diagnosis.**
  - Abdominal ultrasound,
    - Is the imaging of choice in patients with pain located in the upper abdominal quadrant,
    - Accuracy of 95%,
    - Gallstones appear as echogenic foci with a hypoechoic distal shadow,
    - Mobility differentiates stones from polyps and should be proven by examining the patient in different positions (left lateral decubitus or upright),
    - Biliary sludge is detected as sand-like small echogenic foci,
    - Older patients with atypical abdominal pain, immuno-compromised patients with unclear site of infection, or patients with bacteremia suspicious for an abdominal septic focus may also be evaluated by abdominal ultrasound for the presence of (complicated) gallstones,
    - In case of inconclusive abdominal ultrasound and strong clinical suspicion of gallbladder stones, endoscopic ultrasound (EUS) or magnetic resonance imaging (MRI) may be performed,
    - EUS.
    - Has a high sensitivity of 94–98% to detect cholecystolithiasis in patients with biliary pain but normal abdominal ultrasound (Fig. 45.1a, b).

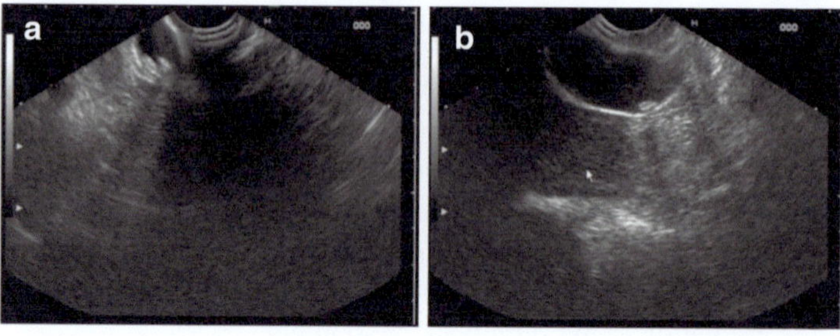

Fig. 45.1 Linear echoendoscopy highlighting images with posterior shadow cone (calculi) (**a**), respectively unique mobile calculus in the gallbladder (**b**), with the echoendoscope placed at the antral level

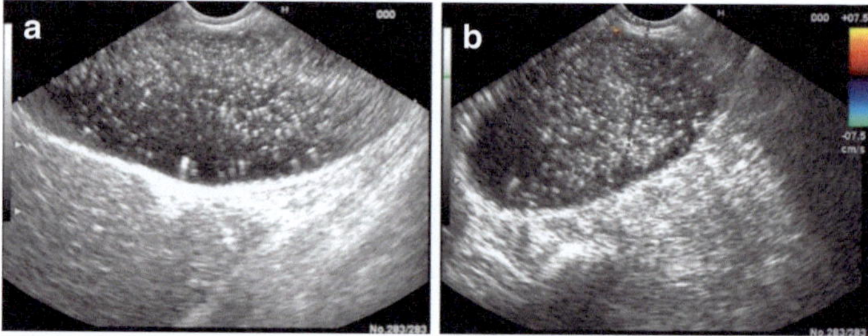

Fig. 45.2 Linear echoendoscopy that reveals gallbladder full of sludge and microlithiasis (**a**), without Doppler signal (**b**), in a patient with tumor of the head of the pancreas

- Might be particularly helpful in patients with unexplained acute and acute recurrent pancreatitis caused by malignant tumors (Fig. 45.2a, b).
- Therapy of gallstones.
  - Litholysis using bile acids alone or in combination with extracorporeal shock-wave lithotripsy is not recommended,
  - Cholecystectomy is reserved for the subgroup of patients with symptomatic gallstones or abnormal gallbladder findings (e.g., chronic cholecystitis, tumors).

45.4 Cholecystitis [3–5]

- The most common type of gallbladder disease.
- Acute or chronic inflammation of the gallbladder.

45.4.1 Acute Cholecystitis (AC)

- The most common complication of gallstone disease.
  - It may have other etiologies (tumors, etc.)
- Presentation.
  - Severe pain located in the upper right quadrant of the abdomen, fever, nausea, vomiting, jaundice,
  - Leukocytosis,
  - Tenderness on palpation (Murphy's sign).
- Classification.
  - Acalculous AC: typically seen in critically ill patients,
  - Xanthogranulomatous AC: irregular thickening of the gallbladder wall, rarely parietal calcifications,
  - Emphysematous AC: intraluminal air or within the gallbladder wall, caused by anaerobes that form gases,
  - Torsion of the gallbladder: seen most frequently in the elderly, compromises the vascular supply, and may result in life-threatening consequences if not promptly treated with cholecystectomy.
- Diagnosis.
  - Abdominal ultrasound.
      The initial imaging modality,
      It has a good diagnostic accuracy (sensitivity 81%, specificity 83%),
      Accurately detects: gallstones, thickened (>4 mm) gallbladder wall and/or a distended gallbladder, pericholecystic fluid and a sonographic Murphy's sign.
  - Scintigraphy using 99mTc-hepatic iminodiacetic acid (HIDA) is the most accurate test to rule in and to rule out AC (sensitivity 96%, specificity 90%).

- CT can accurately visualize gallbladder distention and wall thickening and identify complications of AC (emphysema, abscess formation, perforation).
- MRI may be helpful when obesity or gaseous distention limits use of ultrasound.
- Management.
  - Intravenous fluids,
  - Analgesics:
    NSAIDs (e.g., diclofenac, indomethacin) are first-line therapy.
    Spasmolytics (e.g., butylscopolamine),
    Opioids (e.g., buprenorphine) for severe symptoms.
  - Antibiotics in mild acute cholecystitis (without cholangitis, bacteriemia/sepsis, abscess or perforation) are not constantly recommended,
  - Classic/laparoscopic cholecystectomy,
  - Gallbladder decompression.
    Percutaneous transhepatic gallbladder drainage: standard drainage procedure, should be considered the first alternative to surgical intervention in surgically high-risk patients..
- Endoscopic gallbladder drainage.
  - Is suitable especially for patients with severe coagulopathy, thrombocytopenia, or an anatomically inaccessible location.
    Can be performed using either a transpapillary or transmural approach,
    Can be divided into two different methods: endoscopic naso-gallbladder drainage (ENGBD) or gallbladder stenting (EGBS) under ERCP guidance,
    Prolonged or unsuccessful procedures may lead to serious complications (post-ERCP pancreatitis, perforation of the cystic duct or gallbladder).
- Endoscopic ultrasound-guided gallbladder drainage.
  - The gallbladder is punctured from the body/antrum of the stomach/duodenal bulb under direct EUS visualization, then a lumen-apposing metal stent (LAMS) is inserted.

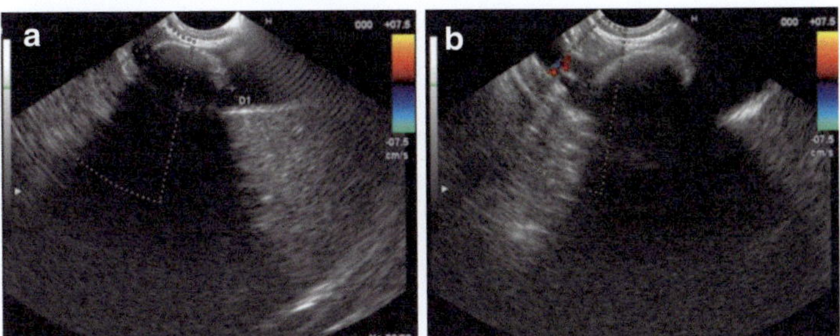

Fig. 45.3 Linear echoendoscopy showing low volume gallbladder with large calculus with posterior acoustic shadowing (**a**), without Doppler signal within the wall (**b**), with the echoendoscope placed at the antral level

45.4.2 Chronic Cholecystitis

- Occurs after recurrent episodes of AC,
- The gallbladder can shrink and lose its ability to store and release bile (Fig. 45.3),
- Symptoms: abdominal pain, nausea, vomiting,
- Cholecystectomy is often the needed treatment.

45.5 Biliary Dyskinesia (BD) [1, 3, 5]

- Functional disorder of the biliary tree.
  - Occurs when the gallbladder has a lower than normal motility,
- Might be related to chronic gallbladder inflammation.
- A controversial group including:
  - Gallbladder dysfunction (GBD),
  - Sphincter of Oddi dysfunction (SOD).
- The symptoms of SOD and GBD do overlap hence making a distinction between the two can be challenging for the clinician, both entities should be considered in evaluating a patient.
- GBD and SOD are diagnoses of exclusion.
  - The incidence of these disorders has increased from 5% to 25%, resulting in an increase in the number of cholecystectomies performed,

- Usually there are no gallstones in the gallbladder with biliary dyskinesia.
- Diagnosis.
    - The pain attributed to BD is generally similar in nature to biliary colic caused by gallstones,
    - The Rome IV diagnostic criteria for BD describe pain as:
        Usually located in the right upper quadrant or epigastric area,
        Episodic character, usually lasts for at least 30 min or longer,
        Recurrent, but generally not daily,
        Progressive, constantly increasing,
        Intense enough to interrupt the patient's daily activities,
        Not relieved by bowel movement, postural changes or antacids,
        Cannot be explained by other organic disease.
- Investigations.
    - The initial work-up,
        Liver function tests, lipase, conjugated bilirubin tests, ultrasound to rule out structural causes (gallstones or tumor),
        Tests are normal in patients with BD.
    - Specific investigations,
        HIDA scans to estimate gallbladder ejection fraction.
        If the gallbladder can only release ≤35–40% of its content, then the BD diagnosis can be established.
    - SOD manometry.
        The gold standard for assessing SOD,
        Invasive procedure,
        Rarely performed because of lack of availability and the risk of complications.
    - Other noninvasive tests to diagnose SOD,
        Ultrasonographic measurement of CBD diameter,
        HIDA scan.
        MRCP or preferably EUS.
- Treatment.

- Variable options, often inefficient,
    i.v. opiates are still the drug of choice with inpatient treatment,
    Muscle relaxers and calcium channel blockers are ineffective,
    Smoking cessation, eating more frequent meals, avoidance of foods high in fat, weight loss, increased physical activity, lying on the right side after meals.

45.6 Gallbladder Polyps [1, 5, 6]

- Represents a broad spectrum of gallbladder wall elevations protruding into the lumen.
- Prevalence is estimated between 0.3 and 9.5%.
- Pseudopolyps.
    - Are more common than true polyps,
    - Might be cholesterol pseudopolyps (most commonly), focal adenomyomatosis, inflammatory pseudopolyps,
    - Do not carry in themselves a malignant potential,
- True gallbladder polyps can be:
    - Benign polyps, most commonly adenomas,
    - Malignant polyps, usually adenocarcinomas,
- Risk factors for gallbladder polyps malignancy: age > 50, primary sclerosing cholangitis (PSC), Indian ethnicity, sessile polyp.
- Investigations.
    - Primary investigation should be abdominal US,
        Hyperechoic structure of the gallbladder wall protruding into the lumen,
        It should not be mobile or demonstrate posterior acoustic shadowing,
        It may be sessile or pedunculated,
        If there is clear reverberation or "comet tail" artifact present posterior to the lesion this should be identified as a pseudopolyp (focal adenomyomatosis or a cholesterol polyp).

- Routine use of alternative imaging modalities is not recommended.
  - Particularly EUS may be useful to aid decision-making in difficult cases,
  - CEUS increased diagnostic accuracy for the characterization of gallbladder polypoid lesions >10 mm but not <10 mm.
- Treatment.
  - Management of polyps <10 mm depends on patient and polyp characteristics,
  - Cholecystectomy.
    - Should be performed in patients with gallbladder polyps ≥10 mm without or with gallstones regardless of symptoms,
    - Recommended for patients with gallbladder polyps of 6–10 mm and risk factors for gallbladder malignancy or in case of growing polyps (increase ≥2 mm),
    - Recommend for patients with PSC and a gallbladder polyp, irrespective of size,
    - Is not indicated in patients with gallbladder polyps ≤6 mm (follow-up by ultrasound),
    - A clearly infiltrating or large mass should be treated as a gallbladder cancer.

45.7 Gallbladder Cancer (GBC) [5–7]

- Aggressive malignancy with poor prognosis.
- Affects over 140,000 patients worldwide and over 100,000 will die each year.
- Risk factors: chronic cholecystitis, gallstones, familial adenomatous polyposis syndrome, inflammatory bowel disease, porcelain gallbladder and gallbladder polyps (>1 cm that are sessile and solitary), choledochal cysts, primary sclerosing cholangitis.
- Symptoms may be similar to those of AC (pain, indigestion, weight loss and/or jaundice), but it may be completely missing.

45.7.1 Gallbladder Carcinoma

- It affects older patients over 50–60 years of age, especially women.
- The most usual is the adenocarcinoma (90%).
- Normally are asymptomatic until an advanced stage, the early detection is crucial to avoid a potential poor prognosis.
- In cases with hyalinizing cholecystitis, with minimal to no calcifications ("incomplete porcelain gallbladder"), the incidence of subtle invasive carcinoma seems to be very high, hence these cases must be carefully examined.
- The minimum staging evaluation of patients with suspected or proven GBC includes imaging methods and diagnostic laparoscopy.
  - Abdominal ultrasound.
    - First tool of choice due to its excellent temporal and spatial resolution, cost-effectiveness, easy manipulation, and no radiation.
  - Contrast-enhanced ultrasound (CEUS).
    - Increases the diagnostic accuracy,
    - The contrast agent applied allows the depiction of small vessels and their blood flow,
    - Vascularization pattern differs from the liver perfusion (the gallbladder is perfused by the cystic artery only and not by branches of the portal vein).
  - EUS.
    - Is an effective method for the differential diagnosis of focal lesions: tumors, sludges, or polyps (especially by using elastography and contrast-enhanced examination),
    - Has limitations demonstrating malignant features (gallbladder wall destruction or infiltration) (Fig. 45.4).
  - Contrast-enhanced abdominal CT.
    - The most accurate modality to determine resectability,
    - Capacity to interrogate portal nodes, peritoneal metastasis, and vascular invasion,

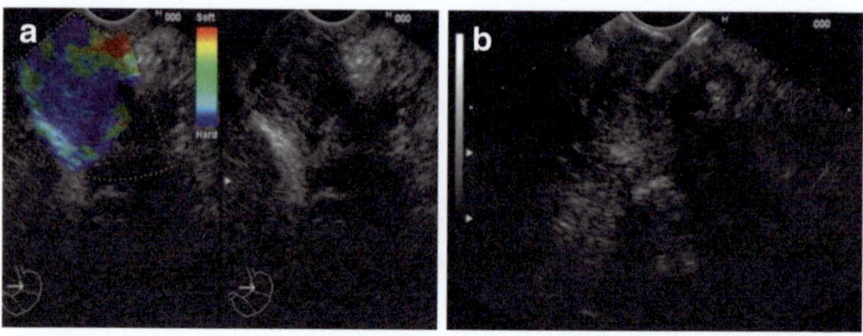

Fig. 45.4 Linear echoendoscopy showing gallbladder with hypoechoic formation inside, with hard elastographic appearance (**a**), confirmed by fine aspiration puncture as adenocarcinoma (**b**)

> Display differential diagnosis such as xanthogranulomatous cholecystitis, inflammation, adenomyomatosis, hepatobiliary malignancies, and metastatic disease.

- Diagnostic and staging accuracy of CT may be augmented by gadolinium-enhanced magnetic resonance imaging.
- Treatment.
    - Management can be difficult as most patients are diagnosed at an advanced stage of disease,
    - For patients with advanced gallbladder cancer, a multidisciplinary approach is recommended, preferably in "tumor board",
    - The combination regimens of chemotherapy, radiotherapy, targeted therapy, and immunotherapy have shown promise in improving prognosis,
    - Surgical resection.
        > Has as much of a role as a staging modality as it does as a therapeutic effort,
        > In early-stage disease offers potential cure, but only a minority of patients (10%) are candidates for these procedures.

References

1. Goussous N, Kowdley GC, Sardana N, Spiegler E, Cunningham SC. Gallbladder dysfunction: how much longer will it be controversial? Digestion. 2014;90:147–54.
2. European Association for the Study of the liver (EASL). Electronic address: easloffice@easloffice.eu. EASL clinical practice guidelines on the prevention, diagnosis and treatment of gallstones. J Hepatol. 2016;65:146–81.
3. Wilkins T, Agabin E, Varghese J, Talukder A. Gallbladder dysfunction: cholecystitis, choledocholithiasis, cholangitis, and biliary dyskinesia. Prim Care. 2017;44(4):575–97.
4. Mori Y, Itoi T, Baron TH, et al. Tokyo guidelines 2018: management strategies for gallbladder drainage in patients with acute cholecystitis (with videos). J Hepatobiliary Pancreat Sci. 2018;25:87–95.
5. Negrão de Figueiredo G, Mueller-Peltzer K, Armbruster M, Rübenthaler J, Clevert DA. Contrast-enhanced ultrasound (CEUS) for the evaluation of gallbladder diseases in comparison to cross-sectional imaging modalities and histopathological results. Clin Hemorheol Microcirc. 2019;71:141–9.
6. Wiles R, Thoeni RF, Barbu ST, et al. Management and follow-up of gallbladder polyps: joint guidelines between the European Society of Gastrointestinal and Abdominal Radiology (ESGAR), European Association for Endoscopic Surgery and other interventional techniques (EAES), International Society of Digestive Surgery - European federation (EFISDS) and European Society of Gastrointestinal Endoscopy (ESGE). Eur Radiol. 2017;27:3856–66.
7. Aloia TA, Járufe N, Javle M, et al. Gallbladder cancer: expert consensus statement. HPB (Oxford). 2015;17:681–90.

Part IX

Liver Diseases

Liver Cirrhosis

46

Larisa Săndulescu
and Elena Codruța Gheorghe

Abbreviations

AFP	Alpha-fetoprotein
ALP	Alkaline phosphatase
AMA	Antimitochondrial antibodies
ANA	Antinuclear antibodies
BP	Blood pressure
EGD	Esophagogastroduodenoscopy
EV	Esophageal varices
GGT	Gamma-glutamyl transferase
INR	International normalized ratio
Plt	Platelet
SAAG	Serum-ascites albumin gradient
SMA	Smooth muscle antibodies
SVC	superior vena cava

L. Săndulescu
Department of Gastroenterology, Research Center of Gastroenterology
and Hepatology, University of Medicine and Pharmacy Craiova, Craiova,
Romania

E. C. Gheorghe (✉)
University of Medicine and Pharmacy Craiova, Craiova, Romania

© The Author(s), under exclusive license to Springer Nature
Switzerland AG 2023
A. Săftoiu (ed.), *Pocket Guide to Advanced Endoscopy in
Gastroenterology*, https://doi.org/10.1007/978-3-031-42076-4_46

46.1   Definition and Classification

Liver cirrhosis is the end stage of chronic liver disease; it is characterized by advanced fibrosis, nodular transformation of the liver, and decreased number of functional hepatocytes. In evolution, cirrhosis can be:

- **Compensated** (generally asymptomatic).
- **Decompensated** (ascites, jaundice, esophageal varices, upper gastrointestinal bleeding (UGIB), encephalopathy).

46.2   Epidemiology

- The overall incidence is around 20/100 000
- The prevalence in the general population is 4.5–9.5%

46.3   Etiology and Pathogenesis

- Viral hepatitis (B, C),
- Chronic alcohol abuse,
- Nonalcoholic steatohepatitis,
- Genetic/congenital diseases: hemochromatosis, Wilson'sdisease, α1-antitrypsin deficiency,
- Autoimmune: primary biliary cirrhosis, primary sclerosing cholangitis, autoimmune hepatitis,
- Toxic: methotrexate, isoniazid, amiodarone.

46.4   Diagnostic

- **Signs and symptoms.**
  - Patients with **compensated** cirrhosis are usually asymptomatic or with nonspecific symptoms (asthenia, loss of appetite, bloating),

- Patients with **decompensated** cirrhosis have features of the two major syndromes:

  Hepatic failure syndrome: jaundice, spider naevi in the SVC territory, palmar erythema, white nails, muscle wasting, gynecomastia, decreased libido, gonadal atrophy, hemorrhagic syndrome, altered mental status, asterixis, sleep inversion, fetor hepaticus, parotid hypertrophy, and Dupuytren's contracture in alcoholics, ascites, edema,

  Portal hypertension syndrome: splenomegaly, ascites, collateral circulation, hydrothorax.

- **Laboratory tests.**
  - Hematological: anemia (mixed pathogenic mechanisms), thrombocytopenia, and leukopenia (hypersplenism),
  - ALT and AST serum levels are normal/moderately elevated; hyperbilirubinemia, slightly elevated ALP and γGT.
  - Later stages, hypoalbuminemia; prolonged prothrombin time and elevated INR,
  - For genetic conditions – ferritin, ceruloplasmin, α1-antitrypsin,
  - In case of autoimmunity – autoantibodies ANA, AMA M2, SMA,
  - AFP >200 – suspicion of HCC.
  - Ascitic fluid analysis: cytology (neutrophils >250/mm^3- SBP, lymphocytes predominate - bacillary ascites), SAAG>1,1 - portal hypertension,
  - For noninvasive staging of fibrosis: APRI score, FibroTest.
- **Imaging tests.**
  - Abdominal ultrasound can reveal:

    Liver changes (hepatomegaly/atrophy, irregular contour; heterogeneous, nodular echotexture),

    Typical changes for **portal hypertension** (dilated portal vein and reversal of PV flow, round ligament recanalization, dilation of splenic veins at the splenic hilum, splenomegaly, ascites).
  - Elastography (FibroScan)—for noninvasive staging of fibrosis and severity of portal hypertension.

46.5 The Role of Endoscopy

46.5.1 Standard Endoscopy

- Assessment of esophageal varices.
  Endoscopy every 2 years in the absence of esophageal varices or annually for grade 1 varices,
  Small (grade 1), medium (grade 2) or large (grade 3) varices (Fig. 46.1a, b),
  Primary (nonselective beta-blockers (NSBB)) and secondary (NSBB + ligatures) prophylaxis of UGIB, until eradication (Fig. 46.2a, b).
- Treatment of variceal UGIB.
  A combination of Terlipressin and ligatures (Fig. 46.3a, b),
  TIPS for rebleeding.
  Self-expandable stents in refractory cases.
- Assessment of portal hypertensive gastropathy,
  Typical aspect - "snake skin",
  NSBB treatment, argon plasma coagulation, or TIPS (for severe forms).

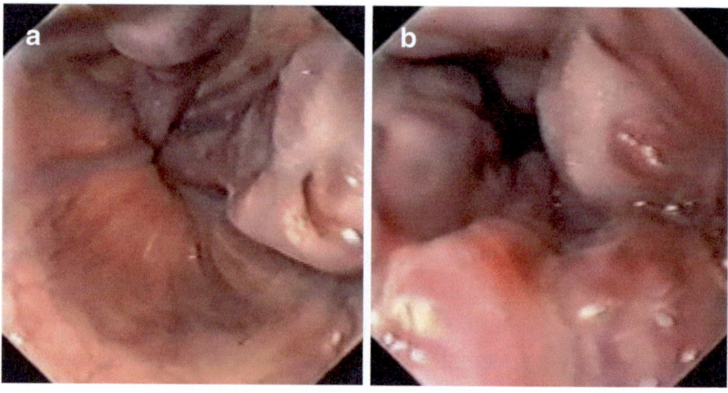

Fig. 46.1 Upper digestive endoscopy revealing varices of grade 2, (**a**), respectively grade 3 (**b**), with red marks on the surface

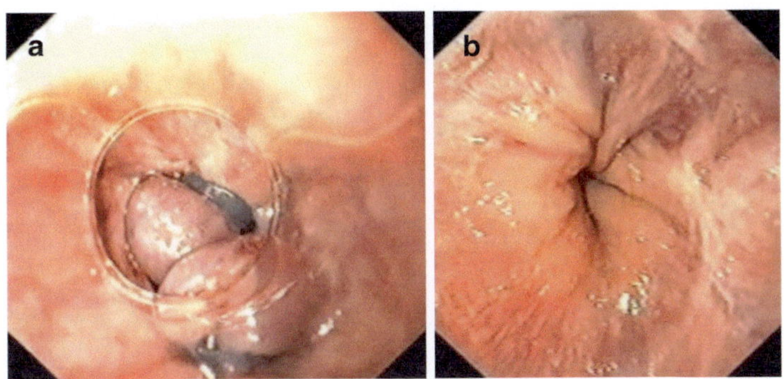

Fig. 46.2 Upper digestive endoscopy with prophylactic ligatures (elastic bands) (**a**) until the eradication of esophageal varices (**b**)

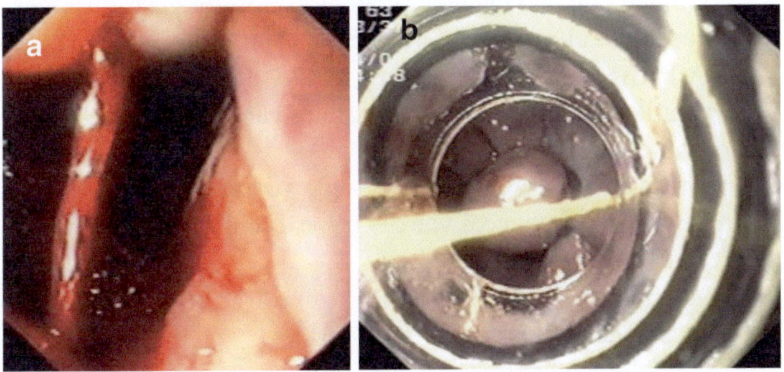

Fig. 46.3 Variceal UGIB (**a**) stopped by placement of ligatures (elastic bands) (**b**)

- GAVE syndrome assessment (gastric antral vascular ectasia): "watermelon stomach").
  Argon plasma coagulation,
  Band ligation.

46.5.2 Endoscopic Ultrasound (EUS)

- Color Doppler examination (Fig. 46.5a, b).
  Assessment of periesophageal and perigastric collaterals, including perforating veins,

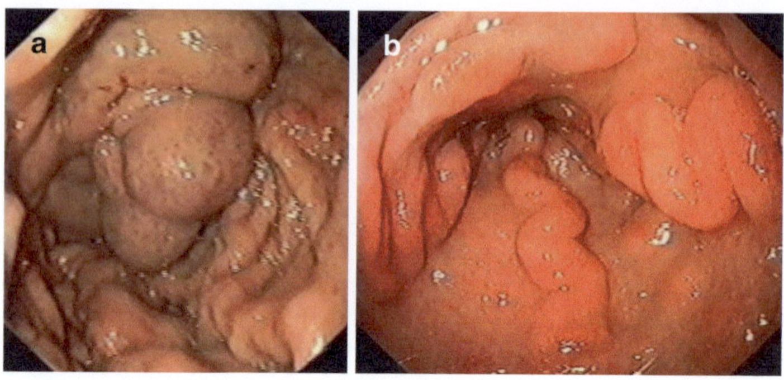

Fig. 46.4 Isolated gastric varices (**a**) and antral varices (**b**)

Guided coil and cyanoacrylate injection for gastric varices,
- Endoscopic ultrasound fine-needle aspiration/biopsy (EUS-FNA/FNB) has similar accuracy to percutaneous biopsy,
- Evaluation and visualization of ascites can also be done ecoendoscopically (Fig. 46.6a, b).
  - Assessment of gastric and ectopic varices.
    Gastroesophageal varices (type 1 and 2) or isolated gastric varices (Fig. 46.4a),
    Antral varices (Fig. 46.4b),
    Duodenal, jejunal, or ileal varices,
    Colorectal varices.

46.6 Complications

- UGIB (Fig. 46.3a, b), ascites (Fig.46.5a, b), hepatorenal syndrome, spontaneous bacterial peritonitis, encephalopathy, hepatocellular carcinoma, malnutrition, infections, etc.

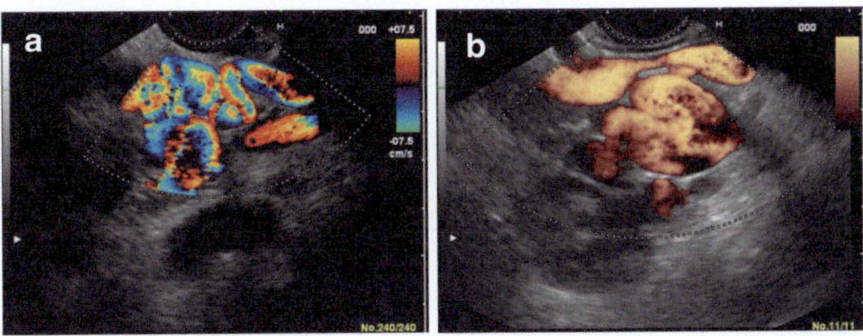

Fig. 46.5 Perigastric collaterals visualized endoscopically in color Doppler (**a**) and power Doppler mode (**b**)

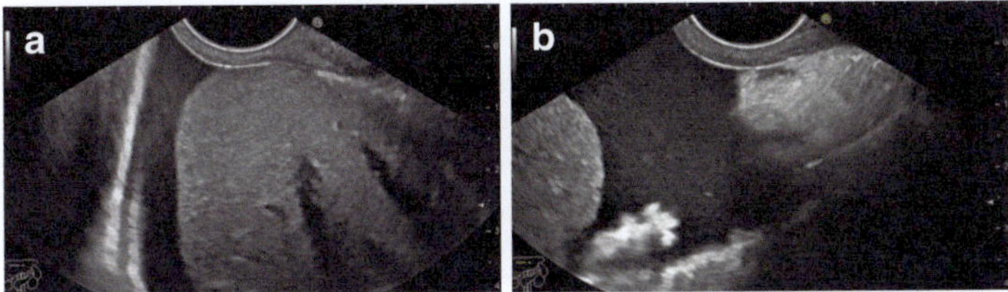

Fig. 46.6 Perihepatic ascites fluid visualized by EUS, liver with inhomogeneous structure and irregular border

46.7 Evolution and Prognostic

- Child-Pugh score (Table 46.1).
- MELD score (Table 46.2).

Table 46.1 Child–Pugh score is used to assess the prognosis of patients with cirrhosis

Measure	1 point	2 points	3 points
Total bilirubin, mg/dL	< 2	2–3	> 3
Serum albumin, g/dL	> 3.5	2.8–3.5	< 2.8
INR or Prothrombin time prolongation (s)	< 1.7 4	1.7–2.3 4–6	> 2.3 >6
Ascites	None	Mild (or suppressed with medication)	Moderate to severe or refractory
Hepatic encephalopathy	None	Grade I–II	Grade III–IV

Points	Child–PughClass	1 year survival	2 years survival
5–6	A	100%	85%
7–9	B	81%	57%
10–15	C	45%	35%

Table 46.2 MELD score estimates mortality at 3 months; it is used to prioritize liver transplant allocation

MELD Score = $3.78 \times \log[\text{bilirubin(mg/dl)}] + 11.2 \times \log[\text{INR}] + 9.57 \times \log[\text{creatinine (mg/dL)}] + 6.43$

Score	90-day mortality
> 40	71.3–100%
30–39	52.6%–74.5%
20–29	19.6–45.5%
10–19	6–20%
<9	1.9–3.7%

[a] If the patient has been dialyzed twice within the last 7 days, then the value for serum creatinine used should be 4 mg/dL

[b] Any value less than 1 of bilirubin and creatinine is given a value of 1

46.8 Treatment

- **General.**
  - Caloric intake adapted to the nutritional status, reduction of salt, 3–5 meals/day, vitamin and mineral supplements,
  - Prohibition of alcohol consumption regardless of the etiology,
  - Bed rest in the decompensated stage.
- **Etiological treatment.**
  - Antiviral treatment for B or C hepatitis,
  - Chelation therapy for hemochromatosis; penicilamine for Wilson's disease; ursodeoxycholic acid for primary biliary cirrhosis.
- **Pathogenic treatment.**
- Diuretic,

  Usually a combination of K-saving (spironolactone) and loop diuretics (furosemide),

  The doses are adjusted according to response (weight loss 500 mg/day for patient without edema, 1000 mg/day for patient with edema), serum ionogram and BP measurements,

  Maximum doses: 160 mg furosemide, 400 mg spironolactone.
- NSBB (propranolol, carvedilol) for the reduction of portal hypertension (primary and secondary UGIB prophylaxis) in case of EV grade 2/3. Doses: propranolol—initially 20 mg × 2/day up to 160 mg; carvedilol 6.25–12.5 mg/day.
- Corticosteroid therapy for active compensated autoimmune cirrhosis,
- **Liver transplant.**
- **Treatment of complications.**
  - **UGIB** of variceal origin.

    i.v. fluid resuscitation,

    Active bleeding control using pharmaceutical agents (terlipressin 2 mg every 4–6 h), endoscopy (variceal band ligation - (Fig. 46.5a, b)) or surgery (porto-cavernous shunts),

    Prophylactic antibiotics.

- **Encephalopathy**: management of precipitating factors,
    Lactulose initially 10–20 mL/day, then dose adapted for 1–2 semisolid stools/day,
    Rifaximin 400 mg × 3/day,
    L-ornithine-L-aspartate (Hepa-Mertz 1 sachet × 3/day or 4–8 a/day iv infusion),
- **Spontaneous bacterial peritonitis,**
    Antibiotic (cefotaxime 4 g/day, 5–7 days),
    Prophylactic treatment for high-risk patients (norfloxacin),
- **Hepatorenal syndrome,**
    Terlipressin 0.5–2 mg/day + human albumin 20–40 g/day,
- **Hepatocelluar carcinoma,**
    Depending on the stage of liver disease, the number, size, and dissemination of the tumor: resection, transplantation, local ablation techniques, systemic treatment.
- **Prophylaxis of infections.**
  - Vaccination against hepatitis A, B, influenza, and pneumococus,
  - Antibioprophylaxis in UGIB and ascites with proteins <1.5 g/dL [1–3].

46.9 Patient Surveillance

- **Screening for HCC.**
  - Ultrasound +/− AFP every 6 months,
- **Screening for portal hypertension.**
  - Patients without indication for EGD (compensated cirrhosis, hepatic stiffness <20 KPa and Plt >150,000—baveno VI): are monitored by platelet count and FibroScan,
  - Patients with indicaton for EGD (compensated cirrhosis with hepatic stiffness >20 KPa and Plt <150,000—baveno VI, decompensated cirrhosis): EGD is repeated every 1–3 years depending on the persistence of the etiological factor, the detection of EV [4].

References

1. Angeli P, Bernardi M, Villanueva C, Francoz C, Mookerjee RP, Trebicka J, Krag A, Laleman W, Gines P. EASL clinical practice guidelines for the management of patients with decompensated cirrhosis. J Hepatol. 2018;69(2):406–60.
2. Garcia-Tsao G, Abraldes JG, Berzigotti A, Bosch J. Portal hypertensive bleeding in cirrhosis: risk stratification, diagnosis, and management: 2016 practice guidance by the American association for the study of liver diseases. Hepatology. 2017;65(1):310–35.
3. European Association for the Study of the Liver. EASL clinical practice guidelines on the management of ascites, spontaneous bacterial peritonitis, and hepatorenal syndrome in cirrhosis. J Hepatol. 2010;53(3):397–417.
4. De Franchis R. Expanding consensus in portal hypertension: report of the Baveno VI consensus workshop: stratifying risk and individualizing care for portal hypertension. J Hepatol. 2015;63(3):743–52.

Liver Tumors

47

Irina Mihaela Cazacu and Adrian Săftoiu

47.1 Definition and Classification

- **Malignant tumors.**
  - Hepatocellular carcinoma.
  - Intrahepatic cholangiocarcinoma.
  - Metastasis (the liver is a common site for metastasis from solid tumors).
- **Benign tumors.**
  - Hepatic hemangioma.
  - Focal nodular hyperplasia.
  - Hepatocellular adenoma.
  - Regenerative nodules (typically seen in the setting of cirrhosis).

I. M. Cazacu (✉)
Department of Oncology, Fundeni Clinical Institute, Bucharest, Romania

Faculty of Medicine, Carol Davila University of Medicine and Pharmacy, Bucharest, Romania

A. Săftoiu
Department of Gastroenterology and Hepatology, Elias Emergency University Hospital, Carol Davila University of Medicine and Pharmacy, Bucharest, Romania

473

A. Săftoiu (ed.), *Pocket Guide to Advanced Endoscopy in Gastroenterology*, https://doi.org/10.1007/978-3-031-42076-4_47

47.2 Hepatocellular Carcinoma (HCC)

47.2.1 Epidemiology

- Sixth most frequently diagnosed cancer worldwide [1].
- Third leading cause of cancer-related mortality worldwide [1].
- Men > women (3:1) [1].
- Risk factors [2]:
  - Cirrhosis.
  - Hepatitis B virus.
  - Hepatitis C virus.
  - Environmental toxins (act synergistically with other risk factors): aflatoxin B1, contaminated drinking water, iron overload.
  - Lifestyle factors (alcohol, cigarette smoking).
  - Metabolic factors (nonalcoholic fatty liver disease, diabetes mellitus, obesity).
  - Genetic susceptibility (hereditary hemochromatosis, alpha-1 antitrypsin deficiency, acute intermittent porphyria).

47.2.2 Pathology

- HCC may present as a single mass, multiple nodules, or as diffuse liver involvement [3].
  - Variants:
    Sclerosing/fibrosing form – associated with hypercalcemia,
    Fibrolamellar carcinoma—young patients, without cirrhosis; has a favorable prognosis and it is not associated increased serum AFP levels.

47.2.3 Diagnostic [2–4]

- Symptoms.
  - Upper abdominal pain/pain in the right subcostal area or on top of the shoulder (phrenic irritation).

- – Fatigue, anorexia, weight loss.
- – Unexplained fever.
- – Early satiety.
- Physical exam.
  - – Hepatomegaly.
  - – Splenomegaly.
  - – Jaundice.
  - – Cachexia.
  - – Ascites.
- Paraneoplastic syndromes.
  - – Hypoglycemia.
  - – Erythrocytosis.
  - – Hypercalcemia.
  - – Diarrhea.
  - – Dermatomyositis, pemphigus foliaceus, Pityriasis rotunda.
  - – Leser–Trélat sign (multiple seborrheic keratoses).
- Laboratory test.
  - – Liver function test may be normal or elevated (elevated serum bilirubin and LDH and lowered serum albumin are associated with poor prognosis).
  - – AFP usually elevated (but it is also increased in benign chronic liver disease).
  - – AFP is not longer part of the diagnostic algorithm.
- Imaging tests:
  - – Transabdominal ultrasound: HCC is usually well circumscribed, hyperechogenic, and associated with diffuse distortion of the normal hepatic parenchyma.
  - – Contrast-enhanced US: HCC shows diffuse internal enhancement during the arterial phase of contrast administration and mild, late (≥ 1 min after injection) washout.
  - – Contrast-enhanced CT: HCC typically appears as an area of low attenuation on CT.
  - – MRI: superior to CT and ultrasound for detection of liver tumors.
  - – Classic radiographic findings of HCC:
    Arterial hyperenhancement.
    Portal venous washout.

- Biopsy (CT/US-guided) is necessary in a non-cirrhotic liver.
- Biopsy is not indicated in cirrhotic liver if:
  Two classic radiographic findings PLUS,
  >1 cm.

47.2.4 Role of Endoscopy [4, 5]

- Upper endoscopy: evaluates the grade of esophageal or gastric varices if any.
- EUS (contrast-enhanced EUS and EUS elastography): increasing role in the diagnosis of indeterminate and small lesions; it can detect hepatic lesions smaller than 1 cm in the left lobe of the liver (Figs. 47.1, and 47.2).
- EUS-FNA/FNB: alternate strategy for histologic confirmation in case of small lesions, accessible by EUS (Fig. 47.2).
- EUS-FNA/FNB: allows the sampling of hilar nodes (non-feasible by traditional imaging methods) (Fig. 47.3).
- Role of EUS and endoscopy in the general management of a patient with HCC:
  - Esophageal varices: endoscopically treated with band ligation/sclerotherapy.
  - Gastric varices: endoscopic injection of cyanoacrylate glue/EUS-guided coil embolization and glue injection.

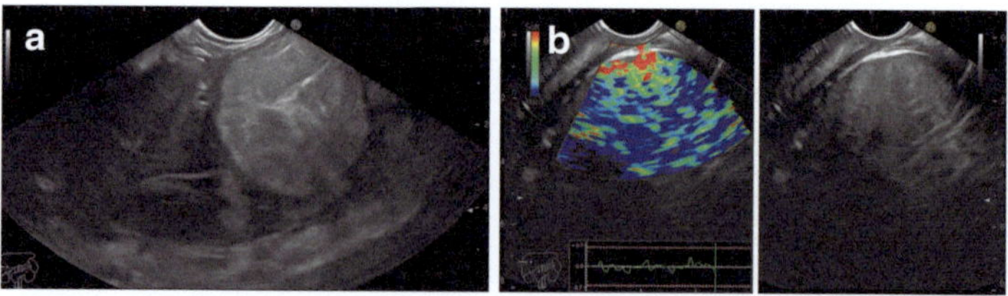

Fig. 47.1 EUS elastography—hyperechogenic lesion in the left lobe of the liver (**a**) "hard" appearance on EUS elastography (**b**), visible from the stomach on EUS

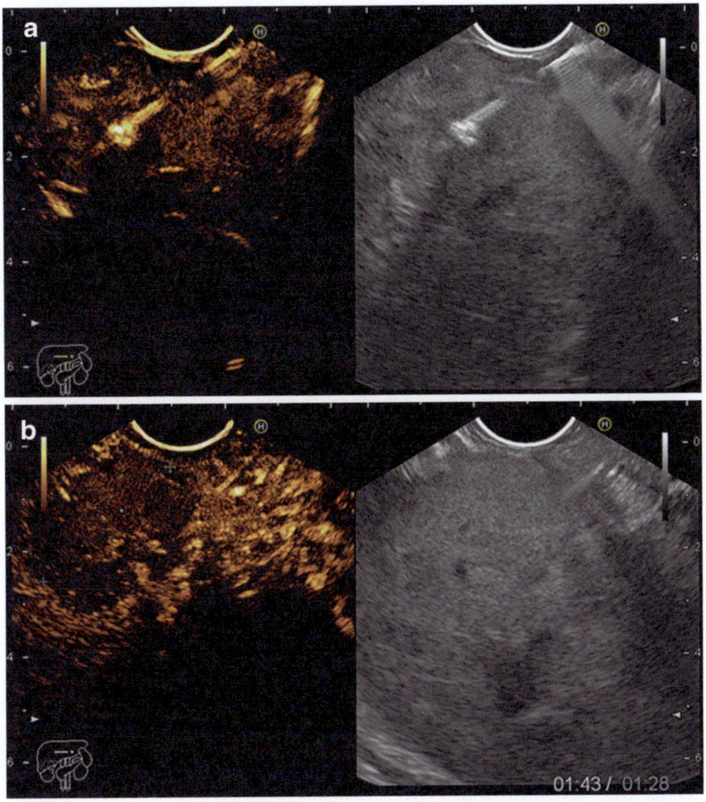

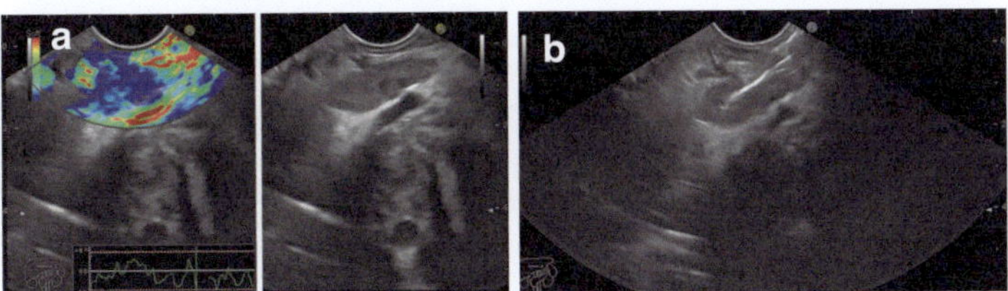

Fig. 47.2 Contrast-enhanced EUS—liver lesion with hyperenhancement in the arterial phase, and washout in the venous phase (**a**), with EUS-guided fine-needle aspiration performed during contrast-enhanced EUS (**b**)

Fig. 47.3 Lymph node in the hepatic hilum, visible on transgastric EUS, with "hard" appearance on EUS elastography (**a**), with EUS-guided fine-needle aspiration for differential diagnosis (**b**)

- Obstructive jaundice: endoscopic biliary drainage (palliation in case of jaundice caused by tumor fragments and/or protruding into the CBD lumen) or EUS-guided biliary drainage; endoscopic retrograde cholangiography (ERC) can relieve jaundice via biliary stenting.

47.2.5 Staging [4]

2.5.1 TNM Staging

- **Tumor (T).**
  - TX—Primary tumor cannot be assessed.
  - T0—No evidence of primary tumor.
  - T1—Solitary tumor ≤ 2 cm, or > 2 cm without vascular invasion.
  - T2—Solitary tumor >2 cm with vascular invasion, or multiple tumors, none >5 cm.
  - T3—Multiple tumors, at least one of which is >5 cm.
  - T4—Single tumor or multiple tumors of any size involving a major branch of the portal vein or hepatic vein or tumor(s) with direct invasion of adjacent organs other than the gallbladder or with perforation of visceral peritoneum.
- **Regional lymph nodes (N).**
  - NX—Regional lymph nodes cannot be assessed.
  - N0—No regional lymph node metastasis.
  - N1—Regional lymph node metastasis.
- **Distant metastasis (M).**
  - MX—Distant metastasis cannot be assessed.
  - M0—No distant metastasis.
  - M1—Distant metastasis.

47.2.6 Prognostic Staging Scores

- Child–Pugh score.
- Okuda.
- Barcelona Clinic Liver Cancer (BCLC).

Following the initial workup, patients are classified into one of the following four categories:

1. Potentially resectable or transplantable, operable by performance status or comorbidity.
2. Unresectable disease.
3. Inoperable by performance status or comorbidity with local disease only.
4. Metastatic disease.

47.2.7 Treatment [4, 6]

- **Resectable disease.**
    - Hepatic resection/liver transplantation are the only curative treatments.
    - Hepatic resection (10%): solitary lesion (no strict size limit as long as liver remnant >25–30%) and preserved liver function.
    - No role for neoadjuvant or adjuvant therapy.
    - Liver transplantation: Milan criteria—unresectable, 1 tumor <5 cm or $\leq$ 3 tumors ($\leq$3 cm), no macroscopic vascular invasion, no extrahepatic disease.
- **Unresectable, localized disease.**
    - Radiofrequency ablation (RFA).
    - Transarterial chemoembolization (TACE).
    - Stereotactic body radiotherapy (SBRT).
- **Advanced disease (vascular invasion and/or extrahepatic disease).**
    - **First line.**
        - **Atezolizumab + bevacizumab**: new standard of care, performance status 0–2, preserved liver function, Child–Pugh A.
        - **Sorafenib**: performance status 0–2, preserved liver function, Child–Pugh A/B.
            - Toxicity: diarrhea, hand-foot reaction, hypophosphatemia.

Lenvatinib: noninferior to sorafenib; for Child–Pugh A only.

- **Second line.**

  Regorafenib.

  Cabozantinib.

  Ramucirumab (if AFP > 400 in Child–Pugh A).

  Pembrolizumab (FDA approved for Child–Pugh A).

  Nivolumab + ipilimumab (Child–Pugh A only).

References

1. Sung H, Ferlay J, Siegel RL, Laversanne M, Soerjomataram I, Jemal A, et al. Global cancer statistics 2020: GLOBOCAN estimates of incidence and mortality worldwide for 36 cancers in 185 countries. CA Cancer J Clin. 2021;71(3):209–49.
2. Casciato DA, Territo MC. Manual of clinical oncology. Philadelphia, PA: Lippincott Williams & Wilkins; 2009.
3. DeVita VT, Lawrence TS, Rosenberg SA. Cancer: principles & practice of oncology: primer of the molecular biology of cancer. Lippincott Williams & Wilkins; 2012.
4. Benson AB, D'Angelica MI, Abbott DE, Anaya DA, Anders R, Are C, et al. Hepatobiliary cancers, version 2.2021, NCCN clinical practice guidelines in oncology. J Natl Compr Cancer Netw. 2021;19(5):541–65.
5. Girotra M, Soota K, Dhaliwal AS, Abraham RR, Garcia-Saenz-de-Sicilia M, Tharian B. Utility of endoscopic ultrasound and endoscopy in diagnosis and management of hepatocellular carcinoma and its complications: what does endoscopic ultrasonography offer above and beyond conventional cross-sectional imaging? World J Gastrointest Endosc. 2018;10(2):56.
6. Vogel A, Cervantes A, Chau I, Daniele B, Llovet J, Meyer T, et al. Hepatocellular carcinoma: ESMO clinical practice guidelines for diagnosis, treatment and follow-up. Ann Oncol. 2018;29:iv238–iv55.

Elena Codruța Gheorghe

48.1   Definition and Classification

The liver has a dual blood supply, hepatic artery and the portal vein. The hepatic veins drain the blood from the liver. Due to this fact, vascular disorders of the liver are rare, the causes being:

- **Ischemia** (hepatic infarction, ischemic colangiopathy),
- **Insufficient venous drainage** (congestive hepatopathy, Budd–Chiari syndrome, sinusoidal obstruction syndrome),
- **Specific vascular lesions** (hepatic artery occlusion, hepatic artery aneurysm, portal vein thrombosis, congenital vascular malformations, schistosomiasis, sarcoidosis).

Supplementary Information The online version contains supplementary material available at https://doi.org/10.1007/978-3-031-42076-4_48. The videos can be accessed individually by clicking the DOI link in the accompanying figure caption or by scanning this link with the SN More Media App.

E. C. Gheorghe (✉)
University of Medicine and Pharmacy Craiova, Craiova, Romania

A. Săftoiu (ed.), *Pocket Guide to Advanced Endoscopy in Gastroenterology*, https://doi.org/10.1007/978-3-031-42076-4_48

48.1.1 Portal Vein Thrombosis

48.1.1.1 Epidemiology

- The incidence in non-cirrhotic patients is between 5-10%, in cirrhotic patients increases up to 64%.
- Prevalence <1% in patients with compensated cirrhosis.

48.1.1.2 Etiopathogeny

- Portal vein thrombosis (PVT) represents the partial or total obstruction of the portal vein flow due to the presence of a thrombus in the vascular lumen.
- The natural history depends on the size, extent, and degree of thrombosis, as well as comorbidities.
- The causes are multifactorial, but in a third of cases they remain unknown:
  - In newborns, umbilical cord infection,
  - In children, appendicitis,
  - In adults:
    Surgery (splenectomy, gastrectomy, colectomy, cholecystectomy),
    Hypercoagulability (myeloproliferative diseases, C or S protein deficiency, factor V Leiden mutation, pregnancy),
    Cancer (hepatocellular carcinoma, pancreatic, renal, adrenal),
    Cirrhosis,
    Trauma.

48.1.1.3 Diagnosis

- Signs and symptoms.
  - Most often, asymptomatic,
  - Rarely, may manifest acutely with acute or progressive abdominal or lumbar pain, abdominal distension due to ileus but with no signs of intestinal obstruction,

- More frequently, it occurs secondary to portal hypertension with splenomegaly and variceal hemorrhage, less often ascites (when cirrhosis is also present),
- PVT should be suspected:
  - Acute PVT in patients with abdominal pain of more than 24 h,
  - Chronic PVT in patients with portal hypertension manifestations in the absence of cirrhosis or slightly altered liver tests + risk factors,
- Laboratory tests.
  - Inflammatory response in the absence of sepsis in acute PVT,
  - Liver tests are generally normal or slightly altered,
- Imaging tests.
  - Color Doppler ultrasound is usually diagnostic – reduced or absent portal vein flow +/– thrombus.
  - MRI and CT scan – can be used for more complex cases, to assess thrombus extension.
  - Angiography – can guide surgery for intrahepatic transjugular portosystemic shunt (TIPS).

48.1.1.4 The Role of Endoscopy

- **Upper gastrointestinal endoscopy**
  - Allows the evaluation of segmental portal hypertension: esophageal, gastric, ectopic varices + portal hypertensive gastropathy,
- **Endoscopic ultrasound**
  - Allows the assessment of the portal vein, the splenomesenteric confluence, and the superior mesenteric vein + splenic vein,
  - Color Doppler examination (Fig. 48.1; Video 48.1a),
  - Evaluation with contrast substance in low mechanical index mode (Fig. 48.2; Video 48.1b),
  - Assessment of collateral circulation as an indirect sign of deep venous thrombosis,

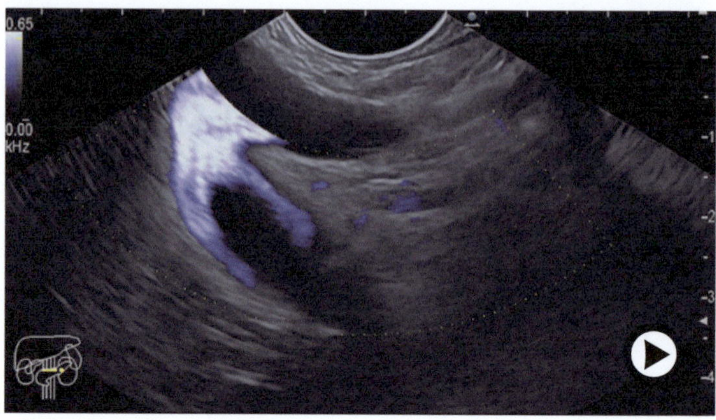

Fig. 48.1 Benign thrombosis of the superior mesenteric vein visualized in power Doppler mode. (▶ https://doi.org/10.1007/000-b6m)

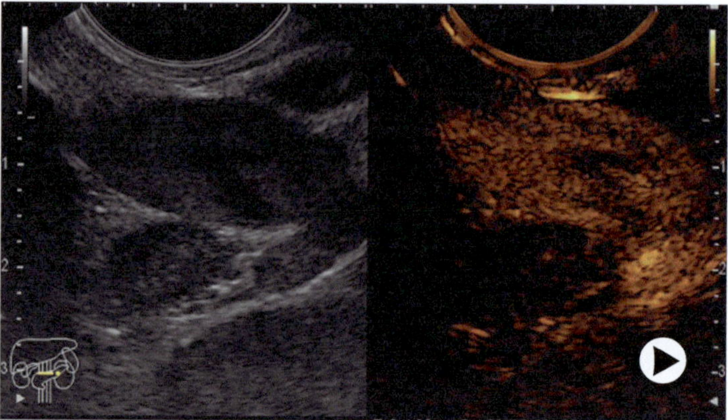

Fig. 48.2 With turbulent flow in the portal vein (hepatic hilum), visualized with contrast substance in specific harmonic mode with low mechanical index. (▶ https://doi.org/10.1007/000-b6k)

- Allows performing fine-needle aspiration/biopsy (EUS-FNA/FNB) when malignancy is suspected,
- Differential diagnosis between benign and malignant thrombosis (Fig. 48.3a, b; Video 48.2).

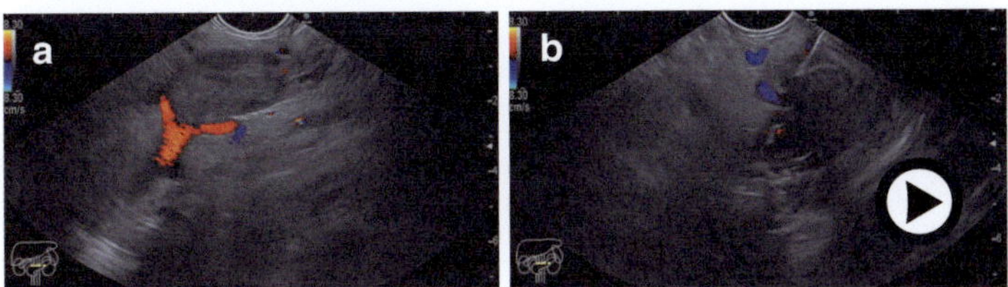

Fig. 48.3 Malignant thrombosis of the portal vein expanding the lumen, visualized in color Doppler mode (**a**), with EUS-FNA which confirmed the diagnosis of primitive hepatocellular carcinoma with direct invasion of the portal vein (**b**). (▶ https://doi.org/10.1007/000-b6n)

48.1.1.5 Treatment

- For acute cases (especially with proven hypercoagulability) thrombolysis is recommended.
- Long-term anticoagulant treatment (for patients with hypercoagulability, patients with cirrhosis + symptomatic acute PVT).
- Management of portal hypertension and its complications (octreotide i.v. and endoscopic band ligation to control variceal bleeding, beta-blockers to prevent variceal rebleeding).

References

1. DeLeve LD, Valla DC, Garcia-Tsao G, American Association for the Study Liver Diseases. Vascular disorders of the liver. Hepatology. 2009;49(5):1729–64.
2. Sanyal AJ. Epidemiology and pathogenesis of portal vein thrombosis in adults. In: Post TW, editor. UpToDate. Waltham, MA: UpToDate; 2023.
3. Basit SA, Stone CD, Gish R. Portal vein thrombosis. Clin Liver Dise. 2015;19(1):199–221.

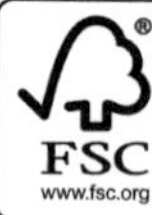

If you have any concerns about our products,
you can contact us on
ProductSafety@springernature.com

In case Publisher is established outside the EU,
the EU authorized representative is:
Springer Nature Customer Service Center GmbH
Europaplatz 3, 69115 Heidelberg, Germany

Printed by Libri Plureos GmbH
in Hamburg, Germany